Physician Location
and Specialty Choice

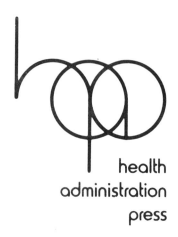

health
administration
press

Health Administration Press was
established in 1972 with the
support of the W.K. Kellogg
Foundation and is a nonprofit
endeavor of The University of
Michigan Program and Bureau of
Hospital Administration.

The Press gratefully acknowledges
the support of The Robert Wood
Johnson Foundation in the
publication of this book.

Physician
Location
and Specialty
Choice

Richard L. Ernst
Donald E. Yett

Health Administration Press
Ann Arbor, Michigan
1985

Library of Congress Cataloging in Publication Data

Ernst, Richard L., Ph. D.
   Physician location and specialty choice.

   Bibliography: p.
   Includes index.
   1. Medical offices—United States—Location.
2. Physicians—United States—Supply and demand.
3. Medicine—Specialties and specialists—United States.
4. Medical education—United States. I. Yett, Donald E.
II. Title. [DNLM: 1. Career Choice—United States—
statistics. 2. Physicians—supply & distribution—
United States. 3. Specialties, Medical—United States—
statistics. W 76 E71p]
RA410.7.E75   1985   331.11'1   85-5469 ISBN 0-910701-03-2

The authors gratefully acknowledge the support of The Robert Wood Johnson Foundation for a grant to support the research on which this study is based.

Health Administration Press
School of Public Health
The University of Michigan
1021 East Huron
Ann Arbor, Michigan 48109
(313) 764-1380

Contents

Preface

This book is the outgrowth of our long-term interest in constructing a model of physicians' specialty and practice location choices. In developing such a model, the logical first step was to undertake a literature review. Our intent was to identify the studies that were the strongest methodologically, summarize their findings, and determine to what extent these findings could be used as the basis for an integrated model of physicians' career decision making.

What we did not realize when we began the study is how much scholarly attention has been devoted to physicians' specialty and practice location choices. The issue has evoked a prodigious number of studies in the past 30 years, and new results are being produced continuously. Consequently, it was necessary to select a cutoff publication date for including material in the book. More or less arbitrarily, we decided on early 1982. Subject to that condition, we believe this to be a reasonably comprehensive and critical summary of the research on physicians' career decisions.

We have tried to structure the material in a manner that will make it useful to economists, sociologists, and other researchers concerned with the process of, and the important influences on, career decision making. At the same time, we recognize that a major audience will be medical care researchers, some of whom are unfamiliar with economics. Although we have tried to make the material comprehensible to such readers, parts of Chapters 6 and 7, which deal with econometric studies of physicians' specialty and location choices, are inherently difficult.

Hence, some readers may wish to skip the technical details in these two chapters in favor of the general information and chapter summaries. In this respect, we should also mention that we are both economists, and our opinions, approach, and even the form we have given the book are inevitably affected by our academic backgrounds.

When we set out on the study, it was widely felt that the medical education system was producing too few primary care physicians, and too few physicians willing to practice in rural and inner-city locations. In that context, we attempted to identify the most effective kinds of policies for remedying these special problems. However, events of the last decade —notably the huge and continuing increase in physician supply—have greatly lessened the pressures to address specialty and geographic "shortages" of physicians. Indeed, as this is written, far more attention is being given to the likely effects of increasing competition for patients among physicians, particularly insofar as it bears on national health care costs. This shift in policy emphasis has reinforced our original view that research in this field has tended to place too much stress on studies of specific policies and programs addressing issues of immediate concern. We believe that in the future more attention should be given to the development of models that can be used better to predict and analyze long-term trends and assess policies in terms of their long-term as well as short-term consequences. Accordingly, we sought to organize the material presented here within a framework that could serve as the basis for structuring such a model. We used this framework as a guide in formulating our summaries and analyses of the policy concerns of the 1980s as well as those of the 1970s and earlier.

Three of our former colleagues, Leonard Drabek, Kathryn M. Langwell, and Daniel S. Levine, assisted in the early phase of the project. We gratefully acknowledge their contributions, a number of which appear in the final product. Above all, we wish to thank The Robert Wood Johnson Foundation for its support. Without that support, the book would literally not exist.

RICHARD L. ERNST
DONALD E. YETT

Human Resources Research Center
University of Southern California

ONE

Introduction

As major providers of medical care, physicians have long been the objects of health manpower policy debate in this country. From the end of World War II to the early 1970s, attention focused on what was widely regarded as a shortage of physicians. The shortage was commonly attributed to secularly rising demands for medical care and physician-population ratios that were either stable or only gradually increasing over time. Beginning in the mid-1960s, concern over the situation led to federal and state legislation that provided massive subsidies to medical schools to encourage them to increase the supply of new medical graduates. The subsidies enabled many new medical schools to be built, and stimulated existing schools to enlarge their class sizes greatly. By the early 1970s, as a consequence of those efforts (as well as large inflows of alien physicians from foreign medical schools), the supply of physicians relative to population began to increase dramatically. The growth rate of physician supply was so high that concern about a shortage of practitioners had all but ended by the mid-1970s; in fact, many authorities began to warn of a serious "glut" of physicians by the year 1990 and beyond.

At about this time policy attention shifted away from the aggregate supply of physicians to the *functional distribution* of physician manpower—that is, the distribution of physicians among specialties and practice locations. Health care authorities argued that physicians were maldistributed both by specialty and by geographic location. There were, it was said, too few "first-contact" or primary care practitioners,[1] and too few physicians in all fields willing to practice in "medically underserved" or "physician-shortage" areas—chiefly rural and inner-city localities whose populations were composed, not atypically, of large percentages of the poor, the aged, and racial minorities. Congress itself defined the maldistribution issue in the Health Professions Educational Assistance Act of 1976 (PL 94-484), which declared that, although the total supply of physicians "is no longer insufficient . . . specialization has resulted in inadequate numbers of physicians [providing] primary care," and "many areas of the United States are unable to attract adequate numbers of [physicians]." Underlying Congress's declaration was the prevailing opinion that educational institutions and the marketplace had failed to assure society's access to primary care practitioners, and that they had also failed to assure equal access to physicians' care in all geographic areas by all patient populations.

One expression of federal involvement with the issue was the creation in 1976 of the Graduate Medical Education National Advisory Committee (GMENAC). Under a mandate from the Secretary of Health, Education, and Welfare, GMENAC was charged, among other things, with determining "the number of physicians . . . required to meet the health care needs of the Nation, . . . the most appropriate specialty distribution of these physicians," and ways of achieving "a more favorable geographic distribution of physicians" (GMENAC 1981c, p. 1). In short, the committee's mission was to assess the dimensions of the maldistribution problem and make recommendations to correct it.

As it happened, GMENAC's tenure coincided with the first evidence of a large increase in the number of physicians entering the primary care fields. Despite some disagreement on the question, a matter to which we will return shortly, there also appeared to be at least the start of an alleviation of physician shortages in rural areas. As a result, the sense of urgency regarding the physician "maldistribution" problem had mostly abated by the time GMENAC completed its report. Indeed, after four years of work, GMENAC (1981a) announced that shortages of primary care practitioners would be eliminated during the 1980s, and that considerably more physicians than "required" would be practicing in most fields by 1990. It put the total surplus of supply over "requirements" in 1990 at roughly 20 percent, thereby reinforcing fears that the shortage of physicians had become a glut. Although the committee concluded that geographic imbalances in physician supply would persist, it advocated a go-slow strategy for correcting them on grounds that standards were insufficient for setting appropriate physician-population ratios and, in any case, that too little was known about how physicians make their practice location choices. (It is hard to avoid speculating that the strategy was probably also prompted by the predicted manpower surplus.) GMENAC went on to recommend cutbacks in medical school class sizes, severe limitations on the immigration of foreign-trained physicians, and a ban on the development of new programs to support the training of primary care practitioners.

Critics have challenged the realism of the assumptions on which GMENAC's estimates of physician requirements crucially depend. However, essentially the same conclusions have also been reached by other experts. For example, the Bureau of Health Professions (BHPr) in the U.S. Department of Health and Human Services, which is also charged with estimating future physician supplies and requirements, projected a small surplus of physician manpower by 1990 (U.S. Department of Health and Human Services 1982).

As we have indicated, it is not yet certain whether physicians are moving into medically underserved areas to a significant degree. Research conducted at the Rand Corporation found that specialists—i.e., physicians other than general and family practitioners—settled into the larger rural areas in increasing numbers in the 1970s (Schwartz et al. 1980; Newhouse et al. 1982a, 1982b). However, other reports have failed to show an increase in overall rural physician-population ratios (Fruen and Cantwell 1982). All the same, there are no signs that physician density is declining in small rural communities, and there is some reason for believing that it may soon increase (see below).

One can interpret these trends as bringing to an end the "maldistribution" of physicians, but that is probably an overly facile conclusion. As will be shown in later chapters, a shift in medical students' career preferences appeared to occur in the late 1960s and early 1970s. Compared with previous generations, many more medical students expressed interest in the primary care fields, and there were some indications of increased interest in shortage-area practice locations. This shift in career preferences could have played a part in moderating the manpower deficits associated with the physician "maldistribution." Nevertheless, the extent to which the reported changes in students' preferences were translated into actual career decisions is not clear. In any case, the functional distribution of physicians seems to have changed very little since 1970. Thus, if the stock was maldistributed a decade ago, there is little justification for claiming that it is satisfactorily distributed today.

A stronger argument can be made that current and future corrections of distributional shortages can be attributed to increases in the total supply of physicians. That is, even if the functional distribution of physicians is stable over time, a rise in the total number of practitioners is bound to increase the numbers of physicians in what were shortage fields and practice locations. The trend that has been observed in the past decade may well be this kind of "spillover" phenomenon, rather than a dramatic change in the functional distribution of physicians itself.

The purpose of this book is to review the empirical evidence re-garding physicians' choices of specialty and practice location, to identify the forces that govern those choices, and, in essence, to examine how the functional distribution of physicians came to be. One area to which our findings apply is physician manpower policy. In light of the events just described, it would be difficult to advocate costly programs to produce more primary care, rural, or inner-city practitioners. Even so, it may still be desirable, as a matter of public policy, to promote the selection of cer-tain specialties or practice sites. In addition, if the emerging resolution of the physician "maldistribution problem" is really an outcome of the in-crease in total physician supply, any serious curtailment of the number of new medical graduates (a suggestion gaining in popularity) will, in time, cause the problem to resurface. In this sense, too, the occasion may arise when programs to influence physicians' career decisions are justifia-ble and appropriate. Hence, it is essential to understand why physicians choose the specialties and locations they do, because only with this knowledge can successful programs be implemented to alter the choices in prescribed ways.

It is also fair to say that physicians' career decisions have been the subject of more study than those of any other profession or occupation. The issues involved have been explored by investigators in all of the be-havioral sciences, by physicians, medical educators, health care planners and policy agencies, and others in the health care professions. Many hy-potheses have been advanced to explain why physicians choose their par-ticular fields and locations, and a variety of different methodologies and approaches have been used to test these hypotheses. As a result, the siz-able literature on physicians' career choices provides important substan-tive information for a general understanding of occupational choice, ar-rays the important issues, and provides us with the techniques for studying occupational choice. We do not claim that the literature is in all respects a model of completeness or rigor, but anyone who wants to know how professionals choose their careers should be familiar with it.

By "physicians" we shall ordinarily mean graduates of U.S. medical schools. We do not explicitly consider the career choices of graduates of foreign medical schools (including Americans who study outside the U.S.) or osteopaths, but this is not to say that either group is an insignifi-cant component of U.S. health manpower. Even though the fraction is expected to fall, in light of the tightening of restrictions on foreign physi-cian immigration in 1978–80, foreign medical graduates currently repre-sent one-fifth of all U.S. physicians. Likewise, osteopaths are important providers of primary medical care in many rural areas, despite their small numbers overall. We excluded these two groups of practitioners only because of the scarcity of existing evidence on their career choices. Relative to the enormous volume of research on the career decisions of U.S. medical school graduates, very little is known about how foreign-trained physicians or osteopaths select specialties and practice locations. Indeed, the career decisions of both groups deserve much more attention than they have been given to date.[2]

Much of our discussion of specialty choice centers on selection of the primary care fields. We take these to include general and family practice, internal medicine, and pediatrics.[3] So as to exclude subspecialists, many physician manpower authorities would prefer to include only general and family practitioners, general internists, and general pediatricians in the definition. (Subspecialization is particularly common among internists, much less so among pediatricians.) However, the literature does not ordinarily distinguish between generalists and subspecialists in internal medicine and pediatrics. Here, physicians not in the primary care fields will be called either referral specialists or nonprimary care practitioners.

In government programs for influencing physician location, the phrases "physician-shortage area" and "medically underserved area" have specific meanings. They are counties or portions of counties designated by the administering agencies as having too few physicians. Researchers tend to use the phrases somewhat loosely to denote rural and inner-city localities where physician-population ratios are much below average. We shall follow this convention. Hence, in this book, a "physician-shortage area" is any community or area where the physician-population ratio is very low. Unfortunately, nearly all of the research on such areas has focused on rural communities. Far less is known about physician location patterns in urban or inner-city shortage areas, and inevitably, this limits our discussion of physician location in inner cities.

The remaining sections of this chapter contain, respectively, a survey of trends in the distribution of physicians, an overview of the medical educational process through which physicians pass before entering practice, and a review of findings on the timing of physicians' career choices. Each section provides background for subsequent chapters. The first documents historical patterns of physician supply. The second describes the factors that influence physicians as they make their specialty and location decisions. The third presents a schema of career stages at which these decisions are made. Because institutional and other forces may operate on physicians either before or after the actual choices are made, this schema affords a framework for evaluating hypotheses that particular factors significantly affect the choice outcomes.

TRENDS IN THE FUNCTIONAL DISTRIBUTION
OF PHYSICIANS

At least in the recent past, the functional distribution of physicians was important because of its implications for access to care. In particular, rising physician-population ratios mean an increase in the availability of physicians and access to care, and falling physician-population ratios mean the opposite. This, of course, is a considerable simplification. "Access" really applies to the availability of physicians' services and not to the availability of physicians. Whether one is trying to evaluate access to physicians' care cross-sectionally (that is, at different locations at the same time) or intertemporally, treating the number of physicians as equivalent to the volume of physicians' services provided can produce erroneous conclusions.

To give an example, suppose the population at locality A is healthier than the population at locality B, but that physician-population ratios are the same in both communities. Other things being equal, one might surmise that locality A needs fewer physicians than locality B because of its higher health status. On those grounds it could be argued that the given physician-population ratio signifies greater access to physicians' care in locality A than in B. On the other hand, if health status and physician-population ratios are the same in the two communities, but for cultural or other reasons people in A tend to utilize more physician services than people in B, it might be argued that access to those services is greater in B than in A.

To give another illustration, it is well known that, on average, physicians in nonmetropolitan counties provide more hours of direct patient care—about 10 percent more per year—than physicians in the most heavily populated metropolitan counties (e.g., Glandon and Shapiro 1980). Hence, comparisons of physician-population ratios in the two types of counties tend to understate access to care in nonmetropolitan counties because they do not take account of differences in the lengths of physician workyears. Even intertemporal comparisons of physician-population ratios may convey misleading impressions. The U.S. Department of Health and Human Services (1982) has reported that the intensity (i.e., the service content) of physician office visits increased by nearly 23 percent from 1970 to 1978. It also reported that the average number of office visits per capita was almost constant during the same period. It is not clear whether the input of physician time in office visits rose commensurately with intensity, but the general implication is that more physicians were required to produce a given number of office visits in 1978 than in 1970. Hence, in view of the changing content of an average office visit, the rise in the national physician-population ratio from 1970 to 1978 overstates the increase in the population's access to these units of care. (Proponents of the supplier-induced-demand hypothesis see these figures as evidence that the increasingly ample physician supply "caused" the greater intensity of an average office visit. Evidence with respect to this possibility is considered in a later section.)

These examples, which can be multiplied, tell us that headcount measures of access to physicians' care must be interpreted cautiously. Ideally, it might be preferable to forgo using headcount measures altogether, but most of the available relevant data are in this form. While historical, area-specific, and specialty-specific records of the numbers of physicians are relatively abundant from such sources as the American Medical Association (AMA) and the U.S. decennial census, data on the quantities of physicians' services are much scarcer, and all but nonexistent for long time series and small geographic units such as counties. Therefore, physician-population ratios are commonly employed as proxies for access to physicians' care, but it is worth stressing that they may be somewhat rough approximations of the actual levels of service availability.

Still another issue is how to measure the number of physicians. Because all censuses of physicians utilize the survey technique and information reported by the survey respondents, they are inevitably susceptible to some degree of reporting error. For instance, a physician can report himself as a general surgeon or an orthopedic surgeon regardless of the amount of training he has had in either specialty. Only when he is credentialed in the field—i.e., certified by the appropriate specialty board —can his specialty status really be documented. This can cause differences in the reported number and functional distribution of physicians depending upon the source. AMA and U.S. census estimates of the numbers of physicians disagree, for example. The AMA tracks physicians from the time they graduate from medical school (or in the case of foreign medical graduates, from the time they enter residency training); and, through its annual activity surveys, classifies physicians by activity status, employment, specialty, and location. The U.S. census merely requests respondents to report their occupations. The AMA data are regarded as the more accurate of the two sets of figures, and they have the marked advantage of being published annually. Regrettably, the annual data have been published only since 1963, although prior to that the AMA's directories were used for developing occasional censuses of physicians.

Another, but more minor, problem is defining what is meant by an "available physician." The oldest relevant time series give only the total numbers of self-designated medical graduates. Newer time series also contain the number of active physicians—i.e., the roughly 90 percent of all medical graduates who are not retired or otherwise inactive.[4] They also separate physicians who provide patient care from those who do not. The latter, who are engaged in teaching, research, or administration, represent about 15 percent of the number of active physicians. A further distinction is often made between federally and nonfederally employed practitioners, the thesis being that federally employed physicians should be excluded from proxies for access to care because they are not available to the population at large. Finally, some analysts distinguish between office- and hospital-based physicians. They do so because the services of office-based and hospital-based practitioners (60 percent of whom are residents in training) are not equally available to the area's population.

Thus, there are at least five possibilities for measuring the number of available physicians: (1) all physicians, (2) active physicians, (3) physicians who provide patient care, (4) nonfederal physicians who provide patient care, and (5) nonfederal office-based physicians. Since measures 1 and 2 include persons who do not take care of patients, they are probably less meaningful than 3, 4, and 5. In constructing the first of the three tables that follow, we used measure 2—the number of active physicians —to construct a time series of physician supplies. This was necessary because data for measures 3, 4, and 5 have been published only in the past two decades.

Table 1-1 depicts long-term trends in the supply of active physicians, in physician-population ratios, and in the percentage of primary care practitioners. Unfortunately, no single data series exists for the 50-year period covered by the table. The four sources that were drawn upon utilize different definitions of "active physicians"; and breaks in the series resulting from different data sources or changes in physician classification occur between 1960 and 1965, 1965 and 1970, and 1980 and 1990. Nonetheless, four significant trends are discernible.

First, the number of active physicians per capita was essentially constant from 1940 to 1960, and not much lower in 1931 than in 1940. Then, in the mid-1960s—but before state and federal efforts to expand physician supplies took effect—the national physician-population ratio began to rise. From 1970 to 1980 the ratio increased by 25 percent, and according to projections by the BHPr, it is expected to increase by nearly 40 percent more between 1980 and 2000. It should be noted that both the GMENAC and the BHPr forecasts are contingent upon the continuation of present medical school class sizes. In any case, barring drastic cutbacks in the annual number of new medical graduates, the increase in physician supply should be a lasting one.

The second significant trend apparent in Table 1-1 is the secular decline in the percentage of physicians engaged in general and (after

TABLE 1-1   The Supply of Physicians in Selected Years, 1931–80, and Physician Supply Projections, 1990–2000

Year	Active Physicians		General/Family Practitioners as Percent of Active Physicians*	Primary Care Practitioners as Percent of Active Physicians†	Primary Care Practitioners per 100,000 Population
	Number	Number per 100,000 Population			
1931	152,400	123	74‡	78‡	95‡
1940	168,800	128	na	na	na
1949	196,600	132	37	46	60
1955	212,300	128	30	42	54
1960	237,700	130	26	39	51
1965	277,600	138	26	45	65
1970	311,200	153	19	38	58
1975	366,400	174	15	36	62
1978	401,400	185	14	36	66
1980	435,600	192	14	37	76
1990	567,900§	233	12	35	82
	561,200¶	231	12	36	84
1995	611,100¶	242	na	na	na
2000	655,400¶	266	na	na	na

Sources: 1931–60 data are from Peterson and Pennell (1962). 1965–80 data are from the American Medical Association (Theodore and Sutter 1967b; Haug et al. 1971; Goodman 1976; Wunderman 1979; and Bidese and Danais 1982). 1990–2000 supply projections are by GMENAC (1981a) and the BHPr (U.S. Department of Health and Human Services 1982). See the text for comments.
na: Figure not available from source.
* Family practice did not become a recognized specialty until 1969.
† Primary care practitioners defined as general/family practitioners, general internists, and general pediatricians.
‡ Part-time specialists combined with general practitioners in source; the figure is over-stated to some unknown degree.
§ Projection by GMENAC.
¶ Projection by Bureau of Health Professions (BHPr), Health Resources Administration. The BHPr included subspecialists in its 1990 forecast of the supply of internists, and the estimates of primary care physicians given here are therefore overstated.

1969) family practice. We will have occasion to speak of this trend later on as "the trend toward physician specialization." Most observers date its beginning about the time of World War I. However, owing to deficiencies in historical data on physician specialists, it is difficult to document the dimensions of the trend precisely. Even so, its character is evident in the table. The percentage of family/general practitioners in the active physician stock fell disproportionately during the 1950s and continued to fall during the 1960s and 1970s. It stabilized in the late 1970s, and both GMENAC's and BHPr's forecasts project its 1990 value at only 15 percent below the level in 1980.

The third significant trend—a decline in the percentage of physicians practicing in the primary care fields—parallels the second. This decline however, is much less marked than the decline in the percentage of physicians in general and family practice, and thus appears to have been due to the decreasing numbers of physicians entering and remaining in general practice. As late as 1949, 80 percent of the active physicians in primary care were general practitioners, but by 1980 less than 40 percent were general or family practitioners. The pattern within the primary care fields has been a pronounced shift away from general practice toward internal medicine and pediatrics. In that sense, the trend toward specialization has favored the other two primary care specialties as well as the referral fields.

The final noteworthy trend is the rise in the availability of primary care physicians since 1970. The number of primary care practitioners per capita rose by 30 percent between 1970 and 1980, and—according to the GMENAC and BHPr forecasts—it is expected to continue to rise at least until 1990. In 1980, access to primary physicians' care was higher for the nation as a whole than at any time since World War II. However, in view of the nearly constant ratio of primary care to referral specialists, this improvement can be attributed to the growth in overall physician supply rather than to shifts in the specialty distribution of physicians.

Table 1-2 presents physician-population ratios classified by census division, practice setting, and specialty grouping. The table demonstrates that these ratios vary widely along all three dimensions, and that the degree of variation changed little during the 1970s. In both 1969 and 1978, the New England, Middle Atlantic, and Pacific regions had much the highest numbers of physicians per capita, while the East South Central and West South Central regions had the lowest. In both years, the New England, Middle Atlantic, and Pacific regions also had the highest numbers of primary care practitioners per capita, while the East South Central and West South Central divisions had the lowest. These disparities are due in part to the uneven distribution of hospital-based physicians, the majority of whom are residents in hospital training programs. Since

TABLE 1-2 Nonfederal Patient Care Physicians per 100,000 Population by Census Division and Specialty Grouping, 1969 and 1978

Census Division	All Physicians	Office-Based Physicians				Hospital-Based Physicians*	Primary Care Physicians†
		General/Family Practitioners	Medical Specialists	Surgical Specialists	Other Specialists		
1969							
New England	148.2	23.6	26.9	33.4	20.8	43.5	55.1
Middle Atlantic	156.5	25.2	27.4	31.3	21.0	51.6	58.3
East North Central	107.7	24.6	16.6	23.8	14.9	27.9	44.1
West North Central	103.4	26.7	15.4	22.5	13.0	25.8	45.0
South Atlantic	106.4	20.6	18.7	26.1	14.4	26.5	42.1
East South Central	83.2	22.3	12.9	21.9	10.1	16.1	36.3
West South Central	94.1	24.1	15.1	23.8	13.1	17.9	39.1
Mountain	110.5	26.8	18.3	29.1	16.2	20.2	45.1
Pacific	145.2	31.9	26.8	35.3	24.6	26.6	58.9
Total U.S.	121.6	25.2	20.6	27.7	17.1	31.0	48.6
1978							
New England	183.0	16.5	40.7	38.9	30.3	56.6	69.9
Middle Atlantic	175.8	17.9	36.7	35.7	27.2	58.3	66.7
East North Central	132.1	19.6	24.9	28.5	22.5	36.6	53.0
West North Central	126.7	23.1	22.6	26.9	19.7	34.5	54.8
South Atlantic	142.6	19.0	28.6	35.0	24.0	36.0	53.9
East South Central	110.0	19.2	19.2	28.1	17.1	26.4	44.3
West South Central	119.7	20.6	21.1	29.5	20.3	28.1	45.9
Mountain	137.8	22.5	27.7	34.1	25.2	28.3	53.6
Pacific	173.9	25.4	36.7	40.8	35.8	35.2	65.8
Total U.S.	148.2	20.5	29.4	33.5	25.3	39.5	57.6

Sources: Haug and Roback (1970); Haug et al. (1971); Wunderman (1979).

* Comprised chiefly of interns and residents.

† Defined as general/family practitioners, general internists, and general pediatricians.

the largest concentrations of teaching hospitals are in the Middle Atlantic and New England states, these areas account for heavy concentrations of physicians in hospitals. Another factor that contributes to the unequal geographic distribution of physicians is the concentration of foreign medical graduates. Both as residents and as practicing physicians, foreign medical graduates tend to cluster in the Middle Atlantic and certain Midwestern states. Nevertheless, many influences other than the dispersions of teaching hospitals and foreign medical graduates are responsible for the very uneven geographic distribution of physicians, and they will be examined in succeeding chapters.

Table 1-3 presents the distribution of nonfederal patient care physicians by county group in 1969 and 1978. Again, the figures are physician population ratios subclassified by specialty and practice setting. The county classification is the AMA's "demographic county classification," in which counties labeled "1" are the most rural and those labeled "9" are the most urban. Three features of the data deserve special comment. The first is the enormous variation in the total number of physicians per capita between the most rural and most urban counties. The second is the association between the specialty composition of physicians and the degree of ruralness or urbanness of the county. General and family practitioners constitute the great majority of patient care physicians in the most rural counties, but only a small minority of them in the most urban counties. Historically, the rural physician has tended to be a general practitioner, and this is still true to a large extent, although the general practitioner is gradually being replaced by the family practitioner. Nonetheless, data suggest that county specialty patterns are due much less to the uneven distribution of general and family practitioners than to the uneven distribution of specialists. Nongeneral practitioners have long shown strong propensities to settle in metropolitan areas and to avoid communities where populations are small and thinly scattered.

The third characteristic of the data is the stability of physician-population ratios in the most rural counties between 1969 and 1978. Counties with populations greater than 25,000 benefited substantially from the growth of total physician supply during the 1970s. Those with populations of 25,000 or less did not. Indeed, other data compiled by the AMA show that the percentage of all nonfederal patient care physicians located in counties with populations of 25,000 or less fell from 3.3 to 3.1 between 1970 and 1980 (Haug et al. 1971; Bidese and Danais 1982). At least in regard to the *total* number of physicians, there is no evidence that the growth of aggregate physician supply in the 1970s improved access to care in the most rural counties. Whether the same was (or was not) true for inner cities is not clear. No data on physician distributions below the county level are regularly published, and none on inner-city communities are routinely available.

TABLE 1-3 Nonfederal Patient Care Physicians per 100,000 Population by AMA County Group Classification and Specialty Grouping, 1969 and 1978

| County Group* | All Physicians | Office-Based Physicians | | | | Hospital-Based Physicians† |
		General/Family Practitioners	Medical Specialists	Surgical Specialists	Other Specialists	
1969						
9	187.6	28.4	33.5	35.1	27.7	62.9
8	152.7	22.4	27.1	33.8	22.6	46.8
7	159.8	27.3	28.9	39.5	23.0	41.0
6	112.0	22.4	19.5	31.4	17.3	21.2
5	101.2	22.6	18.1	27.6	14.2	18.7
4	85.5	26.0	13.4	23.1	10.8	12.1
3	64.8	29.9	8.1	14.8	6.5	5.5
2	49.2	32.9	3.1	6.9	2.9	3.4
1	41.1	33.1	1.4	3.4	1.2	2.0
Total U.S.	121.6	25.2	20.6	27.7	17.1	31.0
1978						
9	214.7	20.9	45.4	39.8	36.9	71.6
8	183.8	18.3	38.1	39.5	32.8	55.1
7	159.9	17.1	32.4	37.4	26.2	46.8
6	137.1	19.5	26.9	35.9	24.7	30.2
5	132.3	18.6	26.8	36.9	23.2	26.8
4	98.5	21.4	18.6	28.2	16.2	14.1
3	75.6	25.2	12.0	19.7	11.0	7.6
2	52.5	28.1	4.9	8.5	5.3	5.7
1	41.2	27.7	2.4	4.3	3.3	3.5
Total U.S.	148.2	20.5	29.4	33.5	25.3	39.5

Sources: Haug and Roback (1970); Haug et al. (1971); Wunderman (1979).

*County Groups are defined as follows:
9—Counties in SMSAs with 5 million or more inhabitants;
8—Counties in SMSAs with 1 to 5 million inhabitants;
7—Counties in SMSAs with 500 thousand to 1 million inhabitants;
6—Counties in SMSAs with 50 to 500 thousand inhabitants;
5—Counties considered potential SMSAs;
4—Non-metropolitan counties with 50 thousand or more inhabitants;
3—Non-metropolitan counties with 25 to 50 thousand inhabitants;
2—Non-metropolitan counties with 10 to 25 thousand inhabitants;
1—Non-metropolitan counties with less than 10 thousand inhabitants;
† Comprised chiefly of interns and residents.

Table 1-3 does indicate that access to *specialists'* care increased in the most rural counties during the 1970s. In fact, as the Rand study observed, specialist-population ratios grew fastest in the most rural communities. However, as the table also shows, the number of general and family practitioners per capita in rural counties dropped by almost 20 percent between 1969 and 1978. Since family/general practitioners constituted most of the rural physician stock, this decline offset the rise in specialists per capita. The end result was the virtually constant overall physician-population ratio in the most rural counties between 1969 and 1978. Commenting on the constancy of the ratio, Fruen and Cantwell (1982) have suggested that it is at odds with Rand's finding of an improvement in the access of rural populations to physicians' care. However, the Rand investigators were careful to point out that their results applied only to specialists, and they noted that the constancy of the overall rural physician-population ratio was essentially the consequence of the continuing decline of general practice (Newhouse et al. 1982b).

The great inequalities in access to physicians' care between metropolitan and nonmetropolitan areas go back for decades,[5] and it is unlikely that they will be eliminated or even materially lessened in the foreseeable future. All the same, there are grounds for expecting that rural physician-population ratios may soon increase. In particular, assuming the percentage of physicians in family/general practice levels off—as it appeared to in the late 1970s—and provided the functional distribution of physicians otherwise remains constant, growth in the national physician-population ratio ought to assure positive growth in rural physician-population ratios. The secular decline in family/general practitioners per capita may well be coming to an end. That fact, coupled with further growth in the supply of rural specialists, should improve access to physicians' care in the most rural areas. Such an improvement could be counted as a benefit of the government's expansionist policy toward physician manpower. However, in light of the still low rural physician-population ratios, it may be regarded by rural populations as less than a signal achievement.

To summarize these observations: the most significant historical trend affecting the distribution of physicians among specialties has been the trend toward greater specialization. By greatly reducing the percentage of physicians engaged in general practice, it also reduced (by a somewhat lesser amount) the percentage of physicians practicing in the primary care fields. The dominant historical pattern in the geographic distribution of physicians has been one of inequality between regions of the country, between urban and rural areas, and between inner cities and suburbs. The distribution of physicians among specialties and locations has changed little in the recent past, and there are no signs that it will change greatly in the next decade or so. On the other hand, the intertemporal stability of this distribution—along with the growth in total physician supply—has produced larger numbers of physicians in the primary care fields and most geographic locations. There can be little doubt that access to primary care physicians and to physicians as a whole improved in the 1970s for most segments of the U.S. population. There is also little doubt that it will continue to improve during the 1980s. However, to the extent that the problem of unequal or inadequate access to care was brought about by a functional maldistribution of physicians, its amelioration has not been the result of a functional *redistribution* of physician manpower. The implications of this fact are examined in detail in subsequent chapters.

THE MEDICAL EDUCATIONAL PROCESS

Typically, the physician's choice of a specialty and a first practice location takes place during his or her medical education. The medical education system operates on physicians' specialty and practice location choices in two basic ways. First, it acts as a filter, admitting preferred types of individuals into medical school, graduate training hospitals, and specialty programs within both types of institutions. Second, it communicates information and a structure of values to those individuals it accepts. Formally, the system provides the physician with an outline of career alternatives, and with scientific knowledge, professional standards, and practical experience in patient care. Informally, it may provide faculty role models in various specialties, concepts of specialty status, exposure to training locations as possible places of practice, and information with respect to practice working conditions.

The medical education process can be viewed as a series of stages culminating with the physician's entry into practice. These stages are: (1) medical school; (2) first-year graduate training (formerly called internship); and (3) residency training. Each of these stages is preceded by the physician's decision as to which educational institution to attend. The decision involves the selection of a training location and, in the final stages, the selection of a training specialty. Since the supply of positions is controlled by the training institutions, the specialties, locations, and other characteristics of physicians at each stage are determined by a combination of physicians' choices and the admissions decisions of the institutions.[6]

The stage-wise nature of the medical education process, which forms the basis of later chapters, is illustrated schematically in Figure 1-1. Also shown in the figure are the various influences acting on physicians as they undergo this process.

FIGURE 1-1   The Effect of the Medical Education Process on Individual Physicians' Specialty and Location Choices

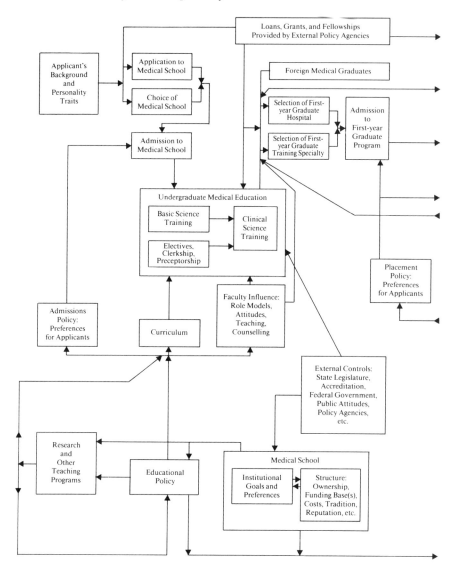

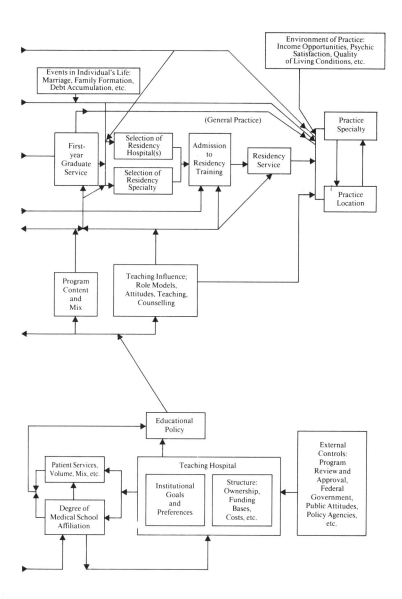

Descriptive evidence suggests that physicians ordinarily decide on a career in medicine by the first or second year of undergraduate college (e.g., Kritzer and Zimet 1967; Geertsma and Grinols 1972; Yancik 1977). During their junior or senior year, students apply to one or more medical schools. At this time they carry with them endowments of abilities, skills, educational experience, personal experience, and tastes. In research on the choice of medicine as a career, these endowments are usually represented by the collection of an individual's personality and background traits.[7]

The applicants to a medical school constitute its applicant pool, which can number many hundreds of candidates. Out of this pool—with its aggregate endowment of abilities and tastes—the school selects a limited number of individuals to fill its first-year places. These students then undergo a four-year program leading to a doctor of medicine degree.

The curriculum in the first two years consists primarily or exclusively of required course work in the "basic" or biological sciences such as anatomy, biochemistry, biophysics, and physiology. The final two years give medical students their first exposure to the "clinical" sciences —supervised course work in direct patient care. During these two years the students gain experience in the diagnosis and treatment of illnesses in a "teaching" hospital affiliated with the medical school.

In the two years before graduation, medical students are also given the opportunity of taking elective courses in the specialties. They are often required to take a special short program called a *clerkship* in a hospital, where they become familiar with hospital procedures and learn from practicing hospital physicians. They may have the option (or be required) to take another short program called a *preceptorship*, in which they serve as apprentices to office-based practitioners.

In most states a year of postgraduate hospital training is a prerequisite for licensure. Accordingly, in the senior (or even junior) medical school year, the student applies for a position in a postgraduate training program.[8] This program, which is given in a teaching hospital and lasts one year, used to be known as an internship and is presently called the *first graduate (or residency) year*. Students who are unsure of their specialty or desire experience in more than one field may elect a program in which they train for short periods in several different specialty departments. This type of program, formerly known as a *mixed* or *rotating* internship (the first type involving a greater specialty emphasis than the second), is now called a *flexible* first year.[9] Students who are reasonably sure of their specialty may choose a program entirely devoted to it. Until 1975, this was called a *straight* internship; it is now termed a *categorical* first-year program.

After being accepted into a program,[10] physicians must decide whether to continue training beyond the first year. Those who decide not to continue enter practice as general practitioners—usually after having taken a flexible first-year residency (rotating internship). Those who elect to continue must choose a specialty and make arrangements to go on with their residency in the same or another teaching hospital.

The purpose of residency training is to furnish physicians with an in-depth knowledge of, and competence in, a specialty.[11] The length and content of a completed residency program are determined in accordance with the requirements of the 20-odd specialty boards—professional associations that confer specialty certification on physicians who meet certain standards of competence. Among these standards are a minimum length of residency training (which varies by specialty) and a prescribed scope of training. Even though specialty board certification has no legal standing as a measure of competence in a field, it is recognized as such both inside and outside the medical profession.

Physicians can terminate their medical education at any of three points: after completing the first-year residency; after completing a full-term residency in a specialty; and after completing part, but not all, of a residency in a specialty. Except in the first case—which results in their becoming general practitioners—physicians normally designate themselves as specialists in their residency field.

Physicians may change their planned specialties or training locations during any stage of the educational process. Although little is known of later changes, physicians may, of course, change locations or specialties after entering practice. For example, a physician may begin as a general practitioner, but later resume full- or part-time residency training and become a specialist. Or a specialist may resume training and take up a subspecialty in his or her field.

As shown in Figure 1-1, a great many institutions and other factors can affect the development of the physician's career preferences during the educational process. The foremost of these is the medical school. Like other educational institutions, the medical school maintains a set of goals which are partly determined by its structure. In turn, these goals form the basis of its production of medical teaching services, research, teaching services for biological scientists and other nonphysician health professionals, patient care, etc. In some cases, the school may have an institutional "mission," such as the production of primary care practitioners, medical missionaries, or black physicians. Or its goals may interact: for example, its research policy may affect its teaching policies and the types of students it seeks to recruit. Its reputation for producing research may also significantly affect the types of applicants it attracts.

The medical school and the teaching hospital (whether affiliated with a medical school or not) are themselves subject to many external controls. We have already remarked on the influence of the specialty boards at the graduate level. In association with other professional groups, the boards regularly review hospital teaching programs for accreditation. Undergraduate teaching programs are also regularly reviewed by professional committees to assure that they meet minimum standards of quality.[12]

If the medical school is publicly owned, the state government may exercise considerable influence over its admissions and curricular policies and other aspects of its long-run management. Even public attitudes can have an impact on its policies. Whether publicly or privately owned, medical schools tend to regard themselves as public service institutions, and they are often sensitive to criticism of their policies and products.

At present, however, the major external controls are those of the federal government, which has been the largest single source of medical schools' income for the past two decades. The incentives embodied in, and regulations attached to, federal payments strongly affect medical schools' teaching capacity, research commitments, undergraduate curricula, mix of residency programs, and investment behavior. Further, federal and state education policies may influence the individual physician's career choices through a variety of loan and scholarship programs encouraging research, teaching, and the selection of medically underserved practice communities.

Forces outside the medical education system—largely those of the medical marketplace—also directly affect the physician's specialty and location decisions. Presumably, physicians select fields and practice locations that maximize the long-run utility they expect to receive as practitioners. This utility (or utility function) depends on the pecuniary and psychic rewards the physician assigns to prospective career alternatives. In turn, these rewards depend on both the markets for physicians' services and the actual conditions of practice.

Even so, the career alternatives the physician perceives—and the "shadow prices" he or she attaches to them—can be strongly influenced by medical education.[13] For instance, the choice of specialty ordinarily occurs well before entry into practice, and at the time it is made physicians may have little personal knowledge of the probable earnings or working conditions of practitioners. Hence, in selecting a field, they may rely heavily on the information conveyed to them by the medical education system. Educational values can affect this choice as well. If physicians learn from their teachers and colleagues that one field is particularly satisfying or prestigious and another is unsatisfying or suited only for the minimally competent, they may select the first over the second on these grounds alone.

This overview of the medical education process is meant to highlight its extraordinary complexity. However, in order to explain how physicians make their career choices, a careful sorting out of the numerous educational and other factors operating on those choices is essential. The chapters which follow are devoted to this by no means trivial effort.

THE TIMING OF SPECIALTY AND PRACTICE LOCATION DECISIONS

A knowledge of the timing of final specialty and practice location decisions is important for several reasons. First, it helps narrow the list of potential influences on career choices. If physicians are known to select specialties or locations before entering a given educational stage, all factors acting on them during that and later stages can be rejected as causes of their choices. Second, it provides a means of testing the reliability of career-choice predictions made in some studies at early educational stages. That is, no matter how well one can forecast career preferences at one stage in physicians' education, the predictions are of little value if most final decisions occur in later stages. Third, it furnishes a general guide for policy intervention. The longer career choices are delayed, the greater is the range of opportunities for altering them by policy action.

The evidence concerning the timing of final specialty choices is of two kinds: *ex ante* and retrospective. The former applies to findings in which physicians in training are simply asked if they have reached final decisions as to their specialties. The latter refers to results in which practicing physicians are asked when they selected their practice fields. Physicians in training may, of course, believe their current preferences are final whether this is true or not. Hence, one would expect the *ex ante* evidence to indicate that the choices occur at an earlier stage than is indicated by retrospective findings—which, of course, does not "prove" that they actually do.

Indeed, as would be expected, *ex ante* studies at several medical schools indicate that 20 percent to 30 percent of medical students choose their specialties before matriculation, and that 85 percent or more do so by graduation (Calahan et al. 1957; Saunders 1961; Boverman 1965; Wasserman et al. 1969; Breed 1970; Oates and Feldman 1971). But most such studies do not evaluate the degree of uncertainty in students' current specialty plans. Not surprisingly, two studies which took into account the uncertainty of specialty preferences both found much lower percentages of students with definite choices. They reported that only 10 percent of the freshman and 50 percent to 75 percent of the seniors at two medical schools were reasonably sure of their final fields (Zimny and Senturia 1974; Held and Zimet 1975).

The retrospective evidence is confined to studies of past generations of physicians by Weiskotten et al. (1960) and Lyden et al. (1968). The former covered all specialists in the graduating classes of 1935, 1940, 1945, and 1950, while the latter dealt with 1,200 graduates of 12 medical schools in 1950 and 1954. Together, the results indicated that 4 percent to 10 percent of the physicians had chosen final fields before entering medical school, 38 percent to 55 percent had done so by graduation, and only 75 percent had done so at the end of their first year of postgraduate training. These findings agree fairly well with the "uncertainty-adjusted" *ex ante* evidence.

The lateness of specialty choices is also reflected in the reported instability of specialty preferences during medical school. Most studies show that, after their freshman or sophomore years, 50 percent to 70 percent of medical students switch out of the fields they originally indicated as most preferred (Boverman 1965; Kritzer and Zimet 1967; Wasserman et al. 1969; Donovan et al. 1972; Geertsma and Grinols 1972; Held and Zimet 1975; Zimet and Held 1975; Cuca 1977). A few report marked shifts into or out of certain fields, but with one exception—internal medicine—the shifts exhibit no systematic pattern. Several studies have found that preferences for internal medicine increase during medical school, particularly in the final two years when students receive their first clinical training (Calahan et al. 1957; Wasserman et al. 1969; Zimny and Senturia 1974; Held and Zimet 1975; Cuca 1977). However, the overall distribution of students by their preferred specialties appears to remain relatively stable during medical school (Calahan et al. 1957; Wasserman et al. 1969; Roos and Fish 1974). The stability of the distribution disguises the volume of switching by individuals, but indicates that, on balance, there are no major shifts favoring or opposing given specialties.[14]

Historical evidence shows that some degree of specialty switching continues even after entry into practice. Studies of U.S. and Canadian physicians by Monk and Terris (1956), Weiskotten et al. (1961), and Weiss (1971) reported a substantial number of specialty changes among medical graduates from the classes of 1915 through 1950. The changes were predominantly from general to specialty practice, and may have been related to the long-run decline in popularity of general practice.

Among samples of 1935, 1940, and 1945 U.S. medical graduates, Weiskotten et al. (1961) found that more than a quarter of those entering general practice had switched to a specialty within 9 to 25 years after graduation. They also discovered a significant number of changes in the opposite direction. Roughly half of the loss of general practitioners was offset by switches into general practice from the specialty fields. A more recent study of U.S. graduates in the classes of 1960, 1964, and 1968 by Holden and Levit (1978) suggests that attrition in the primary care fields is continuing to take place after physicians enter practice. The sampled physicians' specialties in 1976 were compared with those in 1971, and in all three cohorts there were significant net losses of primary care practitioners between the two years. In percentage terms, the 1960 class lost 17 percent of its primary care physicians, the 1964 class lost 20 percent and the 1968 class (part of which was still in residency training in 1971) lost 32 percent. Unlike the findings of earlier studies, the largest net losses occurred in internal medicine—amounting to 26 percent, 28 percent, and 40 percent, respectively, of the physicians in the three cohorts who listed the field as their specialty in 1971. Unfortunately, the data did not indicate the directions of individual specialty switching, but the referral fields as a group attracted many new members. For example, in the 1968 cohort the number of referral specialists increased by 29 percent between 1971 and 1976.[15]

Although little research has examined the timing of location decisions, two salient characteristics of location choices tend to emerge from it. First, the selection of a practice location tends to take place later than the choice of a specialty. Second, rural-reared physicians generally select locations somewhat sooner than do urban-reared physicians.

Both findings are important because of what they suggest about cause and effect in specialty and location planning. The first implies that the choice of location is likely to be contingent on the choice of specialty, rather than vice versa. However—as will be shown in later chapters—rural general and family practitioners are especially likely to have had rural upbringings. In addition, general or family practice is more viable in rural areas than other specialties because it requires a relatively small population base. As a consequence, the second finding suggests that the choice of a rural practice community often precedes the choice of specialty and is accompanied by the selection of general or family practice.

The strongest evidence on the timing of location choices comes from a retrospective study of 1965 medical graduates by Heald et al. (1974).[16] Regrettably, it applies only to the choice between an urban or a rural area. But since the choice of community size precedes the decision as to the specific practice site, it nonetheless establishes approximate lower bounds on the timing of the choices of specific sites. Using a large national sample of physicians, Heald et al. found that 13 percent of the group had determined what size community they wanted to practice in by the time they were admitted to medical school, and only 21 percent had done so by graduation. More than half made the decision during graduate training, and one-fifth delayed it until their military service. Rural-reared physicians were about 50 percent more likely than urban-reared physicians to have decided on community size both at admission to medical school and by graduation.[17]

The few remaining results tend to corroborate these findings. A small-sample study of students at western medical schools by Taylor et al. (1973) reported that 40 percent had tentatively selected specialties but not locations, while only 17 percent had selected locations but not specialties. Again, this indicates that specialty choice usually precedes location choice. The timing of community-size decisions by rural practitioners was also explored by Hassinger (1963) and Parker and Tuxill (1967). In each instance, the percentages of physicians making early decisions to enter rural locations were higher than those for all physicians described by Heald et al., but they were of the same order as the percentages given by Heald et al. for rural-reared physicians.[18]

Little is known of the stability of physicians' location preferences during their medical education, although there are indications that preferences for rural locations decline during medical school (Taylor et al. 1973; California Medical Association 1976). Likewise, almost nothing is known of movements from first to subsequent practice locations. Fragmentary descriptive reports imply that one-third or more of all physicians leave their first locations,[19] but no important efforts have been made to determine the timing, directions, or magnitude of the migration.

On the whole, the available evidence indicates that approximately 90 percent of all final specialty choices and first location choices are made after admission to medical school. Perhaps half of all specialty choices, and three-quarters or more of all location choices, occur after the start of graduate training. These results lead to two conclusions regarding methodologies for explaining physicians' career choices. First, early career preferences *and* their correlates are unreliable predictors of most final career choices. Second, educational and other forces can affect the choices of a substantial proportion of physicians throughout nearly the entire educational process. Similarly—with respect to policy options —the major implication is that some latitude exists for influencing these choices in all but the terminal stage of the process.

SUMMARY

For most physicians, selecting a specialty and a practice location is a dynamic process lasting perhaps many years. In principle, the process can be influenced by a congeries of factors, including individuals' tastes, the medical education environment, and market or other external stimuli. The evidence on the timing of career choices makes it difficult to rule out any of these factors as irrelevant to the decision process.

The manner in which physicians choose specialties and locations has been the subject of extensive empirical research—more than that devoted to any other occupational group. Educators, sociologists, psychologists, and economists have participated, each bringing their special knowledge, interests, and (one must add) prejudices.

One result of the diversity of study approaches is a highly compartmentalized set of findings. For example, a wealth of detail exists about the personality correlates of specialty choices, yet little is understood of the importance of personality traits in relation to other predictors of specialty choices. The research is also of uneven quality. Much of it is purely descriptive, and even a substantial portion of the analytical work is marred by the use of relatively crude statistical methods. Differences in sampling, test instruments or questionnaires, explanatory variables, and statistical tools all contribute to inconsistencies in the empirical findings. Therefore, any discussion of the evidence is incomplete without a review of the study methodologies. In writing the chapters that follow we sought to evaluate the methodologies, as well as to summarize the findings, of studies of physicians' career choices. Often it proved impossible to reach definitive judgments as to the reliability of the findings. Nevertheless, we sought to identify the major hypotheses explicit or implicit in the empirical work, and to distinguish those which can be accepted with reasonable confidence from those which should be exposed to further testing.

NOTES

1. Actually, the expression *primary care* is not confined to first physician contact by a patient seeking treatment. Typically, it refers to generalized or principal care received by a patient on a continuing basis. The paradigmatic primary care physician is one who normally treats a patient; is the provider first seen at the onset of an illness; gives routine care; and, when necessary, supplies referrals to other physicians. See Aiken et al. (1979) for a further discussion and history of the term.
2. The interested reader should see Stevens and Vermeulen (1972), Stevens et al. (1978), and Ernst et al. (1978). At present, no surveys of osteopaths' career choices are available.
3. These are the same as the primary care fields designated by present federal programs. Some authorities argue that obstetrics-gynecology and psychiatry should be added to the list. Others have pointed out that primary care services are often provided by physicians not ordinarily classified as primary care practitioners. For example, a study at the University of Southern California has reported that in 14 referral specialties, 20 percent to 72 percent of all patient visits are for "principal" or primary care (Aiken et al. 1979).
4. The percentages cited in this paragraph are taken from recent AMA tabulations of the number of physicians (e.g., Wunderman 1979).
5. For some evidence, see Stewart and Pennell (1960) and Fruen and Cantwell (1982).

6. Virtually nothing is known of how physicians select educational institutions. In later chapters it will be shown that a knowledge of these choices is crucial for understanding the effects of the medical education system on career decisions. For example, the graduates of a given medical school may display a particular career-choice pattern, and this could be due to applicant self-selection (i.e., to applicants' latent career preferences), admissions filtering by the school, or the particular learning environment. Without knowledge of the demand for the school's positions and its admissions preferences, it cannot be determined which of these factors causes the observed pattern.

7. Personality traits are customarily measured as scores on personality tests. Background traits consist of age, sex, race, marital status, family income, place of upbringing, etc. Obviously, personality and background traits may be interrelated.

8. In 1975, internship and residency programs were integrated into single units in all teaching hospitals. The entire postgraduate specialty program is now called a residency, but, at least informally, the first year is usually differentiated from subsequent years.

9. The rotating internship normally involved short periods of training in each of several specialty departments. The mixed internship entailed up to several months of training in one department with brief periods in others.

10. Most students and teaching hospitals with residency programs participate in the National Resident Matching Program (NRMP) (formerly the National Intern and Resident Matching Program [NIRMP]). Students and hospitals submit lists of their preferences for one another to the program. The two sets of preferences are then centrally matched, although neither students nor hospitals are necessarily awarded their first choices.

11. Both first- and subsequent-year residents are salaried contractual employees of the teaching hospital. As such, they are partly students, partly apprentices to the teaching staff with teaching responsibilities of their own, and partly practicing physicians. They learn by supervised, on-the-job treatment of patients, study of the pertinent medical literature, and formal or informal discussions with the teaching staff. Their performance is continuously monitored, evaluated, and corrected by the senior staff. As residents progress through the program, their responsibilities for patient management increase, and they become members of the teaching staff with a duty to teach and supervise first-year and other junior residents. During residency, physicians many obtain their first license to practice, without which they are legally forbidden to treat patients except under the direct supervision of a licensed practitioner.

12. Indirectly, the state licensing boards have a part in enforcing these restrictions on educational institutions. Graduation from an approved medical school and training in an approved graduate program are requisites for licensure. Hence, any institution that loses its approval runs the risk of losing its students or trainees.

13. A shadow price is the resource value of the opportunities that are forgone by making a specific choice. Even when individuals do not know the clearly de-

fined pecuniary prices of their alternatives, the act of making a choice implies the forgoing of some alternative and, by extension, the value of that alternative.

14. At some medical schools a decline in interest in general practice has been observed (Chipman et al. 1969; Kraus et al. 1971). However, by the late 1970s, there were indications that the percentage of students preferring family practice increases between matriculation and graduation (Cuca 1977).

15. The reasons for this volume of specialty switching are not well understood. A paper by Matteson and Smith (1977) reports that as few as 65 percent to 85 percent of medical students may "select" a specialty that they prefer over all others. If the conclusion is correct, it suggests that many physicians—i.e., those starting practice in fields they do not most prefer—may switch to other specialties as soon as they have the opportunity to do so. Although they are small in number and may not be representative of the physician population as a whole, physicians in public health seem to exemplify this pattern. At least historically, public health has been a low-prestige specialty and one subject to a high rate of turnover. Physicians who choose the field tend to do so late in their careers, and many appear to view it as either a second choice or an interruption in their preferred careers. According to the available evidence, the reasons for choosing public health include indecision about a specialty and/or about a long-term commitment to private practice, the desire to finance graduate training in another field, temporary opportunities for broadening career experience, and even considerations of health and semiretirement. See Coker et al. (1966), Kosa et al. (1966, "Novice Physicians"; 1966, "Transiency of Physicians"), and Miller et al. (1966, "Comparison of Career Patterns"; 1966, "Toward a Typology").

16. Similar results from the same data set were obtained by Cooper et al. (1975) and Steinwald and Steinwald (1975).

17. The choice of a practice location, like the choice of a specialty, appears to occur in two phases—"general" and "specific." The general choice consists of narrowing preferences to a group of desired or acceptable alternatives. The specific choice consists of the selection of an actual location and field. The results by Heald et al. (1974) and the others cited in the subsequent paragraphs refer to one dimension of the general choice of location, while those bearing on specialty decisions refer to specific choices. In this sense, existing research does not provide a clear picture of the process by which location and specialty preferences are narrowed during medical education. Thus, the apparent lateness of career decisions may exaggerate the flexibility of career preferences during the early educational stages.

18. Hassinger (1963) found that, among Missouri practitioners, 25 percent had selected their practice-community sizes before medical school, and 45 percent had done so by graduation. Parker and Tuxill (1967) reported that the percentages were 16 and 26, respectively, for upstate New York physicians. Both studies defined community size as the size of the physician's current practice community, which was generally not the same as the first practice community. For example, 6 percent of the Hassinger sample and 22 percent

of the Parker-Tuxill sample chose community sizes after completing their graduate training. Both studies—and particularly the second—therefore understate the percentages of early decisions as to a *first* practice community size.

19. Further discussion of these reports is found in Chapter 8.

TWO

Personality Traits, Attitudes, and Physicians' Career Choices

Economists regard measures of personality characteristics or attitudes as surrogates for individuals' preferences in analyses of decision making, and they are usually taken as given. By contrast, the individual's personality traits play a much more active part in sociologists' and psychologists' theories of choice—especially those of occupational choice. Regardless of the discipline in which they originate, empirical models of specialty choice may merely postulate an association between individuals' personality traits and their selection of a field without specifying causal relationships. This is particularly true of the economic theories, about which we will have more to say in Chapter 6. However, the theories advanced by noneconomists typically make an effort to delineate the causal linkages between personality traits and the choice of a field. A good illustration is provided by the role-model theory of choice, in which the physician-to-be is postulated to select the field that most nearly resembles the professional identity he or she prefers to take on. This type of theory underlies most of the discussion of specialty choice in the present chapter, since nearly all of the research in the area has been done by sociologists, psychologists, medical educators, and others who employ basically noneconomic methodologies.

Role-model theories of occupational choice are themselves aspects of more global theories of professional development or "professionalization." The latter deal with the process by which individuals who train for a profession come to take on the identities, attitudes, habits, and other characteristics of practitioners in the profession. This process is commonly thought to involve role modeling, but it may also entail many other elements such as the content of training programs or the manner in which it is presented, the values exhibited by teachers or trainees' peer groups, and the prior experience and innate characteristics of trainees.[1] Here, we consider the effects of role modeling in their narrower application to the choice of a specialty, and not to the process of professionalization once a field has been selected.[2] The factors acting on the professionalization process may, of course, influence the way physicians-to-be perceive or select their preferred specialty role. This possibility will be addressed specifically in discussing the educational environment in Chapters 4 and 5.

The roles physician trainees seek may be based on the personalities of one or more real people, on some idealization of what a physician is, or on their own particular abilities, skills, and preferences. In any case, however specialty roles originate in trainees' minds, role-model methodologies must accomplish three objectives if they are to predict specialty choices. Specifically, they must: (1) identify a set of personality traits by which to classify physicians, (2) define a taxonomy of specialties that represent the physician's potential roles, and (3) associate given personality traits with the roles defined by the taxonomy. Hypothesis testing can then take the form of demonstrating the existence and nature of the relationships between personality traits and specialty choices. Clearly, both the outcomes of the tests and the predictive capabilities of the methodology depend on the accurate identification of personality traits and the validity of the specialty taxonomy.

Because roles cannot be assigned to practice locations, the usual methods of determining physicians' locational preferences have not involved this type of theory of choice. Instead, physicians or medical students are typically asked to list the factors that influenced their actual or planned location choice, or to indicate their motives for making the choice. The responses are then arrayed in order of importance to construct a model explaining general location behavior.

Many of the findings discussed in this chapter are either descriptive or based on simple (most often univariate) statistical tests. They can be evaluated in terms of their ability to predict choice outcomes, their qualitative implications for choice behavior, and their fruitfulness for generating further behavioral hypotheses.

PERSONALITY TRAITS AND SPECIALTY CHOICES

More than a dozen different personality tests have been used in studies attempting to associate personality traits with specialty choices.[3]

Unfortunately, no systematic efforts have been made to compare the findings or to evaluate the capabilities of the tests themselves.[4] This makes it difficult to summarize the results and to determine what they mean.

Another problem is that sample characteristics vary enormously. While most studies are confined to small samples at single medical schools, some treat large groups of students or graduates from as many as two dozen different schools. In addition, there is little uniformity in the choice of subjects' ages. Researchers have attempted to correlate personality traits with specialty preferences at virtually all stages of the career-choice process, from entry into medical school to 10 or more years after graduation. The customary hypothesis is that the traits identified by personality tests are stable; but even if the hypothesis is true, it does not, of course, follow that specialty preferences are stable during the early stages of the physician's medical education. As a consequence, the instability of early preferences, is probably an important source of variation in empirical results.

A third problem is differences in methodology. The common procedure is to compare personality test scores across groups of individuals who express preferences for or choose different specialties. Most often the comparisons are made using pairwise or multiple-comparison significance tests on the mean scores (e.g., Myers and Davis 1964; Schumacher 1964; Livingston and Zimet 1965; Davies and Mowbray 1968; Canning et al. 1974), but other methods such as factor and cluster analysis, analysis of variance, discriminant analysis, and regression analysis have also been used (e.g., Schumacher 1963; Paiva and Haley 1971; Donovan et al. 1972; Otis and Weiss 1973; Hadley 1977). Few attempts have been made to assess the accuracy of scores for predicting specialty choices, and the comparison-of-means approach makes it impossible to do so.

Finally, there is considerable variation in the specialty taxonomies used by researchers. Classifications have involved as few as 3 or as many as 10 or more specialty strata. Some authors segregate academic physicians from practitioners while others do not, and most studies aggregate two or more specialties into combined fields. Moreover, recent work has raised doubt about the meaningfulness of the standard specialty definitions in terms of specialty preferences. Otis and Weiss (1973) and Gough (1975) reported that medical students at the University of New Mexico and the University of California at San Francisco, respectively, did not recognize distinctions among certain specialties which correspond to the standard definitions. For example, both studies found that students regarded internal medicine as a referral specialty, unlike the other primary care fields. Gough claimed that pediatrics has no marked characteristics that distinguish it in terms of students' preferences from such diverse fields as family practice, allergy and immunology, psychiatry, and hematology. By contrast, both studies reported that medical students do perceive differences among the surgical specialties, implying that aggregation of the surgical fields into one grouping may obscure the relationships between them and personality traits. Taken together, their results indicate that personality traits may be of restricted usefulness for predicting the choices of specialties as they are conventionally defined.

Subject to the foregoing qualifications, certain personality patterns appear to be associated with particular specialties or fields. Roughly speaking, the stereotypes are as follows. Psychiatrists have been variously described as intuitive, introverted, nonauthoritarian, and uncompulsive. They have been found to exhibit high aesthetic, social, and theoretical values, but low religious values[5] and low economic motivation. They have also been reported as ranking high in thought complexity, preferences for abstract thinking, and death anxiety (Schumacher 1963; Myers and Davis 1964; Livingston and Zimet 1965; Davies and Mowbray 1968; Walton 1969; Yufit et al. 1969; Paiva and Haley 1971).

In many ways, the stereotype of the surgeon is the polar opposite of that of the psychiatrist. According to most findings, the surgeon's personality type is sensing and materialistic (as opposed to intuitive), aggressive, dominating, authoritarian, action-oriented, and extroverted. Surgeons have been found to display low social values relative to other specialists, a high degree of practicality, and low death anxiety (Myers and Davis 1964; Livingston and Zimet 1965; Yufit et al. 1969; Zimny and Thale 1970; Paiva and Haley 1971; Otis and Weiss 1973; Collins and Roessler 1975).

The third field which has been reasonably well identified is academic medicine. The distinguishing traits of academic physicians appear to be low economic motivation; high theoretical, investigative, and social interests; and (unlike psychiatrists) a need for dominance or the assumption of a leadership role (Schumacher 1963, 1964; Myers and Davis 1964; Sanazaro 1965; Weil and Schleiter 1981).

Results for other specialties, including the primary care fields, are far less conclusive. Some researchers have found that general practitioners resemble surgeons more than other physicians, except that they appear to lack surgeons' preferences for dominance. The general practitioner stereotype is said to show low theoretical and aesthetic values, low leadership preferences, high compulsiveness, and high economic and religious values. General practitioners are described by personality tests as sociable, person-oriented, and practical (Schumacher 1963; Paiva and Haley 1971; Hadley 1975). Little is known of the traits of family practitioners, but studies at Baylor (Collins and Roessler 1975) and the University of Utah (Canning et al. 1974) reported that medical students preferring family practice were more sociable and less aggressive, materialistic, and authoritarian than students preferring other specialties. Pediatricians have been characterized as nonaggressive, extroverted, warmhearted, and high in death anxiety (Myers and Davis 1964; Livingston and Zimet 1965; Zimny and Thale 1970; Collins and Roessler 1975), while internists purportedly exhibit high theoretical and intellectual interests, low economic motivation, and strong preferences for leadership (Schumacher 1963, 1964; Zimny and Thale 1970).[6]

Very few attempts have been made to discriminate primary care practitioners as a group from referral specialists on the basis of personality traits. However, Weil et al. (1981) and Weil and Schleiter (1981) have compared the personality traits of residents in internal medicine who were planning either generalist or subspecialty careers. Utilizing a 1977 national sample of resident internists, Weil et al. found that future generalists and future subspecialists had rather similar constellations of personality characteristics. Consistent with the findings just described, both groups tended to rank high in terms of investigative and artistic interests. Nevertheless, the generalists scored significantly higher than subspecialists in social interests, and significantly lower in investigative and artistic interests. The results seem to confirm the indications that general practitioners—the paradigmatic types of primary care physicians—are more socially oriented than referral physicians and less concerned with investigative, theoretical, and aesthetic pursuits.

In a companion study of internists in residency training, Weil and Schleiter (1981) employed an index of investigative vocational interests to predict the residents' preferences for primary care practice. Employing a multiple regression methodology, they found that their measure of primary care preferences was significantly negatively related to the investigative-interests index, even after standardizing for the effects of other variables. The result corroborates the evidence obtained by Weil et al., but the index was less important as a predictor of primary care preferences than other taste and background variables discussed below.

As we have remarked, attempts have been made to construct specialty taxonomies and to link personality traits with them. Based on subjective judgments, Yufit et al. (1969) and Wasserman et al. (1969) defined three specialty groupings—"surgical-technical," "person-oriented," and "mixed"—and three broad personality types—"intimate," "isolate," and "neither intimate nor isolate."[7] Among graduates of the University of Illinois, they reported that isolate physicians predominantly chose the surgical-technical specialties, intimate physicians selected both the surgical-technical and person-oriented fields, and physicians who were neither intimate nor isolate chose specialties in all three of the designated strata.

In another study of Johns Hopkins graduates, Monk and Thomas (1970), inter alia, divided their subjects into practitioners, academicians, and physicians in hospital-based positions or preventive medicine. They found that the last group more frequently showed signs of depression or anxiety than either practitioners or academicians, but differences in the incidence of symptoms among the three groups of physicians were not statistically significant.

Following the work of Yufit et al. (1969), Otis and Weiss (1973) and Quenk and Albert (n.d.) also designed new personality and specialty taxonomies, the latter based on work setting as well as specialty. Otis and Weiss constructed a 5-way occupational classification and a 10-way personality typology, while Quenk and Albert devised a 7-way occupational classification and informally matched it with a set of personality characteristics. Both studies claimed success in identifying physicians who chose academic careers (described as intuitive and intellectual) or institutional settings (described as reserved and introverted). However, neither study found one-to-one associations between personality types and preferences for the primary care, surgical, and other specialties, and neither attempted to predict specialty choices from personality traits.

Studies that have reported the capabilities of personality traits to predict specialty choices have shown that the forecasts are at least moderately superior to random selection. The most successful effort was by Donovan et al. (1972). Using discriminant analysis and a six-way specialty classification, they correctly identified the specialties of 51 percent of a sample of Rochester graduates. However, they included several cognitive variables (such as Medical College Admissions Test scores) among their predictors and did not specify the personality measures they employed.

Anderson (1975) used the same methodology but a different six-way specialty classification to analyze a group of graduates of an unnamed southern medical school, and correctly predicted the specialties of 48 percent of his sample. However, like Donovan et al., he specified a mixed set of (four) personality and (six) physician background variables as predictors and did not state the forecasting ability of the personality measures alone.[8] In the study described above, Yufit et al. (1969) reported that their subjective forecasts were only 22 percent accurate when they employed an initial 11-way specialty classification. As would be expected, the success rate rose (to 48 percent) when they condensed their taxonomy to only three strata.

Hadley (1977) specified four personality traits in regressions predicting the probabilities of choosing five specialty fields. Collectively, the four traits were significantly correlated with the choice probabilities, and the signs of the coefficients were generally consistent with previously de-

fined personality stereotypes.[9] Hadley's regressions correctly predicted
the specialties of 58 percent of the physician subjects, but they contained
other significant variables besides the four personality-trait factors. Hadley did not separately report the contribution of the personality-trait factors to the accuracy of his forecasts.

Zimny (1980) designed and employed a 199-item personality test to
predict the specialty choices of medical students at five medical schools.
He then compared the predicted choices with the specialty programs selected by the students in their first graduate training years. Overall, the
test correctly predicted the choices of 51 percent of the students, with the
percentages of correct predictions ranging from 38 in pediatrics to 74 in
medicine. Zimny noted that first-year graduate specialties are not necessarily indicative of final choices, but in another, smaller student sample
his test accurately predicted 55 percent of the second-year graduate specialty choices.

Thus, while most investigators have not claimed perfect success in
associating personality characteristics with specialty choices, the weight
of evidence implies that certain strong correlations do exist. As yet, the
findings are probably not strong enough to justify a rigorous delineation
of specialty stereotypes or the conclusion that choosing a specialty role is
the major behavioral process underlying specialty selection. They are,
however, compatible with the more modest hypothesis that physicians'
tastes have an important effect on specialty choices. In addition, more
convincing empirical results may be forthcoming as the precision of personality-trait and specialty taxonomies improves.

One shortcoming of the findings is that they do not take account of
how educational experiences affect (or may affect) specialty role modeling. For example, if medical school A gives its students a different con-
ception of a specialty than school B does, one ought not to observe the
same associations between students' personality traits and their specialty
choices at the two schools. All the same, the basic appeal of role-model
methodologies *as predictive devices* lies precisely in their generality. In
this respect, one would like to be able to say that a particular configura-
tion of personality traits is always associated with the choice of a particular specialty. Likewise, one would like to be able to say that the association is invariant with respect to training experiences. Otherwise, the
theory of role modeling becomes primarily a description of the mechanism by which physicians-to-be select their fields. A medical student
with a fixed endowment of personality traits may attend medical school
A or B, and in either case choose a specialty in accordance with his or her
preferred professional role. Yet the choice may easily be affected by the
content of the student's educational experience.[10]

To sum up, three points need to be stressed regarding the role-model theory approach. First, there are sufficient grounds to question whether it is an accurate predictive theory of specialty choice. In particular, to the extent that perceptions of specialty roles are influenced by environmental factors, it is these factors that are causatively related to specialty choices. Second—and in the same vein—we should not necessarily expect the same patterns of association between personality traits and specialty choices to emerge at all medical schools or with respect to all types of training environments. Third, there exists a group of theories, which we will examine in Chapters 4 and 5, holding that the training environment is the dominant factor explaining specialty choices. Since role-model methodologies do not and cannot preclude such explanations, conflict between the role-model and environmental theories of choice is, perhaps, unavoidable.

Obviously, these points should not be exaggerated. Different training environments are not likely to convey radically different views of the activities and attributes of specialties. Hence, it would be unrealistic to expect different medical schools and graduate programs to produce radically different patterns of specialty choice by individuals with the same traits. Indeed, many of the results discussed above do, in fact, show stable relationships between personality traits and specialty choices over several or more medical schools. This is perhaps the best testimony to the general validity of the role-model hypothesis. But, to the extent that the hypothesis is generally valid, it undermines the theory that the educational environment significantly influences specialty choices. If the same set of personality traits is always associated with a particular choice, then either the training environment has a negligible impact on the choice or else it is so similar in different schools and training programs that it does not generate the variations in experience necessary to cause different choices.

Another problem with the findings summarized above is that they apply almost exclusively to white male physicians. Since 1970, medical schools have accepted large numbers of female and minority applicants. At present, these groups represent approximately one-third of all U.S.-educated physicians entering practice. There have been no systematic studies of the personality traits of minority physicians, and little is known about the characteristics of women physicians. Conventional wisdom holds that women physicians are much more likely than their male counterparts to exhibit "feminine" or "maternal" attributes which lead them to choose such specialties as pediatrics and psychiatry.[11] Yet Cartwright (1972) has reported that male and female medical students' personality traits are essentially similar. And, in a study at the University of Colorado and the University of California at San Diego, McGrath and

Zimet (1977) found that female medical students regarded themselves as more action-oriented, independent, and aggressive than men. However, since both studies involved small samples and were based in whole or part on medical students' self-evaluation, it would be rash to say that they reveal new behavioral patterns. All in all, the question of how the personality traits of women and minority physicians bear on their specialty choices remains unsettled.

ATTITUDINAL STUDIES OF SPECIALTY CHOICE

Most attitudinal studies of medical students' or physicians' specialty preferences fall into one of two categories. In the simpler of the two types, subjects are merely asked to list or rank their reasons for selecting a specialty, or to assess the importance of various factors acting on their choices. For the most part, the results are what one would expect.

For example, surveys by Monk and Terris (1956) and Lyden et al. (1968) indicated that humanitarian, service-oriented, and intellectual motives were influential in specialty decisions, but income motives were not.[12] Less naively, perhaps, Weil et al. (1981) and Weil and Schleiter (1981) asked residents in internal medicine to evaluate the importance of anticipated working conditions and income in their choices of primary care or subspecialty practice. As in the other studies, income expectations did not seem to affect the choice, but Weil and Schleiter (1981) found that an index of preferences for working conditions was the strongest of four predictors of type-of-practice preferences (the others were personality traits, personal background characteristics, and educational experience). Generalists were significantly more interested than subspecialists in establishing continuing, principal-care relationships with patients, and less interested than subspecialists in research, utilizing technical diagnostic methods, consulting, and controlling their work hours.[13] It is, of course, valuable to know that anticipated working conditions (i.e., one dimension of the attributes of a field) strongly affect attitudes toward primary care as opposed to subspecialty practice. Yet, on balance, the results tell us only that physicians who prefer the working conditions usually associated with primary care practice are especially likely to select primary care practice as a career.

The more sophisticated kinds of attitudinal studies are basically extensions of efforts to correlate personality traits with specialty choices, and they have proceeded in several directions. Namely, they include: (1) attempts to construct physicians' qualitative images of specialists (or specialties); (2) efforts to measure the relative professional status and social attractiveness of specialties; (3) examination of changes in perceived specialty status as physicians progress through the educational system; and (4) tests of the hypothesis that physicians choose specialties whose images are most similar to the images they have of themselves. Most of the work in this area was conducted by Bruhn and Parsons (1964, 1965) at the University of Oklahoma and by Zimet and his colleagues at the University of Colorado (Kritzer and Zimet 1967; Fishman and Zimet 1972; Zimet and Held 1975; McGrath and Zimet 1977).

The findings of these attitudinal studies indicate that physicians' images of specialists largely resemble the basic stereotypes developed from personality tests (Bruhn and Parsons 1964; Coker et al 1966; Zimny and Thale 1970).[14] Surgeons emerge with three distinctive traits—exceptional competence; aloofness toward others; and a forceful, decisive manner often characterized as arrogant or egotistical. Internists appear to be regarded as intellectuals whose approach to medicine is logical, investigative, and detached. General practitioners are considered average, energetic, friendly, and (unlike surgeons and internists) interested in other persons. Pediatricians tend to be perceived as having the most desirable social traits—warmth, compassion, humor and patience—and psychiatrists the least. In contrast to personality studies, attitudinal research has either produced no clear-cut stereotype of psychiatrists or, alternatively, has suggested that psychiatrists are not greatly admired by other physicians. Psychiatrists have been described by other practitioners as intellectual but confused and emotionally unstable (Bruhn and Parsons 1964), or unambitious and aloof (Zimny and Thale 1970).

Because the qualititative stereotypes contain a mixture of traits to which normative judgments can be attached, efforts have been made to develop indices of specialty attractiveness. One, designed by Bruhn and Parsons (1965), gave numerical scores to specialty attributes and weighted them by subjects' assessments of the favorability or unfavorability of the attributes. The other, employed by Zimet et al. (Kritzer and Zimet 1967; Fishman and Zimet 1972; Zimet and Held 1975; McGrath and Zimet 1977), proposed separate measures of the professional status and social attractiveness of specialties. The latter showed systematic, and apparently stable, differences in perceived specialty status and social attractiveness persisting over several medical school classes. Surgery was consistently ranked as the most prestigious of all specialty fields, with internal medicine ranked second, and family or general practice ranked last.[15] In terms of social attractiveness, however, general or family practice was consistently ranked first and surgery last. Psychiatry was perceived to have low status and social attractiveness, while pediatrics was rated intermediate in status and high in social attractiveness. The aggregative Bruhn-Parsons measure awarded the highest overall "image scores" to general practice and internal medicine and the lowest to surgery and psychiatry.

All studies indicate that the perceived desirability of internal medicine increases during medical school, especially in the final two years when students are first exposed to clinical medicine. This pattern is consistent with the increasing popularity of internal medicine as a specialty preference before graduation,[16] and suggests that increased information may affect preferences. The high status of surgery and internal medicine is also compatible with the results of personality studies showing that surgeons and internists are likely to be more prestige-conscious than other practitioners.

Attitudinal researchers have reported that surgery and internal medicine are the most frequently chosen specialties, despite their low or average social attractiveness. Hence, the implication is that professional status is a far more important consideration in specialty decisions than the social attractiveness of the field. Unfortunately, only one attempt has been made to estimate the influence of status seeking on specialty selection, and it was carried out on a small sample. Kritzer and Zimet (1967) surveyed residents at the University of Colorado and found that those from the lowest socioeconomic backgrounds tended to choose the most prestigious specialties.[17]

Despite the general directions of the evidence, its lack of rigor raises doubt about its usefulness for predicting specialty choices. The work of Zimet et al. (Kritzer and Zimet 1967; Fishman and Zimet 1972; Zimet and Held 1975; McGrath and Zimet 1977) has repeatedly demonstrated that medical students believe their self-images more closely resemble the images of their chosen specialties than those of other specialties.[18] This would seem to confirm the hypothesis that the physician searches for a specialty whose image (as measured by his perception of physicians in the field) most nearly matches his perception of himself. Yet study methodologies have not directly tested the existence of cause-effect relationships, and no efforts have been made to predict specialty choices from prior knowledge of students' self-images.

The lack of direct testing leaves open the alternative hypothesis that similarities between believed specialty images and self-images are rationalizations of decisions already made. For example, in the studies noted in the previous paragraph, Zimet et al. also found that, having selected or announced preferences for given specialties, medical students invariably ranked their chosen fields highest in professional status and social attractiveness. Even the fields given low professional status and social attractiveness by students as a whole were rated highest in these attributes by individuals who planned to enter them. Thus, it may easily be that students' descriptions of specialties are biased by their choices, or else that perceptions of specialty attributes vary substantially among individuals. Although there can be little doubt that role modeling occurs in

the specialty-decision process, it is difficult to argue that the existing attitudinal research gives a solid operational framework for predicting the
outcomes of the process.

SHIFTS IN SPECIALTY PREFERENCES: ERA EFFECTS

With one exception—general practice—the distribution of physicians among specialties has remained largely stable over the past generation. AMA data on the specialty composition by year of medical school
graduation (Martin 1975) show that 19 percent of the U.S. medical
school graduating classes of 1945–54 were in general practice in 1973, as
opposed to only 7 percent of the graduating classes of 1965–69. By contrast, little systematic change took place over this same period in the specialty distribution of non-general practitioners. An examination of the
graduating classes from 1945 to 1969 in five-year intervals revealed that
the percentage of medical specialists among non-general practitioners
ranged from 28 to 32, and the percentage of surgeons ranged from 30 to
36. For individual specialties, the percentage of internists among non-
general practitioners fluctuated between 15 and 18, the percentage of
pediatricians held constant at about 7, the percentage of obstetrician-gy-
necologists ranged from 5 to 9, and the percentage of general surgeons
declined from 12 to 7.[19] As a result, the period from World War II to
1969 was marked chiefly by the decline of general practice, and by relatively minor shifts in the specialty distribution of other physicians. However, as mentioned in Chapter 1, the secular losses of primary care practitioners seemed to stabilize in the 1970s, and the number is now on the
rise.

As a way of viewing these trends, Funkenstein (1978) proposed dividing the history of medical education in this century into six eras. The
first, which he called the "general practice era," was characterized by
broad but shallow premedical training, produced chiefly physician generalists, and ended about 1939. The second two eras began, according to
his schema, at the start of World War II and reached their peak in the
mid-1960s. He labeled them the "specialty" and "scientific" eras. Their
hallmark was training in a university environment where first priority
was given to faculty research and great value was placed on competence
in a narrow specialty field. Because general practice was accorded low
status, the two eras witnessed an appreciable decline in the percentage of
new graduates entering the field. Clearly, the data cited above are consistent with this thesis.

Funkenstein called his fourth historical period the "student activism era." He dated its beginning in 1969, when medical students' interests in the primary care specialties suddenly appeared to increase. This increase he attributed to social commitments arising out of the political and cultural movements of the 1960s (e.g., civil rights reform, opposition to the Vietnam war, and general dissatisfaction with impersonal bureaucracy and technology). The social changes of the 1960s were reflected, he argued, not only in students' changed attitudes toward primary care, but also in the creation of family practice as a recognized specialty in 1969, the liberalization of admissions policies and curricula in medical schools, and federal subsidy programs for primary care training.

Funkenstein called the final two periods of his schema, starting in 1971, the "doldrums era" and the "primary care and increasing government control era." The first, he claimed, was characterized by conflict, uncertainty, and caution within medical schools about their new directions, and an indecisiveness brought about by their growing budgetary problems. The second period was defined by the wave of government legislation initiated in the mid-1970s to encourage medical schools to produce more primary care and rural practitioners. Presumably, the cutbacks in government support of medical education since the late 1970s signal an end to this last "era" and the beginning of a new phase for medical education.

Obviously, it is an open question whether secular changes in specialty choices are primarily the results of social phenomena.[20] The latter part of Funkenstein's "specialty and scientific" era was, for example, coterminous with a huge federal subsidy program supporting biomedical research in medical schools. This subsidy program undoubtedly stimulated research interests within medical schools and probably promoted a research-oriented teaching environment on its own. Nevertheless, a significant shift in specialty preferences favoring the primary care fields does seem to have taken place in the late 1960s. Oates and Feldman (1971, 1974), Otis and Weiss (1972), Fishman and Zimet (1973), Herrmann (1973), and the California Medical Association (1976) all reported large increases in preferences for the primary care fields at a number of medical schools, beginning roughly with the entering classes of 1968. Rothman (1972) also found shifts in the measured personality traits of medical school freshman at the University of Toronto during the late 1960s.

More recent data continue to indicate that medical students' interests in primary care, and in rural or underserved practice locations, are much stronger now than in the mid-1960s (Mantovani et al. 1976; Meyer et al. 1976). As was shown earlier in Table 1-1, some 38 percent of all active physicians were practicing in the primary care specialties in 1970. In that year, the same percentage—38—entered internship or first-year residency positions in the primary care fields (Steinwachs et al. 1982). By 1974, the percentage of new graduates choosing first-year positions in the primary care specialties rose to 52, and from 1975 to 1980 it stayed in the range of 58 to 60 (Graettinger 1976, 1979; Steinwachs et al. 1982). In the late 1970s, there were even signs of excess demands for primary care positions, particularly in family practice and internal medicine.[21] These figures suggest that the percentage of physicians practicing in the primary care specialties will exceed GMENAC's forecast of 35 in 1990 (see Table 1-1), but they should be cautiously interpreted. Switching into specialties out of the primary care fields (or into subspecialties within the primary care fields) is known to occur after the first year of graduate training. Indeed, some experts (e.g., Langwell 1980a) have conjectured that the attrition rate may be substantial. Unfortunately, no data documenting the specialty distribution of physicians first entering practice (as opposed to graduate training) in the late 1970s and early 1980s have been published. As a result, it cannot be said with certainty just how much current rates of entry into the primary care specialties exceed those of the 1960s.

ATTITUDINAL STUDIES OF LOCATION CHOICE: PROFESSIONAL DECISION FACTORS

Attitudinal studies of location choice have generally dealt with physicians' reasons for selecting rural or urban practice sites. Ordinarily, they divide location motives into two categories: "professional," referring to the ease or profitability with which the physician believes he or she can carry on a practice; and "personal," referring to the physician's tastes for certain types of living conditions. Data are generated by asking physicians to rank or state the importance of a list of location motives provided by the investigator.

The results obtained in this manner are naturally susceptible to the problems created by subjective responses. In particular, motives the physician believes are important may or may not significantly affect his or her actual behavior, interpersonal comparisons can have limited value, findings may be affected by the phrasing of questions, and so on. In addition, the empirical evidence has been derived from a variety of different geographic samples, age groups of physicians, and methodologies.[22] Thus, predictably, even though broadly consistent patterns of responses emerge, disparities in the directions and strength of the evidence occur as well.

Five basic (and interrelated) categories of professional motives for location choices have been identified. They are: (1) gaining access to hospital facilities and other support facilities or personnel; (2) avoiding professional isolation, maintaining contact with colleagues, and having access to continuing medical education; (3) avoiding an excessive work load and obtaining practice coverage; (4) having opportunities to join a group practice; and (5) securing an adequate income. Nearly all attitudinal studies have reported that these motives are of moderate to paramount importance in shaping community preferences.

Since rural areas, relative to urban areas, typically offer smaller supplies of hospital services, a higher degree of professional isolation, a larger work load, and fewer opportunities to join group practices, professional factors have often been cited as the major impediments to rural practice. Although most data indicate that rural physicians' annual incomes are not systematically lower than those of urban physicians,[23] recent studies by Langwell and Budde (1978) and Langwell (1980b) have suggested that rural physicians' lifetime earnings are lower than those of urban physicians, especially in the referral fields. Accordingly, area characteristics (e.g., population size and the supply of hospital facilities) may critically determine physicians' net income opportunities and thereby reduce the attractiveness of rural practice.

Surprisingly, investigators have rarely inquired about the direct influence of the physician's specialty on rural-urban practice choice. One would expect, for example, fewer referral specialists than primary care physicians to enter rural areas simply because of the large population bases required to support reasonably successful referral practices. In a small sample of New York physicians, Parker and Tuxill (1967) found that urban physicians did, in fact, regard the difficulties of establishing specialty practices as the most important professional deterrent to choosing rural locations, but other findings on the point are inferential.[24]

The proximity of hospital resources and, to a lesser extent, support personnel and facilities (e.g., laboratories) has been described as a major influence on practice location decisions in many studies (Fein 1956; Parker and Tuxill 1967; Bible 1970; Charles 1971; Heald et al. 1974;[25] Diseker and Chappell 1976; Zetzman and Stefanu 1977; Burket 1977; Parker and Sorensen 1978). The few studies which segregated responses by specialty (Parker and Tuxill 1967; Heald et al. 1974) indicate that referral specialists are much more likely than general or primary care practitioners to consider access to hospital services important. However, Heald et al. showed that even primary care practitioners consider nearness to hospitals a significant factor in choosing practice location. They found that 70 percent of the respondents in one sample of primary care physicians preferred office locations where travel time to the nearest hospital was no more than 15 minutes.

Nearness to a medical school, the availability of continuing education facilities, and access to collegial contact have been reported as moderately influential factors, ranking just behind the proximity of hospital resources. Again, however, they seem to be less important to primary care physicians than to referral specialists (Fein 1956; Parker and Tuxill 1967; Martin et al. 1968; Riley et al. 1969; Bible 1970; Charles 1971; Heald et al. 1974; Diseker and Chappell 1976; Zetzman and Stefanu 1977; Parker and Sorensen 1978).[26] In the 1978 study by Parker and Sorensen, physicians ranked limited opportunities for professional growth second in importance to the desire to change practice as a factor leading them to leave rural practice.

Heavy work loads, long and irregular hours, and the lack of practice coverage in small communities are widely believed to characterize rural practice. AMA tabulations at least partly support this view (Balfe et al. 1971; Warner and Aherne 1974; Cantwell 1976; Langwell and Budde 1978). Metropolitan and nonmetropolitan physicians appear to work approximately the same number of weeks per year (47), but nonmetropolitan physicians average 8 to 10 percent longer workweeks (53 to 54 hours as opposed to 49 to 50). Nonmetropolitan practitioners also average about 10 percent more hours of direct patient care per week and 30 percent more patient visits.

The attitudinal evidence regarding rural practice and work-load preferences is confined largely to small-sample studies. Fein (1956), Parker (1970), and Crawford and McCormack (1971) indicated that overwork is the major reason why physicians leave rural primary care practice—and in some instances switch specialties as well. Riley et al. (1969), Bible (1970), and Taylor et al. (1973) reported that physicians believe long hours or disruptions of family life are drawbacks of rural practice. Diseker and Chappell (1976) and Zetzman and Stefanu (1977) stated that physicians rated the availability of practice coverage as the most important locational influence after access to hospital facilities.

However, Parker and Tuxill (1967) obtained a curious anomaly in a study of New York practitioners. Although 85 percent of the urban respondents claimed that large work loads and long hours were important factors in *other* physicians' location decisions, less than 30 percent professed to have been influenced themselves by either dimension. Similarly, Burket (1977) found that, although medical students rated overwork as the most important deterrent to rural practice, practicing physicians judged it to be a relatively minor consideration. This suggests that an element of conventional wisdom enters into opinions toward rural practice. Nevertheless, whether grounded in fact or not, the belief that rural working conditions are strenuous is clearly sufficient to discourage many physicians from choosing rural locations.

Several investigators have reported that income opportunities significantly influence the choice of a community in which to practice (Fein 1956; Martin et al. 1968; Charles 1971; Heald et al. 1974; Diseker and Chappell 1976; Cordes 1978). But results concerning the strength of the influence vary, and physicians have not been asked precisely how perceived earnings opportunities affect their location decisions. As we have observed, income expectations do not seem to influence the choice between urban and rural locations provided the locations offer an adequate population base and the availability of hospital facilities or referrals. Otherwise, it is impossible to infer from attitudinal evidence what forms of income motivation physicians display, or what types of communities income-motivated physicians are likely to select.

The opportunity to join a group practice has been cited as a locational influence by Charles (1971), Heald et al. (1974), Diseker and Chappell (1976), Zetzman and Stefanu (1977), and Parker and Sorensen (1978). Charles and Diseker and Chappell both reported that it is of minor importance, but Heald et al. found that group practice opportunities were rated among the three most significant of all location factors by a large national sample of 1965 medical graduates in the primary care fields. Urban and rural physicians assigned it roughly equal importance. However, non-general practitioners, regardless of their location, rated it as the most influential factor affecting their location choices. Interestingly, Zetzman and Stefanu found that access to a group was described by medical students as an important factor affecting their location choices, but it was ranked less highly by residents and less highly still by physicians in practice.

Two points deserve comment in connection with these findings. First, the popularity of group practice has increased markedly in the past two decades, particularly among young physicians. For example, AMA tabulations have indicated that approximately 18 percent of all active nonfederal physicians (excluding interns and residents) practiced in groups in 1969, and that the percentage rose to 23 in 1975 (Haug and Roback 1970; Todd and McNamara 1971; Goodman 1976; Goodman et al. 1976).[27] Recent tabulations of preferences for type of practice among medical students and residents indicate that 40 percent or more of new physicians plan to enter group practice.[28] Consequently, opportunities to join or establish groups may affect location decisions more in the future than they have in the past.

The second point is that, according to common belief, the desirability and economic viability of group practice vary with community size. Groups are presumably more difficult to set up and maintain in rural than in urban areas because of small or low-density population bases. But for reasons already mentioned—assuring practice coverage, regularity of work hours, collegial contact, etc.—groups are also thought to be more desirable to rural physicians than to urban practitioners. Hence, it has been argued that programs to support rural group practices will attract physicians to rural communities.

Despite their plausibility, neither the foregoing claim nor its underlying hypotheses have been rigorously tested. The results by Heald et al. (1974) do not bear on the attractiveness of rural group practice to urban physicians; and they do not show that groups are more desirable to rural than to urban practitioners.[29] We know little about the magnitude of the difficulties of establishing rural groups, and only one behavioral study of the effect of group practice on rural location patterns has been conducted to date. Using a national sample of 287 nonmetropolitan areas, Evashwick (1976) regressed the change in the physician-population ratio between 1960 and 1970 on a set of predictor variables including the percentage of patient care physicians practicing in groups in 1960. In five of the eight regional subsamples, coefficients on the group percentage were significantly positive, suggesting that existing group practice opportunities do tend to attract physicians into rural areas. However, there were no persuasive explanations for why the coefficients were not significant for three of the subsamples (the South Central, Mountain, and Pacific Coastal regions). Furthermore, no evidence was given as to whether physicians entering the other five regions joined existing groups or formed new ones. Thus, the feasibility of subsidizing groups as a device for attracting physicians into rural communities is not yet fully established.

ATTITUDINAL STUDIES OF LOCATION PREFERENCES: PERSONAL FACTORS

Attitudinal studies have identified a number of personal factors or tastes which affect physicians' location decisions. The broad categories are: (1) unspecified general preferences for urban or rural life-styles; (2) the desire to locate in or near one's hometown; (3) the desire to locate near family and friends; (4) climate or geographic preferences; (5) tastes for recreational, cultural, or social opportunities; (6) preferences regarding involvement in community affairs; (7) the desire for an adequate school system; and (8) the location preferences of the physician's spouse.

Many researchers have remarked on the variability of individual physicians' location choice behavior, and the weights physicians assign to the various taste factors tend to vary across study samples. Nevertheless, most of the findings indicate that personal preferences are at least as important as professional factors in location decisions.

General preferences for urban or rural living conditions (or for a particular community size) have been cited as major determinants of location choices in large national studies of physicians by Heald et al. (1974) and Steinwald and Steinwald (1975). Similar results were reported in smaller studies by Hassinger (1963), Parker and Tuxill (1967), Longnecker (1975), Zetzman and Stefanu (1977), Cordes (1978), and Parker and Sorensen (1978), although one study (Schaupp 1969) described urban-rural preferences as a minor decision factor. Physicians choosing rural practice locations seem to have stronger feelings about the ideal community size than urban practitioners (Heald et al., Steinwald and Steinwald, Parker and Tuxill), but it is not clear how to explain this finding. One possibility is that community-size preferences signify attitudes toward a constellaton of life-style characteristics, none of which may be easy to define. For example, Charles (1971) reported that, for a sample of Alabama physicians, the most influential location consideraton was the individual's overall perception of the community as a pleasant place in which to live and raise a family.

The desire to locate in or near one's hometown has frequently been mentioned as a location factor (Fein 1956; Parker and Tuxill 1967; Schaupp 1969; Champion and Olsen 1971; Charles 1971; Johnson et al. 1973; Diseker and Chappell 1976; Cordes 1978). Its significance differs from sample to sample—possibly reflecting age or regional differences in location tastes—but on the whole it appears to be important only to a minority of physicians. Likewise, the desire to locate near family or friends also seems to influence only a small percentage of practitioners (Brown and Belcher 1966; Peterson 1968; Schaupp 1969; Charles 1971; Heald et al. 1974; Diseker and Chappell 1976; Parker and Sorensen 1978).

Both hometown location preferences and those associated with family ties are (or are arguably) aspects of the influence of prior area contact on location decisions. According to the prior-contact hypotheses (which are taken up in Chapter 3), physicians develop attachments to areas where they have lived before entering practice—e.g., during their upbringing or medical education. Moreover, the strength of the attachment grows with the number and recency of contacts. Behavioral evidence shows that previous contact is a significant predictor of practice location at the state level, but very little work on the issue has been done at the intrastate level.

The climate of an area, its geographic features, or both, are generally ranked among the two or three most influential professional and personal factors (Fein 1956; Charles 1971; Roleston 1973; Heald et al. 1974; Steinwald and Steinwald 1974; Diseker and Chappell 1976; Longnecker 1975). In one small-sample study, Schaupp (1969) found climate preferences to be an unimportant decision factor for graduates of the West Virginia University School of Medicine, but in another, Martin et al. (1968) reported that climate strongly affected the decisions of Kansas graduates to leave or remain in the state.[30] Unfortunately, no substantive attempts have been made to determine what types of climates or geographic characteristics physicians prefer.

The availability of social, cultural, or recreational opportunities also appears to have a moderate or strong influence on location decisions (Fein 1956; Parker and Tuxill 1967; Schaupp 1969; Bible 1970; Charles 1971; Johnson et al. 1973; Roleston 1973; Heald et al. 1974; Diseker and Chappell 1976). Unfortunately, as is true of climate and geographic preferences, no efforts have been made to specify precisely what kinds of such opportunities physicians seek. However, there are some indications that they perceive metropolitan areas to be richer in leisure alternatives than rural areas (Parker and Tuxill 1967; Bible 1970).

Evidence on the remaining personal factors is generally mixed. The opportunity to take an active part in community affairs seems to be a minor influence (Parker and Tuxill 1967; Bible 1970; Johnson et al. 1973; Heald et al. 1974). Parker and Tuxill found that urban practitioners ranked community activity higher in importance than rural practitioners, but Bible implied that the opposite was the case.

Schaupp (1969), Bible (1970), and Burket (1977) described the quality of primary and secondary schools in the community as an important locational factor, but Charles (1971), Heald et al. (1974), and Diseker and Chappell (1976) found it to be of moderate to minor importance. Both Schaupp and Bible indicated that a poor school system was a major reason for *not* locating in a given community or area. This suggests that perceptions of community characteristics—whether they bear on the physician's professional or personal life—may have asymmetric effects on location behavior. Characteristics considered desirable need not necessarily attract physicians, but those considered undesirable may well keep physicians away.

Results regarding the location preferences of the physician's spouse are also variable. Some studies have reported that the spouse's preferences are a major influence (Parker and Tuxill 1967; Martin et al. 1968; Roleston 1973; Taylor et al. 1973; Diseker and Chappell 1976; Cordes 1978), while others have found them to be relatively unimportant (Charles 1971; Longnecker 1975; Parker and Sorensen 1978; Stewart et al. 1980). Heald et al. (1974) obtained what is probably the strongest evidence on this point from large national samples of physicians and physicians' wives. According to their tabulations, only 16 percent of the physicians believed that their wives' attitudes significantly affected their location decisions, and 81 percent of the wives felt that they had little influence on their husbands' choices.[31]

On balance, attitudinal studies indicate that climate and geographic preferences are the strongest personal motives for choosing regions or states of practice. Attitudinal studies also suggest that the strongest personal motives affecting urban-rural choices are general urban-rural preferences, preferences for areas of prior contact (the role of which has not been examined at the intrastate level), and tastes for leisure activities. Unfortunately, except in the case of prior contact, none of these preferences has been well delineated in existing research. Hence, it is at least debatable whether, as a practical matter, they can be used to predict physicians' location choices.

In addition, many related issues still need to be explored. These concern: (1) the effects, if any, of personality traits on location choices; (2) the impact of living conditions such as the adequacy and price of housing, travel time between potential home and office locations, pollution, tax rates, and crime rates; (3) attitudes toward inner-city practice locations; (4) the location preferences of women physicians (for whom spouses' preferences may prove to be a major influence); (5) the location preferences of black and other minority physicians;[32] and (6) the possible effects of malpractice insurance prices, peer review, and other recent changes in the practice environment.

SUMMARY

Studies of personality traits show that certain associations exist between physicians' psychological makeup and their choice of specialty. Results indicate that surgeons, psychiatrists, and academic physicians display the clearest patterns of personality attributes. General or family practitioners and internists are less easy to identify, and the results applying to pediatricians and other physicians are both fragmentary and weak. Nevertheless, it seems reasonable to conclude that physicians in the primary care specialties do not all share a common group of personality traits.

It has been argued, both implicitly and explicitly, that physicians select a specialty—i.e., a professional role—which is most similar to their perception of themselves. According to attitudinal study findings, physicians do, in fact, believe that their self-images correspond closely to the images of the specialties they choose. This can be taken as partial confirmation of the self-image hypothesis, but the hypothesis itself is too general to provide a working understanding of the decision process.

At the broadest level, one can say that each specialty possesses a set of characteristics and that each of these characteristics yields a certain amount of utility to the physician making his or her specialty choice. To-

gether, the set of characteristics associated with each field generates a total amount of utility the physician expects to receive by selecting and
practicing in that field. The decision as to which specialty to select can be
viewed conceptually as a matter of maximizing expected or anticipated
utility. Unless constrained by physical, intellectual, or institutional factors, the physician chooses the specialty which yields the largest amount
of expected utility to him or her as a practitioner.

Unfortunately, there is no widespread agreement as to what the
characteristics are that define a specialty or how to measure them. Neither is there agreement about how to define the dimensions of physicians' personalities which would allow personality types to be matched
with configurations of specialty characteristics. As a result, research on
predicting specialty choices from a knowledge of physicians' personality
types is still in its initial stages. Even so, a few recent studies show that
personality models of specialty choice can—at least in statistical terms—
achieve a reasonably high degree of predictive accuracy. These studies
indicate that the choices can be predicted successfully at rates two to
three times higher than would be the case for random assignment (i.e.,
under the assumption that selection probabilities are equal). While the
results do not demonstrate that personality types or specialty preferences
are the only factors operating on specialty decisions, they imply that physicians' tastes are a strongly significant element in these decisions. Indeed, one might expect that improvements in research methodology will,
if anything, tend to sharpen personality models and their predictive capabilities.

Attitudinal studies of practice location choice indicate that preferences can be grouped into two categories: professional and personal. The
former represent a collection of tastes related to practice working conditions, income opportunities, and attitudes toward medical practice. The
latter signify tastes for living conditions. The attitudinal evidence on location factors is vulnerable to many criticisms, and the findings themselves are variable, reflecting differences in sample composition and
methodology. For these reasons, it cannot be said that attitudinal studies
have produced a coherent theory of location choice.

These qualifications notwithstanding, two important types of results tend to emerge. First, physicians believe personal preferences have
as large a part as professional factors in the selection of a practice location. This, of course, is not surprising in light of the mobility of young
physicians, and the high value they (as high-income professionals) are
likely to place on leisure time. The second type of evidence pertains to
the specific factors physicians see as qualitatively affecting their choice of
location. Among the important professional factors are the accessibility
of hospitals, collegial contact, training facilities, and group practices. The

income potential of the area or community, and an acceptable work load, are probably also influential. The personal factors which physicians most often report as affecting location decisions are climate and geography, access to a variety of leisure opportunities, previous contact with the area, and general tastes for community size.

The findings discussed in this chapter apply primarily to white male graduates of the mid-1960s and earlier. Neither personality nor attitudinal research has focused to any great extent on the generation of physicians who entered medical school after that time. Descriptive reports tell us that a break may have occurred between that generation and its predecessors in terms of physician characteristics. By outward appearances, the break was accompanied by a strong shift in preferences toward primary care fields—and possibly toward rural and inner-city practice. Additionally, since 1970 there have been large increases in the numbers of women and minority students who have entered medical schools. Inevitably, these events bring into question the value of much of the existing research for understanding the career choices of physicians now beginning practice.

NOTES

1. See Zabarenko and Zabarenko (1978) and Bucher and Stelling (1977) for recent research on the professionalization of physicians. Also see Bloom (1979) for a review and history of the literature on professionalization in medicine. We allude to this literature in Chapters 4 and 5, but little of it deals explicitly with specialty choice.
2. See Mitchell (1975) for a conceptual application of role-model methodologies to specialty choice.
3. In one review of the literature, for example, Otis et al. (1973) listed the following tests which have been employed: the Allport-Vernon-Lindzay Study of Values, Minnesota Multiphasic Personality Inventory, Heist Omnibus Personality Inventory, Eysenck Personality Inventory, Maudsley Personality Inventory, Personality Factor Questionnaire, Myers-Briggs Type Indicator, Edwards Personal Preference Survey, California F-Scale, Rokeach Dogmatism Scale, Strong Vocational Interest Blank, and Gordon Survey of Interpersonal Values. Moreover, in a few instances tests or test procedures have been designed specifically for individual studies.
4. In a study of Australian medical students, Mowbray and Davies (1971) measured extroversion on the Eysenck Personality Inventory (EPI) scale and "thinking-introversion" on the Heist Omnibus Personality Inventory (HOPI) scale. They found that students planning to enter psychiatry were about average on the EPI extroversion scale but exhibited the highest scores of all subjects on the HOPI thinking-introversion scale. This result illustrates the difficulty of drawing firm conclusions from the results of different personality tests.

5. Psychiatrists are disproportionately likely to come from nonreligious or Jewish families.
6. Donovan et al. (1972) claimed moderate success in predicting the choice of internal medicine among graduates of the University of Rochester, but they did not list their predictor variables or propose a stereotype of the specialty. Most studies have described pediatricians and internists as displaying "average" personalities.
7. The first specialty stratum consisted of the surgical fields, anesthesiology, pathology, and radiology; the second of internal medicine, pediatrics, and psychiatry; the third of general practice, obstetrics-gynecology, and other medical fields. "Intimate" personalities were defined as those preferring or capable of intimate relationships with persons, work, or objects. "Isolate" personalities were characterized as the opposite of "intimate"—emotionally detached or aloof—and "neither intimate nor isolate" were intermediate between the two extremes.
8. The four personality proxies were apparently designed for the research and consisted of such measures as "difficulty in making friends," "time spent in leisure activity," etc. Anderson (1975) interpreted the results as the individuals' response to the medical school social culture rather than as pure personality traits.
9. The four traits were obtained from a factor analysis (i.e., as factor scores) of additional responses by the sampled physicians to the Career Attitudes Inventory Test. The factors were defined as desires for prestige, intellectual challenge, patient contact, and work pressure. According to the strongest qualitative results, general practitioners desired work pressure but not intellectual challenge. Other primary care physicians desired patient contact but not prestige. Surgeons desired work pressure but disliked patient contact. Medical specialists desired prestige and intellectual challenge but sought to avoid work pressure. And "other" (chiefly hospital-based) specialists desired intellectual challenge but disliked patient contact.
10. Recent work has tended to stress the effects of education on how physicians perceive their professional roles and identities (e.g., Bucher and Stelling 1977). Unfortunately, however, little of it has addressed the question of specialty choice.
11. See Chapter 3 for discussion on this point.
12. This, of course, is not surprising in view of the ideology of medicine which places income goals below service goals. In both studies, general practitioners stated that financial pressures or the desire to begin earning a living soon were influential in their specialty decisions. We shall return to this point in Chapter 3.
13. Weil and Schleiter (1981) also estimated a set of correlates of the residents' interests in following academic careers as opposed to clinical practice. Not surprisingly, perhaps, they found that the same index of preferences for working conditions was the strongest single predictor of these interests. Moreover, the same types of attitudes that were associated with preferences for subspecialization were associated with preferences for academic careers.

This tends to show that personality characteristics associated with preferences for academic medicine are more closely associated with those for subspecialization than with those for primary care.

14. The procedure is to ask subjects to select adjectives which best describe their
impressions of physicians who practice in the specialty. In the case of medical students, the primary (if not exclusive) source of these impressions is presumably the medical school faculty.

15. No attempts have been made to explain why surgery is regarded as the most
prestigious specialty, although one can speculate that it is because the surgical fields demand the longest and presumably most specialized residencies
(e.g., Balfe et al. 1971, Crowley 1975b). This would be compatible with the
low status accorded general and family practice, which ordinarily require the
shortest residencies (or none at all); but psychiatry also requires a long residency and yet is not regarded as a prestigious specialty. Thus, the image of
what a physician "ought to be," the content of graduate training and work,
special ability associated with the specialty, and other factors may all have a
part in determining specialty status.

Interestingly, McGrath and Zimet (1977) reported that female medical students at the University of Colorado and the University of California at San
Diego reversed the status order of surgery and internal medicine, but maintained the same ordering as men of the other major specialties. This may reflect the subtlety with which perceptions of professional status are formed.

16. See Chapter 1.

17. Also see Chapter 3.

18. Linn and Zeppa (1980) have reported that students preferring internal medicine do not fit this pattern, and, indeed, exhibit confusion about their specialty roles.

19. Nearly 10 percent of the 1965–1969 graduates were still unclassified when
the data were collected in 1973. Thus, it is likely that the rates of entry into
all specialties other than general practice were understated for this group of
physicians.

20. Chapter 4 discusses a collection of alternative theories which hold that the
educational system is the primary determinant of specialty choices.

21. The implications of these figures are probably overstated because first-year
"primary care" positions were defined to include those in obstetrics-gynecology and all positions in internal medicine whether or not they led to later
training in subspecialties.

22. As an example of differences in methodology, some researchers ask physicians their preferences regarding general community characteristics, while
others ask the reasons for choosing a particular community. Clearly, some
reasons for selecting a given community—such as family ties—may have little to do with overall location preferences.

23. The evidence on physician net incomes in urban and rural areas is confined
to tabulations and fairly crude regression estimates. Tabulations by the
American Medical Association have shown that metropolitan and nonmetropolitan practitioners earn approximately the same mean annual net in-

comes except in the referral specialties (e.g., Cantwell 1976, p. 165). Because nonmetropolitan physicians tend to work more hours per year, this suggests that net income per hour is lower in rural than in urban areas. However, the tabular data on incomes have not been standardized for such factors as the cost of living or physician characteristics which may affect net income levels. The little available evidence from regression estimates shows no strong associations between annual or hourly net income and the physician-population ratio. For a review of the regression evidence, see Sloan and Feldman (1978).

24. The relationships between specialty and location choices are discussed further in Chapters 3 and 7.

25. Cooper et al. (1975) and Coleman (1976) used the same data as Heald et al. (1974) and reported similar results. Since the three studies are duplicative, the references to Cooper et al. and Coleman are omitted in the text.

26. At this writing, 15 state licensing boards and 12 state medical societies required physicians to take continuing medical education courses as conditions for licensure and membership, respectively. In addition, all 22 specialty boards had established, or were considering, policies calling for periodic board recertification. Assuming that the relicensure and recertification movement grows, it will clearly make the availability of continuing education services a more significant location factor in the future than in the past. Whether this means that medical schools will become the focal points of the geographic distribution of physicians is another matter. In 1976, continuing education courses were given in 44 states, many of them in (apparently) unaffiliated hospitals, and it is possible that efforts will be made to decentralize course offerings. See AMA (1976) for the status of continuing medical education in the mid-1970s.

   Also, the desires for contact with other physicians reported in attitudinal studies cannot be unambiguously determined. They may signify no more than preferences for professional communication, but they may also reflect perceived opportunities for obtaining referrals or the receptivity of established physicians toward the threat of entry in local markets. To the extent the latter is a concern, new physicians would presumably not wish to locate in areas where they were treated as unwanted competitors and, accordingly, their earnings opportunities were seriously jeopardized.

27. These AMA tabulations understate the number of physicians in multiphysician practices because groups are defined as practices including three or more persons with income-sharing arrangements.

28. See, e.g., Breed (1970), California Medical Association (1976), and Mantovani et al. (1976).

29. AMA data show that the percentage of physicians in groups is slightly higher in rural than in urban counties (Goodman 1976, Goodman et al. 1976), but the percentages may be misleading because interns and residents are not segregated from practicing physicians in either county category. Actually, the general motives for entering groups seem to be complex. Specialty evidently has a major role (as the findings by Heald et al. [1974] indicate), and results by Kimbell and Lorant (1977) imply that physicians in small groups earn

higher net incomes than solo practitioners. Tastes for professional autonomy, entrepreneurship, and business management also seem to affect the choice between solo or group practice. See Mahoney (1973) and Sloan (1974) for discussions of the factors motivating the choice of type of practice.

30. More specifically, Martin et al. reported that climate preferences were regarded as important by physicians who left Kansas to practice, and as unimportant by those who stayed. Their study made one of the few attempts to relate location behavior to physicians' stated location preferences. The result cited here also illustrates one of the pitfalls of small-sample research on given subpopulations of physicians. Had the sample been confined to graduates who remained in Kansas, climate preferences would have appeared to be an insignificant location factor. Had it been restricted to those who left the state, the reverse would have been true.

31. The disparities among the findings may only reflect sampling variation; on the other hand, they may exemplify the difficulties of interpreting attitudinal data. For instance, physicians may incorrectly perceive the extent of their spouse's influence, or they may describe it as important only if family conflict occurs over the choice of location and the physician accedes in whole or part to his or her spouse's wishes.

32. The only existing study of black physicians' location preferences suggests that their motivational factors are similar to those of white physicians (Lloyd et al. 1978).

THREE

Physicians' Background Characteristics and Career Choices

       This chapter examines the empirical evidence on the relationships between physicians' background characteristics and their career choices. By background characteristics, we mean such personal or biographic attributes as the individual's ability, age, sex, race, and place of upbringing. These and similar attributes, reflecting the physician's cultural background, aptitudes or limitations, information about career opportunities, and other factors such as economic motivation, represent the physician's tastes and constraints on his or her decision behavior. Most of the evidence is descriptive, since there have been few efforts to model or test the relationships between background characteristics and career choices. In some instances the underlying mechanisms seem clear, but in others they do not, in which case it is only possible to present or suggest plausible explanatory hypotheses.

ABILITY

       The most common measures of medical students' ability are college grade-point averages (GPAs), scores on the Medical College Admissions Test (MCAT), medical school GPAs and class rankings, and scores on the test given by the National Board of Medical Examiners (NBME).[1] A number of efforts have been made to compare one or more of these performance measures with planned or realized specialty choices. The majority of results indicate that the tests distinguish among academic physicians—that is, teachers and researchers—general practitioners, and other practitioner-specialists. Such findings have been viewed as establishing a hierarchy of measured ability in which academicians rank highest, followed by internists, other specialists, and general practitioners, in that order.

The strongest evidence linking measured ability with specialty choices was found in a descriptive study of 1950 and 1954 graduates of 12 public and private medical schools reported by Peterson et al. (1963) and Lyden et al. (1968). They found that: (1) general practitioners were two to three times more likely to be drawn from the lowest third of their class and lowest MCAT group than from the highest; (2) academic physicians were two to three times more likely to rank in the highest third of their class and highest MCAT group than in the lowest; (3) internists were about twice as likely to rank in the highest third of their class and highest MCAT group as in the lowest; and (4) surgeons were overrepresented in the lowest third of their class. No other patterns of association appeared.

Using another large sample of data on 1960 medical graduates, Schumacher (1964) obtained similar results on specialty choices as of the end of internship training. Those who saw themselves as future academicians achieved the highest MCAT scores, while those who planned to become general practitioners had the lowest. In the middle of the range, those planning to enter medical specialties ranked slightly higher than would-be surgeons.

Using a sample of approximately 4,500 British physicians, Last et al. (1967) also found that medical school performance was associated with career choice. Honor students tended to enter academic medicine, internal medicine, or pathology, while the lowest-ranking graduates chose general practice and obstetrics-gynecology.

A number of authors (Levit et al. 1963, Peterson et al. 1963, Sanazaro 1965, Lyden et al. 1968, Oates and Feldman 1971, Perlstadt 1972) have reported that graduates with the lowest MCAT scores or class rankings are those most likely to enter unspecialized internships. However, these findings must be considered somewhat weaker than those of Schumacher and of Last et al. since the type of internship training is not necessarily associated with choice of specialty.

Not surprisingly, studies conducted at individual schools have shown more mixed results. For example, a student ranking in the lowest third of the class at a prestigious and selective school might have ranked near the top of the class at a less prestigious or selective school. In either case, the student may be equally capable of becoming, say, an academician. The available findings tend to confirm this conjecture.

In an early study at the State University of New York at Buffalo, Monk and Terris (1956) showed that, up to the age of 28, seniors in the lowest third of their class were nearly five times as likely as those in the highest third to plan to enter general practice. Similarly, Geertsma and Grinols (1972) reported that low class performance among seniors at the University of Rochester—a selective, research-oriented school which graduated few general practitioners—was associated with the intention to enter general practice. The same results were found at the University of Toronto by Chipman et al. (1969). Conversely, Monk and Thomas (1973) found that at Johns Hopkins—another highly selective school which produced few general practitioners—general practitioners ranked near the top of their class, just below academicians.

Until fairly recently, little has been known of the relative abilities of family practitioners, but some findings indicate that graduates entering family practice exhibit higher measured abilities than general practitioners. In a study of approximately 13,000 graduates participating in the National Intern and Resident Matching Program[2] in 1976, Cuca (1977) reported that those seeking first-year residencies in family practice had MCAT scores and undergraduate GPAs nearly equivalent to the total sample averages. Graduates preferring pathology and internal medicine had the highest average MCAT scores, while those preferring residencies in obstetrics-gynecology had the lowest.[3]

Another, much smaller study at Baylor by Collins and Roessler (1975) also suggests that family practitioners probably do not fit the ability stereotype of general practitioners. Collins and Roessler found that residents in family practice had the highest undergraduate GPAs among five specialty groups (the others were surgery, internal medicine, obstetrics-gynecology, and pediatrics) and, next to internists, the highest average MCAT scores. This finding is reinforced in a study of 1,135 medical graduates by Gough (1978), who reported that the choice of family practice was unrelated to the subjects' scientific aptitudes or preferences. Gough found that internists, pediatricians, and psychiatrists all ranked relatively low in terms of scientific aptitudes and interests, while surgeons, anesthesiologists, and pathologists ranked relatively high. Similarly, in a large national sample of residents in internal medicine, Weil and Schleiter found that "the MCAT was an insignificant predictor in the decision for careers in primary care medicine" (1981, p. 699). However, they also found that residents intending to enter academic medicine rather than clinical practice exhibited significantly higher MCAT scores than those preferring clinical practice to academic medicine.

The only large-sample evidence disputing the contention that ability discriminates between general practitioners as opposed to family practitioners and specialists was obtained by Hadley (1977, 1979) from analyses of the data on 1960 graduates examined by Schumacher.[4] Hadley estimated the probabilities of individuals' choosing general practice and several other specialty fields as functions of MCAT scores, scores on Part 1 of the NBME, and a large number of additional explanatory variables. The probability of selecting general practice was not significantly associated with either of the two performance measures.[5] Hadley (1975) also made an effort to link ability directly with practice location, but found that his ability measures were not significantly related to the choice of state in which to practice.[6]

No substantive hypotheses have been developed which explain the observed associations between measured ability and specialty selection. Several studies have shown that high academic performers receive more faculty attention than low performers. It has also been reported that personality traits are correlated with medical school performance (e.g., Lief et al. 1965; Fredericks and Mundy 1967; Lyden et al. 1968; Haley et al. 1971; Rothman 1973; Turner et al. 1974; Gough and Hall 1975b). Hence, medical school faculty may have a part in directing students into specialties or specialty training for which their abilities or personalities qualify them. But it is not known to what extent this is true, or whether specialty choice is conditioned by barriers to entry or other factors associated with the physician's ability. Interpretation of the empirical results is further obscured by the repeated findings that MCAT scores, undergraduate GPAs, and even medical school GPAs are generally weakly related to clinical aptitude and other measures of practice performance. (See Chapter 4 for further discussion of this point.)

AGE

All studies that have examined relationships between age and specialty choice have found that general practitioners are markedly older than other physicians when they graduate from medical school (Monk and Terris 1956; Coker et al. 1960; Lyden et al. 1968; Monk and Thomas 1973; Hadley 1977).[7] Hadley found that surgeons were significantly younger than other physicians at graduation, but no systematic differences among ages of nongeneral practitioners have been described elsewhere.[8] Tabulations by Cuca (1977), Gordon (1978), and Barish (1979) indicate that the mean age of family practitioners at graduation is virtually the same as those of other specialists, which suggests that age may discriminate between general and family practitioners, but not between family practitioners and other physicians.

The most plausible explanation for the connection between age and entry into general practice is well known—namely, that it reflects the effect of the expected earning span on the length of graduate training the physician chooses to take.[9] That is, at the end of first-year residency

training, the physician must decide between immediate entry into practice as a general practitioner and continuing residency service to train for
a specialty. Physicians selecting a specialty may expect their annual net
income eventually to exceed the annual net income they could have
earned as general practitioners, but during residency training they must
forgo the amount of earnings that is equal to the difference between net
income as a practicing physician and net income as a resident. Thus, in
order for the present value of *lifetime* specialty earnings to be larger than
the present value of lifetime general practice earnings, the physician
must expect to have a reasonably long working life.[10] The longer the physician's anticipated earnings span, the larger is the probability that its
present value will exceed that of the income forgone during residency
training. Conversely, the older the physician is at the end of first-year
residency, the more attractive he or she will find the lifetime earnings
potential of general practice compared with that of a specialty. Consequently, to whatever extent physicians' choice of specialty is motivated
by anticipated income, we would expect to observe larger percentages of
older than younger graduates entering general practice.

Basically, then, age at the time of graduation from medical school
acts as a proxy for the *comparative* lifetime earnings opportunities the
physician attaches to general practice and to the various specialties. In
general, the actual or planned length of residency training should be observed to vary inversely with the physician's starting age—a hypothesis
which, unfortunately, has not been tested. Since the surgical specialties
typically require the longest periods of residency training for certification, it would be reasonable to expect younger graduates to enter the surgical fields. That such a tendency has not been observed systematically in
empirical studies can be attributed to several factors: (1) entering surgery
(or any other field) does not necessarily impose a given length of training
on physicians because they may choose not to become certified; (2) earnings calculations depend on expected income rates as well as on the
length of training; and (3) a variety of preference factors appear to play a
large part in the selection process. These factors undoubtedly differ considerably among individuals, suggesting that associations among age,
length of training, and specialty choice are probably weak for physicians
selecting fields other than general practice.

SEX

Historically, women have represented a small fraction of the supply
of physicians. As late as 1973 they comprised only slightly more than 6
percent of all living graduates of U.S. medical schools,[11] and even by

1980 they made up less than 12 percent of the total number of U.S. physicians (Bidese and Danais 1982). However, as a result of the liberalization of admissions policies and a rapid growth in the number of female applicants, the percentage of women among students entering medical schools rose from 9 to 26 between 1969 and 1979 (AMA 1980). Consequently, the effects of sex differences on career choices will undoubtedly affect the distribution of physicians far more in the future than in the past.

At least in the case of specialty choices, descriptive findings indicate that the effects of sex differences are substantial. Tabulations have shown that women are: (1) more than three times as likely as men to enter pediatrics; (2) twice as likely to enter psychiatry; (3) slightly less likely than men to enter internal medicine, but twice as likely to enter certain nonmedical, nonsurgical specialties such as anesthesiology and pathology; (4) roughly two-thirds as likely as men to enter general and family practice; and (5) only one-fifth as likely as men to enter the surgical specialties other than obstetrics-gynecology (Shapiro et al. 1968; Renshaw and Pennell 1971; Walsh et al. 1972; Haug 1975; Cohen and Korper 1976a; Kehrer 1976; Cuca 1977; Gordon 1978; Wunderman 1980). Only one regression study (Hadley 1977) has treated the effect of sex on specialty choice. It showed that, other factors held constant, women were significantly more likely than men to select pediatrics, psychiatry, obstetrics-gynecology, and the nonmedical, nonsurgical fields.

Until lately, it appeared that the male-female specialty choice differences were stable over time. But recent data on residency specialties by the American Medical Association (AMA 1973, 1980) indicate that a growing percentage of U.S. women graduates are entering the surgical fields. Whether this signals an important shift in the historical distribution of women's specialty choices is not yet clear (e.g., Weisman et al. 1980).

Three predominantly social hypotheses have been offered to explain the historical pattern. They are: (1) women have been deliberately excluded from male-dominated fields such as surgery (Lopate 1968); (2) women tend to select the more "feminine" specialties such as pediatrics and psychiatry, and to avoid the "masculine" fields such as surgery (Kosa and Coker 1965; Lopate 1968; Davidson 1979);[12] and (3) women choose specialties whose training requirements and working conditions interfere least with their actual or planned commitments to marriage and the bearing and rearing of children (Lopate 1968; Davidson 1979).

While all of the foregoing hypotheses may be true to a greater or lesser degree, none of them has been adequately tested and the pertinent evidence is indirect at best. Most of it bears on the third hypothesis, chiefly in connection with the effect of conflicts between marriage and careers on women physicians' participation in the labor force. The general argument is, first, that medical training programs typically make no provision for interruptions due to childbearing or other marital choices and responsibilities, and, indeed, place great demands on students' and graduates' physical and emotional resources (Buzek and McNamara 1968; Lopate 1968; Kaplan 1971; Williams 1971; and Bodel and Short 1972). Thus, if a woman wishes to marry or bear children, she must find some way of continuing her training with minimal interruption, discontinue training altogether, or delay marriage or pregnancy until her training is completed.[13] The overall implication is that curtailment of training is frequently the preferred alternative. It suggests, other things being equal, that women have a higher propensity than men to select general practice because of the shorter period of required graduate training, and a lower propensity than men to select surgery because of the longer period of residency training.

The second part of the argument is that women are more likely than men to choose practice settings where working hours are regular and conditions permit part-time or interrupted employment. Thus, women might be expected to have stronger preferences than men for hospital-based fields such as anesthesiology, pathology, and radiology, and for specialties such as office-based psychiatry. By the same token, they might be expected to have weaker preferences for general practice or surgery, where working conditions are strenuous or hours are irregular because the physician is routinely on call. Some evidence for this hypothesis was found by Davidson (1979). In a small sample of residents at a New York hospital, Davidson found that women listed the opportunity for limiting their work hours as the second most important reason for choosing a general specialty (work challenge was ranked first), and the most important reason for choosing a subspecialty.[14]

These conjectures only partly fit the observed distribution of women among specialties, and it is impossible to test them adequately with data from published sources. However, the role of tastes for marriage and family formation has been amply documented in connection with women physicians' selection of training periods and practice settings, and in their labor force participation rates. In addition, it has been demonstrated that single women most resemble men in these aspects of their career behavior, while married women with children least resemble men. On the whole, women spend substantially less time in graduate training than men, and are less likely to be certified in their specialties.[15] The highest rates of board certification—comparable to those for men— are exhibited by single women, and the lowest by women who bear children during their training (Powers et al. 1969; Westling-Wilkstrand et al. 1970; Kehrer 1974).

Given their specialties, women are more inclined than men to choose institutional practice settings such as hospitals or industrial firms, and to choose institutional careers such as teaching, research, or administration (Dykman and Stalnaker 1957; Powers et al. 1969; Monk and Thomas 1970; Cohen and Korper 1976b; Kehrer 1974, 1976).[16] Women are also more likely to withdraw temporarily or permanently from practice than men, to work fewer weeks per year when they are active, and to have somewhat shorter working lives (Dykman and Stalnaker 1957; Rosenlund and Oski 1967; Powers et al. 1969; Monk and Thomas 1970; Jussim and Muller 1975; Cohen and Korper 1976b; Kehrer 1974, 1976).[17]

Even so, most of the causes of women physicians' career interruptions and reduced work time are due to marriage, childbearing, and child rearing. The labor force participation rates of single women physicians have been shown to be only slightly lower than those of male physicians (Shapiro et al. 1968; Powers et al. 1969; Cohen and Korper 1976b).

Little is known about the behavior of women physicians with respect to their choice of practice location at either the state or intrastate levels,[18] but sample evidence has indicated that 70 percent to 80 percent of women physicians are married, and half of those are married to other physicians (Dykman and Stalnaker 1957; Shapiro et al. 1968; Powers et al. 1969). This suggests that a third or more of all women physicians may select their practice location in concert with the decisions of their physician husbands.

If historical patterns hold, the large numbers of women currently entering medical schools imply that shifts will occur in the specialty distribution of new physicians, notably out of the surgical fields and into pediatrics and psychiatry. In addition, it is likely that the percentage of physicians entering self-employed office practice will decline and that the average work year will diminish. Nevertheless, a major element in the pattern seems to be the traditional marital, professional, and social roles of women. Insofar as the roles themselves are changing toward greater emphasis on careers outside of marriage, women's preferences for specialties and practice settings may be changing as well.[19]

RACE

In comparison with whites, exceptionally little is known about the numbers and career distributions of black and other minority physicians. Indeed, only four contemporary surveys of black physicians have been conducted. Using as a source the membership files of the National Medical Association (NMA), a black professional association, Haynes (1969) placed the number of known black physicians at 4,805 in 1967, but estimated the actual figure at 6,000. The 1970 U.S. census identified 6,100 active and inactive black physicians and osteopaths, and Thompson (1974a) reported the number of active black doctors as 5,478 in 1972. The implication is that in the late 1960s and early 1970s, blacks represented less than 2 percent of the U.S. physician population.

Until recently, the great majority of blacks were graduates of only two medical schools, Howard and Meharry. Haynes (1969) stated that 83% of the NMA members in 1967 had graduated from Howard or Meharry, and Thompson (1974b) indicated the same percentage in 1972. In the early 1970s medical schools began campaigns to recruit blacks and other minorities. By the mid-1970s minority students, of whom three-quarters were black, constituted approximately 8 percent of the total enrollment (Crowley 1975b; AMA 1976). In the four-year period 1973–76, medical schools graduated 2,233 black students, 65 percent of them from schools other than Howard and Meharry (AMA 1973, 1976; Crowley 1975a, 1975b). While total minority enrollments have been steadily increasing, recruitment efforts aimed specifically at blacks have not been notably successful. In 1978–79, although 13 percent of all medical students were minorities, blacks still represented only 6 percent of total enrollment (AMA 1980).

Because of the historical association between race and specific medical schools, it is hard to draw conclusions about the relationships between race and physicians' career choices. Haynes (1969) reported that 39 percent of all NMA members were general practitioners in 1967, as opposed to only 22 percent of the total physician population (Haug and Roback 1968), and Gray (1977) put the figure at 30 percent in the early 1970s. However, these data may well reflect the past admissions or educational policies of Howard and Meharry. Moreover, only 7 percent of the 1965–69 graduates of both schools were in general practice in 1973, a figure equivalent to the percentage of general practitioners graduated by all schools in the same period (Martin 1975).

The recent but fragmentary data on black physicians' specialty choices indicate that they are probably not greatly different from those of white physicians. Johnson et al. (1975) reported that only 8 percent of the black medical students in 1972–73 intended to enter general practice, but they claimed that blacks as a group were more likely than whites to select the primary care fields. However, other studies show that in the late 1970s 40 percent to 50 percent of black medical students planned to enter, or were entering, the primary care fields, and 10 percent to 15 percent were selecting family practice (Lloyd et al. 1978; Long 1980). These rates appear to be only slightly lower than those of white physicians.[20]

Thompson (1974a) tabulated the location patterns of black physicians in the United States and the District of Columbia, and found that the highest concentrations of black physicians occurred—with two notable exceptions—in the same 10 locations as the highest concentrations of all physicians. The two exceptions were the third and eighth most popular locations with black physicians, the District of Columbia, where Howard University is located, and Maryland, which is in close proximity to Howard. Similarly, another tabulation by Wooldridge (1976) of the location patterns of Howard and Meharry graduates showed that the two locations with the highest ratios of office-based black physicians to all office-based physicians were in the District of Columbia and Tennessee—the latter being the state in which Meharry is situated.

It is commonly believed that black physicians are disproportionately likely to settle in inner-city neighborhoods and to serve black patients. Substantive evidence supports that belief. U.S. census figures examined by Gray (1977) showed that 72 percent of the active black physicians practiced in central cities in 1970, in contrast to only 40 percent of the active physician population. A considerably lower percentage (32) was reported from a survey of Howard University medical graduates by Lloyd et al. (1978), but this is probably due to a narrower definition of the central city. Lloyd et al. also presented tabulations showing that an average of 72 percent of the Howard graduates' patients were black. While no comparable data are available on the percentage of black patients treated by white physicians, there is no reason to think that it is greatly dissimilar from the percentage of blacks in nearby populations—or about 20 percent for the U.S. as a whole. The tabulations indicated further that 70 percent of the Howard graduates' patients had average or below-average incomes, and the survey respondents reported that a quarter of their patients were "very poor."

Two statistical studies of physicians' locational patterns tend to confirm the view that black physicians have a much greater tendency than white physicians to serve black populations and, perhaps, to serve poorer clienteles. In a sample confined to five metropolitan areas in the Middle Atlantic and Southern states, Wooldridge (1976) matched the locations of Howard and Meharry graduates with the racial and economic characteristics of the ZIP code areas where they practiced. According to her findings, black physicians were located in ZIP code areas with racial compositions averaging 45 percent black, while white physicians chose ZIP code areas with racial compositions averaging less than 10 percent black. The ZIP code areas of black physicians also appeared to have populations that were poorer and of higher density than those of white physicians.

Using regression methods, Guzick and Jahiel (1976) investigated the distribution of physicians in 73 Health Areas in New York City during 1972–73. They also found that the numbers of Howard and Meharry graduates increased significantly with the percentage of blacks in the population. They did not report the effects of population racial composition on the locations of graduates of other medical schools, but black physicians appeared to be much more likely to practice in predominantly black Health Areas than the sample of white and black physicians as a whole.[21] The available results do, therefore, indicate that blacks have considerably higher propensities than whites to practice in black, inner-city neighborhoods.[22]

RELIGION

Relationships between religious background and specialty preferences have been reported in several studies. However, these findings may not be altogether reliable because they are based on small samples, single medical schools, or data on beginning medical students. Nevertheless, they do tend to display distinct patterns.

Specifically, it has been shown that: (1) actual and potential general practitioners are chiefly Protestant; (2) actual and potential surgeons are predominantly Protestant or Catholic; and (3) psychiatrists and students planning to enter psychiatry are especially likely to have no religious affiliation or to be Jewish (Livingston and Zimet 1965; Kritzer and Zimet 1967; Kosa 1969; Paiva and Haley 1971; Monk and Thomas 1973). Jews and individuals without religious affiliations appear to be most similar. Several studies have shown that both groups are attracted to academic medicine, and both are considerably underrepresented among surgeons and general practitioners. Some of the evidence indicates that Jews are likely to select nonacademic medical specialties as well as psychiatry, while Catholics have been found to avoid general practice, and Protestants are the group least likely to enter psychiatry.

In their studies of residents in internal medicine, Weil and his colleagues (Weil et al. 1981; Weil and Schleiter 1981) reported that Jews and nonreligious individuals were significantly more likely than members of other religious groups to prefer subspecialty careers in clinical practice. Conversely, Protestants were significantly more likely than members of other religious groups to prefer careers in general internal medicine. Weil and Schleiter (1981) further showed that Jews had significantly higher propensities than other physicians to prefer careers in academic medicine. These results suggest that the "Jewish-specialist" and "Protestant-generalist" religious patterns hold within fields (such as internal medicine) as well as between them (general practice versus the specialties).

It is not known whether religious background signifies cultural values which affect tastes for specialties, or whether it is merely associated with other background traits that are linked to specialty choices.[23] Kosa (1969) reported that Jews and nonreligious medical students had stronger intellectual interests and motivation than Protestants or Catholics, and stronger desires for intellectual recognition. Other researchers have reported systematic personality differences among religious groups in terms of dogmatism and aesthetic and intellectual values (Juan and Haley 1970; Haley et al. 1971).[24] It has also been noted (e.g., Hunter 1965; Kosa 1969; Monk and Thomas 1970) that the academic performance of Jews in medical school tends to be higher than that of any other religious or ethnic group.

In addition, in his study of eight medical schools, Kosa (1969) found that Protestants were the religious group most likely to be drawn from rural backgrounds, while Catholics and Jews came almost exclusively from urban backgrounds. As is shown below, the urbanness of a physician's upbringing appears to be separately related to his choice of specialty: a disproportionately large number of physicians from rural areas enter general practice and a disproportionately large number of those from urban areas enter the referral specialties. Hence, the associations between religion and specialty choice may be due to the effect of place of upbringing on specialty choice. Insofar as it applies to the choice between primary care and subspecialty careers in internal medicine, this explanation has been rejected by Weil et al. (1981), who found that Jews had exceptionally high tendencies to enter the subspecialties regardless of the size of their places of upbringing. On the other hand, in his regression analysis of 1960 medical graduates, Hadley (1975) concluded that religious background is not related to the choice of any specialty field. However, he did find that the choice probabilities were significantly associated with personality traits, measured ability, and the size of the physician's hometown.

On balance, the evidence implies that religious background is correlated with certain personality traits, individual ability, and the urbanness of the physician's upbringing. The observed associations between religion and specialty choice may signify tastes for specialties beyond those denoted by these other traits, but that hypothesis has yet to be verified definitively. A further possibility offered by some authors (e.g., Lieberson 1958; Weil and Schleiter 1981) is that Jews are induced more than other religious groups to specialize in order to attract patients. The theory holds that, because the ratio of Jewish physicians to Jews in the general population tends to be large, Jewish physicians must specialize if they wish to attract non-Jewish patients. Presumably, non-Jewish patients visit non-Jewish physicians as long as the latter meet their medical needs, and go to Jewish physicians chiefly to obtain specialty services not otherwise available. This hypothesis also has not been verified empirically.

SOCIOECONOMIC AND MARITAL STATUS

Various researchers have hypothesized that socioeconomic status affects specialty decision making in two ways: (1) directly, insofar as physicians choose specialties to raise or maintain their family economic status; and (2) indirectly, to the degree that socioeconomic status is a proxy for the physician's family wealth and the ability to sustain the costs of training beyond the first year of residency. In the latter case, the implicit argument is that physicians from the wealthiest families are most capable of meeting the opportunity costs of extended residency training. Those physicians are therefore most likely to choose specialty practice, while physicians from the poorest families are most likely to end their training after the first year of residency and to enter general practice.

Marital status serves as a partial proxy for the physician's preferred current rate of family consumption spending (i.e., the rate of current consumption is positively related to the size of the physician's immediate family). Also, the psychic costs of income forgone during residency training may increase with family size. Consequently, physicians who are married and have children before entering residency training are most likely to choose general practice, married physicians without children are the second most likely, and single physicians are the least likely.

The hypotheses that (1) low family income or wealth and (2) large numbers of dependents give incentives to curtail the length of graduate training are well grounded in the general theory of investment in human capital (e.g., Thurow 1970). Both hypotheses hinge on the absence of perfect capital markets in which graduates can borrow against their future incomes as practicing physicians. Consider, for example, a medical student who greatly prefers current to future consumption spending. Technically, this is known as having a "high rate of time preference" for current consumption. Suppose further that the student is unable to borrow enough to satisfy his or her preference for present consumption. Then, economic theory indicates that the student should be especially likely to opt for the minimum residency training and to enter general practice. Such a training pattern yields a higher portion of his or her income stream in the near term than one involving considerable residency training and the postponement of a (higher) future income stream.

Clearly, one likely cause of a "high rate of time preference" is a large number of dependents. That is, other things being equal, the physician's tendency to prefer current consumption spending against future spending should increase with the number of dependents and the size of the family's immediate wants.

With respect to the effects of wealth, the basic argument is that the choice of investment alternatives is influenced by the "diminishing marginal utility" of income. That is, the wealthy individual is ordinarily more willing to forgo a given dollar amount of current consumption (because it is more likely to be "discretionary") than the poor individual in order to add a given amount to future consumption. Thus, among graduates with the same general and specialty income expectations, one would expect to observe more physicians from wealthy families than from poor families opting for specialty practice and extended residency training.

In reality, of course, the associations between choice of general practice and family wealth or marital status will appear less clear-cut than these observations suggest. Substantial borrowing does occur, and the strength of the associations can be obscured by differences in pecuniary or psychic income expectations among physicians, averseness to borrowing, or other factors affecting attitudes toward present versus future consumption.

If status seeking is a motive in specialty decisions, it can be hypothesized intuitively that physicians from poor families—i.e., those with the lowest socioeconomic status (SES)—should tend to choose the most prestigious fields. This hypothesis is at variance with the economic theory outlined above, which argues that poor physicians are more likely to select the least prestigious fields such as general practice because of their shorter postgraduate training requirements. These contrasting predictions provide a way of interpreting the observed relationships between specialty choices and family income or SES.

The strongest evidence supporting the status-seeking hypothesis was reported by Kritzer and Zimet (1967). In a study of residents at the University of Colorado, they found a perfect inverse correlation between the perceived status of specialties chosen by the residents and their family SES. Nevertheless, their results raise a question which the study did not adequately answer—namely, that while physicians of low family SES selected prestigious specialties, physicians of high family SES selected unprestigious specialties. The latter finding implies some type of negative status-seeking behavior on the part of physicians from the highest SES backgrounds.

Most of the other findings either favor the economic hypothesis that there is a relationship between background and specialty choice, or else do not clearly support the status-seeking hypothesis. In his regression study, for example, Hadley (1977, 1979) reported that specialty selection was significantly related to physicians' desires for professional prestige[25] but not to their fathers' occupational status. These results support the thesis that status seeking is a motive in specialty choices, but they also imply that family SES is probably not an accurate proxy for the strength or content of that motive.

Small-sample studies by Oates and Feldman (1971) and Otis and Weiss (1972) also failed to uncover relationships between specialty choices and parental occupations, although both were confined to single medical schools, and the researchers in the second study grouped into one field somewhat dissimilar specialties (family and general practice, pediatrics, and obstetrics-gynecology) in order to test their hypothesis. More recently, Weil and Schleiter (1981) used an index of family SES based on parental education and father's occupation to predict the choice between primary care and subspecialty practice by subjects in their national sample of residents in internal medicine. Like other researchers, they obtained nonsignificant correlations between family SES and the types of careers preferred by physicians.

These results notwithstanding, virtually all other evidence shows that family SES tends to distinguish general practitioners from other physicians. Moreover, contrary to the predictions of the status-seeking theory, the thrust of the evidence indicates that physicians of low family SES are especially likely to enter general practice. Many studies have reported that a disproportionate percentage of general practitioners' parents come from the lowest educational, occupational, and income classes (Monk and Terris 1956; Coker et al. 1960; Lyden et al. 1968; Chipman et al. 1969; Kosa 1969; Paiva and Haley 1971; Monk and Thomas 1973; Gough and Ducker 1977). For instance, Lyden et al. found that, among 1950 and 1954 medical graduates, general practitioners least often described family income as a major source of financial support during medical school, were most dependent on their own earnings during medical school, and most often described financial pressures as influential in their specialty decisions.[26]

By and large, the relationships observed between marital status, current income, and debt on the one hand and specialty choices on the other tend to confirm the predictions of economic theory. With one exception (Monk and Thomas 1973), all studies of the effects of marital status have shown that general practitioners are more likely than other students to be married during medical school or to be married with children (AAMC 1959; Coker et al. 1960; Schumacher 1964; Lyden et al. 1968; Hadley 1975). In their research on future internists, Weil et al. (1981) did report that marital status and number of children were unrelated to the internists' choices between generalist and subspecialty careers. However, the difference in required length of residency training between the two options may not have been large enough to induce the expected associations. In addition, it is worth pointing out that residents' salaries (and, very likely, spouses' participation in the work force) have increased greatly over the past two decades. As a result, the incentives to cut short residency training and to enter general practice or generalized practice within a specialty are undoubtedly weaker now than they have been historically.

A few studies have examined the relationships between the size of the physician's actual or planned debt at graduation and his or her specialty or location choices, but with mixed results. Mantovani et al. (1976) found that medical students with large debts exhibited much stronger "interests" in practicing in physician-shortage areas than those with no debt, regardless of their other background traits. Unfortunately, the students' creditors were not identified, and it is probable that many of the high-debt students had received "forgiveness" loans under which some or all of the loan principal is canceled if the physician-debtor practices for a specified time in a physician-shortage area (see Chapter 8). No clear or consistent relationships have been found between specialty choices and the amounts of students' or residents' debts.[27]

The only direct evidence concerning the influence of family income on the length of residency training was also presented by Mantovani et al. In their sample of medical students, nearly 6 percent of those whose parents had annual incomes of less than $10,000 planned two or fewer years of residency training, and 85 percent planned four or fewer years. The corresponding figures for students whose parental incomes were $30,000 or more were approximately 3 percent and 76 percent, respectively.[28] These differences, while not large, are compatible with the hypothesis that overall length of training increases with the level of parental income. However, it is not known whether parental income influences specialty choices through its effects on length of training.

Weil et al. (1981) found no significant differences in the immediate family incomes (as opposed to parental incomes) of residents choosing between generalist and specialist careers in internal medicine. However, their figures indicate that married residents in the higher income classes ($20,000 per year or more in 1977) were one-third less likely to opt for generalist careers than those in the lower income classes (less than $20,000 per year). The same pattern held for unmarried residents, although different definitions of "high" and "low" income were used. Insofar as generalist careers entail shorter residencies than subspecialty careers, these data confirm the predictions of economic theory. Nevertheless, this finding is weakened by the fact that the observed relationships between income and career choice depended crucially on the specification of the income classes.

Thus, the majority of the available findings point to limited family wealth, high rates of desired current consumption, or both, as important reasons for curtailing the length of graduate training and entering general practice. It is not clear that the same kinds of background traits materially influence physicians' choices among specialties when they do not choose general practice, but this could be due to the relatively small variations in length of residency training among many of the specialties.

It is important to keep certain qualifications in mind in interpreting observed associations between specialty choices and family SES or income, student's or resident's marital status, and similar background traits. First, these traits are, at best, proxies for the underlying economic forces acting on specialty choices. As such, they may not adequately capture the true substance of those forces. Second, the background traits themselves may be related to other characteristics such as ability,[29] age, or place of upbringing, each of which can have its own direct or indirect effect on specialty choices. Although the evidence to date provides qualified support for the economic theory, it is possible that more rigorously specified future versions of the status-seeking theory of specialty choice may be found to have greater predictive power than current versions.

A few studies have reported that physicians' propensities to locate in rural or urban areas are associated with parental occupation. Hassinger (1963), Schaupp (1969), and Champion and Olsen (1971) all found that urban practitioners are more likely than rural practitioners to have fathers who are white-collar or professional workers.[30] However, it remains to be demonstrated what mechanism connects parental occupation with location choice. Thus, the observed relationship may denote links between practice location and other background traits or the choice of specialty.

PLACE OF UPBRINGING: INTERACTIONS BETWEEN SPECIALTY AND LOCATION CHOICES

The relationships between the physician's place of upbringing—whether a rural or an urban community—and both specialty and practice location selection have been investigated at length. Many descriptive studies have shown that general and family practitioners are considerably more likely than other physicians to have been brought up in rural areas (Coker et al. 1960; Weiskotten et al. 1960; Schumacher 1964; Lyden et al. 1968; Kosa 1969; Paiva and Haley 1971; Oates and Feldman 1974; Rushing 1975; Cullison et al. 1976a; Longnecker 1975; Barish 1979). In his regression study of the specialty choices of 1960 medical graduates, Hadley (1975) also reported that general practice was the only field in which rural upbringing was significantly positively related to specialty choice.

Most studies have focused on the size of the physician's hometown, given the choice of specialty. Consequently, it is difficult to conjecture about the probabilities of particular specialty choices given a knowledge of the size of the physician's hometown. Nonetheless, fragmentary evidence indicates that physicians raised in rural areas are two to three times more likely to select general or family practice than physicians raised in urban areas.[31] While general and family practitioners may differ with respect to other background or personality traits, both appear to be drawn heavily from rural areas. For example, Longnecker (1975) has reported that 56 percent of a 22-state sample of residents in family practice had been brought up in communities of 50,000 or fewer persons.

Like other professional groups, physicians migrate away from their places of upbringing in order to establish practices. The majority migrate from both rural areas and cities with high-density populations into communities that can be characterized as moderately urbanized. Most investigators have interpreted this pattern as a movement to the suburbs. In a study of nearly 2,200 medical graduates from the class of 1960, Rushing (1975) found that 454 were raised in counties whose populations were less than 50 percent urban according to the 1960 U.S. census, but that only 261 entered practice in such counties—representing a 43 percent net loss due to out-migration. Counties whose populations were 90 percent or more urban experienced a 9 percent net loss of physicians, but counties whose populations were 50 percent to 90 percent urban gained 24 percent more graduates than they produced. Similar results were published in another study of 1960 graduates by Schwartz and Cantwell (1976) using the same data base.

Yet despite these trends, a reasonably strong tendency exists for physicians to choose practice locations resembling the locations of their upbringing in terms of population size or degree of urbanization. Data tabulated by Rushing (1975) indicated that 40 percent of the Association of American Medical Colleges (AAMC) sample of 1960 medical graduates selected counties having percentages of urban populations similar to those of their counties of upbringing, and 22 percent chose practice communities of similar population size. Not surprisingly, the most highly urbanized counties and largest cities exhibited the highest retention rates (50 percent to 60 percent of the physicians originating in them), while the most rural counties and smallest communities showed the lowest (3 percent to 4 percent).

Large-sample studies of 1965 medical graduates by Heald et al. (1974) and Coleman (1976) also revealed that the population size of the physician's home county is a major correlate of the population size of his county of practice. These two studies estimated the population size of the physician's county of practice by means of regression equations in which a large number of attitudinal and background traits were defined as explanatory variables. Among them, population size of the physician's home county was by far the most significant predictor of practice county population, regardless of specialty.

Virtually all small-sample studies of earlier generations of rural physicians singled out rural upbringing as a trait distinguishing them from urban practitioners (Dinkel 1946; Fein 1956; Hassinger 1963; Peterson et al. 1963; Brown and Belcher 1966; Schaupp 1969; Johnson et al. 1973; Burket 1977; Paul 1978; Becker et al. 1979; Aaron et al. 1980). Data on recent medical students by Carline et al. (1980) indicate that the pattern continues to hold. By contrast, there is no evidence that rural practitioners are drawn to any appreciable extent from urban-reared physician populations. These results seem consistent with the findings that physician migration occurs chiefly from rural places of upbringing to urban practice locations.

In addition to the associations observed between rural upbringing, the choice of family or general practice, and the selection of a rural practice site, it has long been known that general and family practitioners are more likely than other physicians to enter rural practice. For instance, AMA data on the distribution of office-based physicians in 1975 showed that 22 percent of all general and family practitioners lived in counties of less than 50,000 persons, as opposed to 5 percent of all medical specialists, 7 percent of the surgeons, and 5 percent of the remaining specialists. Moreover, 52 percent of the office-based physicians in such counties—in contrast to only 19 percent in all other counties—were general and family practitioners (Goodman and Mason 1976).[32]

It also appears likely that the historical function of general practitioners as the major providers of rural physicians' services will be carried on by family practitioners. Studies of students or residents planning to enter family practice by Taylor et al. (1973), Oates and Feldman (1974), Longnecker (1975), and Barish (1979) all reported that two-thirds or more of their subjects preferred practice locations in rural communities. In addition, Cullison et al. (1976a) cited unpublished results of a survey of family practice residents who completed training in 1974 which showed that 35 percent were practicing in communities of less than 15,000.

The associations between rural upbringing, entry into general or family practice, and the choice of a rural practice location suggest some form of causal relationship. One element is the minimum size of a patient population necessary to support a full-time general or family practitioner on an acceptably profitable basis. Although little empirical evidence exists as to the requisite size of support populations for the various specialties, they are probably much smaller for general and family practice than for other fields.[33] The implication is that for physicians wishing to practice in thinly populated areas, where travel time between patients' homes and the physician's office restricts the geographic size of the market, general or family practice is the most viable field. By the same token, physicians who enter general or family practice have a wider range of profitable market location opportunities, including both rural and urban areas, than other practitioners. It would be expected that a relatively large number of them might select rural locations for that reason alone. Conversely, physicians with weak locational preferences but strong preferences for the hospital-based or referral specialties have considerable income motives to choose urban practice locations.

To what extent prior locational decisions induce specialty choices, and to what extent prior specialty decisions induce practice location choices, are not known. Indeed, the direction of causation remains a subject of speculation. Obviously, the direction may not be the same for all physicians, and both types of causation may occur. The findings on the timing of specialty and practice location decisions reviewed in Chapter 1 indicate that specialty choices tend to precede location choices, but these findings are subject to too many qualifications to be interpreted as proof that the choice of rural or urban practice location is the result of prior specialty decisions.[34]

Likewise, the other causal factors which connect place of upbringing with career choices are not well understood. In cases where practice location is in or near the physician's community of upbringing, it can be surmised that the attachment influences described in Chapter 2—the physician's or spouse's family or friendship ties, opportunities for beginning practice, and so on—account for some part of the association. In instances where place of upbringing and practice location are geographically separate, the influences are less clear-cut.[35] Moreover, rural upbringing is correlated with other background traits such as religion and social class which have been found to be associated with specialty choices. Cullison et al. (1976b) reported that rural students entering medical schools in 1973 had somewhat lower MCAT scores than metropolitan students, which makes them likely candidates, other things being equal, for entry into general practice. Such findings suggest that explanations of the relationships between place of upbringing and career choices may be more complex than is often thought to be the case.

PRACTICE LOCATION AND THE PRIOR-CONTACT HYPOTHESIS

Upbringing is one source of a physician's contact with a community, state, or geographic region before entry into practice. Undergraduate education, medical school education, graduate training, and military service are the other principal sources. The preceding section cited studies which indicate that physicians often choose practice communities of similar size to the communities in which they were reared. But stronger relationships have been observed between the geographic location of the physician's practice and the geographic locations of his or her upbringing and educational experience.

Weiskotten et al. (1960) investigated the effects of four types of area contact prior to entry into practice—residence prior to medical school, during medical school, during internship training, and during residency training. They did not analyze the structure of prior contact and its relationship to place of practice, but they reported that nearly 50 percent of their samples of 1945 and 1950 graduates practiced in cities, and approximately 80 percent in states, with which they had prior contact. They also noted that place of residency training showed the strongest effect, with one-third of the sampled physicians practicing in the cities where their residency hospitals were located and 60 percent practicing in the same states.

More recently, associations between practice location and two or more of the four types of prior contact have been studied by Wiggins et al. (1970), Held (1972), Yett and Sloan (1974), Mason (1975), and Ernst et al. (1978).[36] They have also been confirmed in a number of smaller studies of the practice locations of graduates of individual medical schools and of physicians living in particular states (Fein 1956; Hassinger 1963; Martin et al. 1968; Bible 1970; Charles 1971; Roleston 1973; Balinsky 1974; Brandt et al. 1979; Stefanu and Pate 1978; Stefanu et al. 1979; Watson 1980a, 1980b).[37] Broadly speaking, the evidence has produced two results. First, the mobility of physicians between regions of the country is relatively low, but mobility among states in the same region is fairly high, and mobility within states is higher still. Second, the percentage of physicians who practice in areas where they have had prior contact has declined over the past generation. Taken together, these trends imply that physicians have become more mobile as a group and show decreasing tendencies to practice in areas of prior contact.[38]

Yett and Sloan (1974) attempted to give more precision to the attachment hypotheses by formulating two empirical propositions: namely, that the likelihood of the physician's practicing in a given state increases with (1) the number of previous contacts in the state and (2) the recency of contacts with the state. They tested and confirmed both propositions using data on the population of physicians entering practice in 1966 and the four-way typology of prior contact originated by Weiskotten et al.[39] The results demonstrated that the structure of prior contact must be known in order to predict practice locations accurately, but they left an important question which has not yet been resolved. As Yett and

Sloan (1974) noted, their findings did not necessarily establish a causal connection between prior contact and state of practice. Indeed, physicians may select medical school or graduate training locations because they wish to live and practice in those locations. Yett and Sloan offered evidence against this interpretation by showing that regressions using measures of prior contact as explanatory variables forecasted state physician retention rates markedly more accurately than those using measures of the desirability of the state as a practice location.[40]

However, Lee (1980) has partly challenged the prior-contact hypotheses by arguing that medical students choose residency locations where they plan to practice. Using data on students from five medical schools, he found that the probability they would apply for residency programs near their planned practice communities increased if: (1) they and their spouses agreed on a practice location, (2) they planned to enter full-time clinical practice, and (3) their planned practice locations were near their high schools or medical school communities. Lee interpreted these results as showing that students are especially likely to choose residency locations in their planned practice communities when the latter have been firmly decided. On that basis, he concluded that the selection of a residency community is determined by prior selection of a practice community.

It is difficult to assess Lee's findings for at least two reasons. First, they give no information on what fraction of his sample may have been motivated to choose residency locations on the basis of their practice location plans. Since the prior-contact theory does not claim that prior contact has a causative impact on all physicians' location decisions, it is conceivable that Lee's results may reflect the behavior of the minority of physicians who had indeed chosen residencies near their intended practice locations. Second, as Lee himself observed, his analyses imply that students tend to select practice locations near their places of upbringing or medical school education, and these patterns are consistent with the prior-contact theory.

Nevertheless, the results cast at least some doubt on the proposition that graduate training locations are an important influence on physicians' practice location plans. As we remarked in Chapter 1, the effect of environmental factors on physician's career decisions very likely depends on the timing of those decisions. That the majority of practice location decisions appear to be made during graduate training favors prior contact as a causative factor in most practice location choices. But for physicians who determine their places of practice early in their careers, graduate training or medical school locations are probably more the effect than the cause of practice location choices.

Another question is what causes geographic attachments to occur. Hadley (1975) has suggested that the degree of attachment measures the physician's tastes for mobility—i.e., that some physicians inherently develop attachments to areas while others do not—an issue that is not without policy significance. If physicians' area attachments increase with the amount of contact or the recency of contact, then physician allocation policies based on structuring the locations of postgradute as well as undergraduate medical education have a significant chance of success. If, on the other hand, many physicians' practice location choices are not affected by prior area contact, the geographic distribution of physicians cannot be modified by inducing medical students or residents to train at institutions in physician-shortage areas.[41]

SUMMARY

In Chapter 2 it was argued that the empirical findings on physicians' personality characteristics and career-choice behavior can be evaluated in terms of their qualitative implications, their value for predicting career choices, and their contribution to an understanding of how those choices are made. The same criteria can be applied to findings on background traits and career selection.

With respect to specialty choice, the evidence on background traits —like that on personality traits—indicates that primary care practitioners are not homogeneous and cannot be distinguished as a group from referral specialists. Background traits perform best in terms of identifying general practitioners, who currently represent less than 10 percent of the physician population. They are somewhat less successful in characterizing physicians in the other specialty fields. The stereotypical general practitioner is older than his or her colleagues at graduation from medical school, ranks lower in measures of academic performance, is more likely to have been raised in a rural community, and is more likely to be Protestant, to have working-class parents, and to be married and have a family at graduation. By contrast, family practitioners exhibit traits similar to those of all physicians. The only distinctive trait they share with general practitioners is the tendency to have been raised in rural areas.

Internists rank high in measures of academic ability, a trait they share with academic physicians. This finding is consistent with results of personality studies showing that both groups have above-average intellectual interests. Women have especially strong propensities to enter pediatrics, but potential pediatricians are otherwise poorly identified by background traits. Women also have strong tendencies to choose psychiatry, and there are indications that nonreligious and Jewish physicians are disproportionately likely to choose psychiatry, academic medicine, or internal medicine. Because their numbers are still small relative to the total physician population, however, female, nonreligious, and Jewish physicians do not typify members of any of these fields.

In the main, investigation of background traits and specialty selection is still in the descriptive stage. Many background traits appear to be significantly associated with the outcomes of specialty decisions in the statistical sense, and they seem to be moderately successful in distinguishing between general practitioners and specialists. However, general practitioners currently represent a very small proportion of new medical graduates, so that knowing how to discriminate between them and specialists does not help much in predicting the overall specialty distribution of physicians.

The collective capabilities of background traits as a means of predicting choices among several different specialties have been examined only by Hadley (1975, 1977, 1979). It is doubtful that background traits as a group account for a large part of the variation in outcomes of specialty decisions, and this naturally raises questions as to their predictive power.

The predictive utility of background traits has also been clouded by the directions research methodologies have taken. For the most part, research has centered on identifying background traits given prior knowledge of the physician's specialty choice, whereas the predictive problem is to forecast the physician's choice of specialty given prior knowledge of his or her background traits. The two approaches are formally and methodologically dissimilar, and the first—esentially a matter of classification—is not necessarily useful for predicting specialty choices.[42] At least some background traits are intercorrelated, and some are probably correlated with personality characteristics as well. This raises the possibility that certain observed associations between background traits and specialty choices are spurious.

The existing evidence on background traits does not, in itself, constitute a theory of specialty choice. Rigorous causal hypotheses need to be developed and tested to further our understanding of the process. Although some background attributes may be proxies for tastes, others—such as age at graduation, marital status, and family income—are more likely to be proxies for the influence of economic factors. The physical and intellectual abilities which qualify physicians for certain specialties have not been adequately defined or studied. Hence, it remains conjectural whether they are captured by the customary measures of academic performance. Competing, and weakly tested, hypotheses exist for explaining women's specialty choices, but none has been advanced to account for those of blacks and other minorities.

With regard to practice location choice, it is clear that physicians have high propensities to settle in areas with which they have had prior personal contact. The amount and structure of previous contact are highly significant predictors of state of practice. Indeed, state retention rates of physicians can be reasonably well predicted from a knowledge of prior contact alone.

At the intrastate level the evidence is much weaker and more fragmentary. Consistent with the findings of attitudinal studies on location, physicians are to some degree attracted to communities near their place of upbringing or similar in size to their hometown. However, urban-reared physicians are much more likely to choose urban practice locations than rural-reared physicians are to choose rural locations. Other types of prior community contact—such as during medical school and graduate training—also appear to lead physicians to select the same or similar communities as practice locations. On the whole, however, the effects of intrastate prior contact have been little studied, and existing findings cannot be considered conclusive.

As is true of specialty choice, a number of additional questions concerning practice location need to be resolved: (1) What is the direction of causation in observed relationships between prior contact and location choice? (2) How does prior contact interact with other factors that influence location behavior? (3) Do distinct subpopulations of physicians exist—for example, those with tastes for mobility and those without— among whom the effects of prior contact vary? Can such subpopulations be identified on the basis of other background traits? (4) How do the location choices of women, blacks, and other minority physicians differ from those of white male physicians? (5) What background traits are associated with physicians' permanent choices of underserved rural and inner-city areas? The answers to these questions would materially add to our knowledge of physicians' location behavior and our ability to devise successful policies to influence such behavior.

NOTES

1. The Medical College Admissions Test must be taken before a candidate applies to a medical school. It consists of four parts which measure the applicant's science knowledge, science problem-solving ability, reading skills, and quantitative skills. Before 1977, the MCAT also consisted of four parts, but these tested the applicant's science knowledge, verbal ability, quantitative ability, and knowledge of "general information" (i.e., history, literature, etc.). In 1976, the general information section was dropped and the other three sections were revised so as to better evaluate the applicant's analytical capabilities.

The test of the National Board of Medical Examiners is made up of three parts. Successful completion of the NBME test is accepted by nearly all states in lieu of passing the (state) board examination. Thus, the physician who completes the NBME test is eligible (subject to training requirements) for licensure in almost every state. The first part of the NBME is normally taken at the end of the second year of medical school, the second just before medical school graduation, and the third after the first year of graduate training.

As shown in Chapter 4, premedical measures of performance such as college GPAs and MCAT scores have usually been found to be weakly correlated with measures of performance in medical school, particularly clinical performance. There is some question, then, whether they and NBME scores really measure the same dimensions of ability. Types of ability such as manual dexterity, clinical aptitude, and skill in interpersonal relationships have not been explicitly correlated with specialty choices.

2. See Chapter 5 for a discussion of the National Intern and Resident Matching Program, now known as the National Resident Matching Program.

3. These results should be interpreted with caution. Cuca's tabulations were based only on two-way classifications of specialty and background traits. As she herself observed, interactions among the traits may have distorted the apparent associations. For example, a disproportionately large number of blacks—a large percentage of whom had below-average MCAT scores and were admitted to medical schools under admissions-variance programs (Johnson et al. 1975)—expressed preferences for obstetrics-gynecology. This could have lowered the mean MCAT scores of graduates preferring that field. Also, graduates may be placed in residency specialties which are not their first choices, and many switch fields after their first year of residency. As a result, Cuca's figures may not give a wholly reliable impression.

4. See Chapter 6 for a more detailed discussion of Hadley's work. Paiva and Haley (1971) and Haley et al. (1971) also found no significant differences between the MCAT scores of medical students preferring general and specialty practice at six medical schools. But their subjects were freshmen, and the instability of early specialty preferences casts doubt on the reliability of their conclusion.

5. It is not clear why Hadley's finding on this score conflicts with that of Schumacher. Hadley rejected the hypotheses that medical school and internship characteristics significantly influenced the choice probabilities, so it would appear that the ability measures were correlated with other personal traits or market forces which led to the selection of general practice. However, since he removed from his sample individuals who had not taken the NBME test, it is also possible that editing eliminated the less able students.

6. In a study of medical school graduates in West Virginia, Schaupp (1969) speculated that physicians ranking in the lowest third of their class were most likely to practice in West Virginia. He based his conjecture on the hypothesis that such physicians were especially likely to enter general practice and to remain in the predominantly rural state, but the data did not confirm his conjecture. We shall return to the relationships between specialty and practice location below.

7. As is shown in the next chapter, performance in medical school tends to be inversely correlated with age. Thus, some part of the observed associations between age and the choice of general practice may be attributable to low performance. Nevertheless, Monk and Terris (1956) and Hadley (1977) both reported results that conflict with such an interpretation. Both studies indicated that the high propensity of older students to enter general practice prevailed independently of their medical school performance.

8. Weil et al. (1981) found that residents who planned generalist careers in internal medicine were significantly older (statistically) than those who planned subspecialty careers in the same field—although the average age difference was only about seven months. This could mean that the "old-generalist-versus-young-specialist" paradigm holds within specialties as well as between them, but the finding remains to be replicated.

The evidence relating physician age to practice location choice is sketchy. Hadley (1977) found that age was unrelated to practice location at the state level, and Haug et al. (1980) claimed that age was unrelated to preferences for rural and urban communities among beginning medical students. Heald et al. (1974) used regressions to predict the urbanness of practice locations for a sample of 1965 medical school graduates, and found that age was weakly positively correlated with the choice of an urban location regardless of specialty. With the same data but a smaller set of explanatory variables, Coleman (1976) reported a positive correlation between age and urban location for general and other primary care practitioners, but a negative and nonsignificant correlation for referral specialists. Thus, clear-cut connections between physician age and practice location, if they exist, have not yet been established.

9. For a discussion of the optimal length of occupational training, see, e.g., Becker (1975).

10. The present value of a future net income stream is the sum of each increment (usually taken to be annual) to the stream discounted to the starting date of the stream by the appropriate interest (or subjective discount) rate. Because of discounting, annual incomes in the distant future contribute much less to the present value of the stream than incomes earned in the immediate future. Also see Chapter 6.

11. Women represented approximately 9 percent of the total supply because of the relatively large percentage (17 percent) of women among foreign medical graduates. About 9 percent of all U.S. women physicians were graduates of the Medical College of Pennsylvania (see Martin 1975).

12. The stereotype of women as "mother-healers" seems to be common in medicine, even among those who reject other female stereotypes (Bowers 1968; Scher 1973). This suggests that both professional pressures and self-selection may lead women into pediatrics or psychiatry where subjective qualities such as warmth, understanding, and tenderness are considered especially desirable. For example, Kosa and Coker (1965) argued that the single most important reason women physicians entered public health was to avoid the entrepreneurial competitiveness which they believed to characterize other fields.

Also, according to Lopate (1968), the profession has traditionally assigned women physicians the role of treating children and female adults. The studies cited in the text indicate that approximately 50 percent of women physicians practice in pediatrics, psychiatry, and obstetrics-gynecology. It is not known to what extent women psychiatrists specialize in treating female patients, but otherwise the data tend to support Lopate's position.

13. For example, Matthews (1970), Westling-Wilkstrand et al. (1970), and Williams (1971) all reported considerable anxiety among married women—particularly mothers—in training, evidently based on the fear that they could not meet their competing obligations as physicians, wives, and mothers. Matthews and Williams both cited the total length of training as a concern to women, although the specific reasons for concern were not stated. In some cases it was presumably related to the long delay women perceived before they could marry or bear children. According to Matthews and Williams, some women also expressed worry over accumulating large debts during their training because they felt it would jeopardize their opportunities for marriage.

14. Cohen and Korper (1976a, 1976b) reported that nearly a quarter of their sample of women physicians in Connecticut had changed specialties in response to the conflicts they saw between their careers and marriages, but the directions of the changes were not given. They cited one example of a woman who had chosen a field (psychiatry) because she believed its working conditions would be compatible with her marriage. In a study of Radcliffe alumnae who had entered medicine, Williams (1971) also stated that an undisclosed number switched specialties as a means of resolving marital conflicts.

15. Certification by the specialty boards requires completion of approved graduate programs extending three to seven years beyond the M.D. degree; see Chapter 5.

16. According to 1978 AMA tabulations, 62 percent of all active U.S. women physicians were in office practice, 23 percent practiced in hospitals, and 14 percent held positions in teaching, research, or administration. The corresponding percentages for men were 77, 13, and 10. These figures were derived from Wunderman (1979, 1980), and do not include residents, physicians unclassified by the AMA, or those whose addresses were unknown.

17. For example, Jussim and Muller (1975) estimated that the average working lifetimes of male and female physicians were approximately 90,000 and 56,000 hours, respectively. Population data by Haug and Roback (1970) and Renshaw and Pennell (1971) indicate that (excluding those in graduate training) 19 percent of all female physicians, but only 6 percent of all male physicians, were professionally inactive in 1969. Recently, the figures have converged. Data presented by Wunderman (1980) show that 7 percent of male physicians and only 10 percent of female physicians were professionally inactive in 1978.

Another aspect of female physicians' labor supply was reported by Kehrer (1976). After standardizing for personal characteristics other than sex, Kehrer found that women physicians' hourly earnings were 22 percent lower than men's. She also found that, while the number of working hours supplied by male physicians was significantly positively associated with hourly net income, women physicians' supplies of hours were negatively and not significantly associated with hourly net income. On that basis she conjectured that women physicians have backward-bending labor-supply curves.

18. Tabulations of sample data by Wooldridge (1976) suggest that the geographic distributions of female and male physicians are closely similar. Haug et al. (1980) also found close similarities between the urban-rural distributions of planned practice locations by male and female first-year medical students, although women seemed to have stronger propensities than men to prefer inner-city locations. In contrast to these results, Ernst et al. (1978) reported that women entering practice in 1970 had markedly stronger propensities than men to locate in metropolitan areas. They conjectured that the pattern may have been due to the strong propensity of women to select institutional types of practice settings. Data presented by the AMA (1977), Barish (1979), D'Elia and Johnson (1980), and Wunderman (1980) also suggest that women are somewhat less likely than men to choose rural practice locations.

19. One frequently alleged cause of the high retirement rates for women physicians—the lack of retraining facilities for women who withdraw from practice to bear and raise children (e.g., Jussim and Muller 1975)—should also be less important in the future than in the past. Large numbers of programs in continuing medical education have been introduced since 1970 which, while not specifically designed for women, should make it easier for women who wish to reenter practice to do so.

20. Except in two respects, tabulations by Cuca (1977) also indicated no strong differences between the preferred specialties of blacks and whites entering residency training in 1976. In that year, blacks were five times as likely as whites to prefer obstetrics-gynecology and two and one-half times as likely to prefer public health. Unfortunately, Cuca offered no explanations for these new and surprising results.

21. Guzick and Jahiel also presented two other interesting results. First, the number of black physicians decreased significantly with the percentage of nonblack minorities in the population. Second, the number of non-European (and presumably mostly nonwhite) foreign medical graduates increased significantly with both the percentage of blacks and the percentage of nonblack minorities in the population. Whether the evident propensity of physicians to serve patients of their own races is attributable to tastes or other factors is not clear.

In an earlier study, Lieberson (1958) found a marked tendency for Chicago physicians to choose office locations in neighborhoods where the ethnic background of the population was the same as their own. He argued that the pattern was probably not due to the physicians' ethnic preferences for patients, because many physicians resided in neighborhoods where the ethnic composition of the population differed from their own. He suggested instead that the preference of patients of a given ethnic background for physicians of the same background created income opportunities for the physicians and led them to establish offices where they could serve ethnic demands.

22. Mantovani et al. (1976) surveyed more than 7,000 medical students in 1975 and reported that blacks expressed much stronger "interests" in practicing in physician-shortage areas than whites. Unfortunately, they did not specify whether shortage areas referred to inner-city or rural communities.

23. The relationship may also be due to other factors. For example, it has sometimes been charged that Jews had difficulty in securing training positions in the surgical fields because of discrimination. Conversely, the founders of psychiatry were largely Jewish, so that anti-Semitic discrimination would not have been a barrier to entry into psychiatric training or practice.

24. It is of interest to observe that the religious composition of the student body varies strikingly from one medical school to another. In the sample of seven medical schools examined in 1967 by Haley et al. (1971), the percentage of Protestants ranged from 12 to 82, the percentage of Catholics from 9 to 75, and the percentage of Jews from 0 to 41. It is unknown to what extent this variation is due to admissions policies (e.g., priority for state residents) and to what extent it reflects regional self-selection by medical students (e.g., in one school two-thirds of the students were Mormons). But at least to the degree that religious background is related to specialty choice, the variation indicates that self-selection and admissions screening probably affect the specialty distribution of graduates. Also see Chapter 4 on this point.

25. The variable was defined as the physician's score on the prestige dimension of the Career Attitudes Inventory Test. The score was positively related to the probabilities of selecting surgical and medical specialties, and negatively related to the probabilities of selecting general practice and a partial grouping of other primary care fields. Hence, the variable appears to capture the physician's desire for professional esteem as a motive for choosing a field.

26. In a later study, Gordon (1978) tabulated data on more than 12,000 1975 medical graduates and found that those who entered family practice residencies tended to have lower parental incomes than those choosing other residency fields. It is not immediately evident whether this can be interpreted as a phenomenon parallel to general practitioners' having low parental incomes. Since family practice residencies need not be much shorter than those in other fields, limited financial resources should not necessarily lead a physician to choose family practice as they might general practice.

27. Coker et al. (1960) and Lyden et al. (1968) both stated that general practitioners had larger debts at graduation than other physicians, and Weil et al. (1981) indicated that residents planning generalist careers in internal medicine had significantly higher debts than those planning to practice in subspecialties. However, in other large-sample studies Hadley (1977) and Mantovani et al. (1976) found nonsignificant or quantitatively weak associations between size of debt and actual or planned specialty choices.

28. The data were cross-classified only by size of hometown. The patterns held regardless of hometown size, but they could have been distorted by systematic variation in other important background traits. Mantovani et al. (1976)

indicated that the planned length of residency training was inversely correlated with the size of debt expected at graduation, but they failed to standardize for other student traits. In particular, they found that debt size varied
substantially with certain characteristics such as the physician's sex, race,
marital status, place of upbringing, and parental income. Consequently,
other interpretations of their tabulations are possible besides the one that
large debts induced students to plan short residencies.

29. The conventional hypothesis is that physicians' measured ability increases
with family SES, but empirical evidence on the issue is inconclusive. See,
e.g., Motto (1965), Fredericks and Mundy (1967), Woods et al. (1967), and
Haley et al. (1971).

30. In a study of North Carolina general practitioners, Peterson et al. (1963) rejected the hypothesis that parental occupation affects practice location
choice except when the physician's father is also a physician. Although his
sample was small and geographically restricted, he found a strong tendency
for physicians' offspring to locate in their fathers' practice communities—
presumably to join the parental practices. The relationship has not been explored further, but it may be an important one inasmuch as approximately
15 percent of all physicians are the sons or daughters of physicians (U.S. Department of Health, Education, and Welfare 1974).

31. In one large-sample study of medical students in the 1950s, Coker et al.
(1960) stated that 59 percent of those from rural areas, but only 18 percent of
those from urban areas, planned to enter general practice. Using another
large sample of graduates from the early 1950s, Lyden et al. (1968) found
that 35 percent of the rural-reared physicians, but only 17 percent of the urban-reared physicians, chose general practice. And in a third study of graduates of the University of Missouri from 1957 to 1968, Cullison et al. (1976a)
reported that 47 percent of the rural-reared graduates and 18 percent of the
urban-reared graduates entered general practice or family practice.

Because of the secularly declining fraction of physicians becoming general
practitioners, the foregoing percentages overstate current rates of entry into
general and family practice. They may, of course, also misstate the *relative*
rates of entry by rural- and urban-reared physicians. In addition, some of the
evidence on the effects of upbringing is far weaker. After standardizing for
other background and personality traits, Hadley (1975) estimated that a 10
percent increase in the number of rural-reared medical students would increase the proportion of general practitioners by only 1.3 percent. However,
he defined "rural" hometown somewhat narrowly as a community of less
than 10,000 persons. Using the same data and a different definition of the
urbanness of place of upbringing, Rushing (1975) reported that 24 percent of
the physicians from counties where populations were less than 40 percent
urban entered general practice, whereas the figure was 9 percent for physicians from counties which were 90 percent or more urban. Obviously, estimates of the relationship between place of upbringing and specialty choice
depend upon the specification of "urbanness."

The relationship may also vary among graduates of different medical schools. At two medical schools, Oates and Feldman (1971) and Otis and Weiss (1972) found no association between students' planned specialties and the size of their hometowns, although Oates and Feldman reversed their conclusion in the later paper (1974) cited above. More recently, Weil et al. (1981) indicated that residents' plans to enter generalist or subspecialty practice in internal medicine were unrelated to the size of their hometowns.

32. Surgeons represented 24 percent of the total, and it has occasionally been noted that general surgeons—particularly those with rural backgrounds—have a relatively high probability of settling in rural areas (e.g., Cullison et al. 1976a).

33. One source of evidence is the specialty staffing patterns of prepaid group practices. Data reported by Feldstein (1971) on three of the largest prepaid groups showed that they employ approximately one first-contact physician (a general or family practitioner or a general internist) per 2,200 to 2,700 subscribers, one pediatrician per 4,500 to 7,700 subscribers, and other specialists in the ratio of one to 9,000 or more subscribers. The figures may not be reliable indicators of the exact support populations for typical fee-for-service physicians—especially in the case of pediatricians—but they probably give the order of relative population sizes with reasonable accuracy.

34. More specifically, none of the descriptive evidence disaggregates the timing of decisions by both specialty and the size of community location, so it is hard to tell what relationships exist between the timing of the decisions and their outcomes. Most results bearing on practice location are unclear about the nature of the choice—whether it pertains to the actual practice site or to the general characteristics of the type of site chosen. However, it is reasonable to believe that preferences for community sizes are shaped earlier than those for specific geographic areas or communities. Moreover, some reports have suggested that rural practitioners are especially likely to make early location decisions with respect to their actual practice communities, perhaps even before choosing their specialties.

35. As was discussed in Chapter 2, physicians appear to develop pronounced tastes for urban or rural life-styles, but it has not been shown that these tastes are unambiguously related to their background experience. Most of the studies mentioned in this section revealed strong preferences for rural life-styles among rural practitioners. Even so, physicians have migrated in large numbers out of the rural areas where they were brought up, from which it may be concluded that rural upbringing does not necessarily produce decisive rural attachments. Thus, it would seem to be the case that the physicians who remain exhibit unusually strong tastes for rural living.

36. Hadley (1975), in a study discussed at length in Chapter 6, segmented his sample of the class of 1960 and estimated the probabilities of settling in areas in which the physician (1) had no prior training contact, (2) attended medical school, (3) did graduate training, and (4) both attended medical school and did graduate training. Among his explanatory variables was an indicator of whether the physician was born and reared in the area. The results were generally not consistent with the findings of studies that use all four prior-con-

tact attributes as explanatory variables. The exception was subsample 4, in which Hadley found that birth and upbringing in a state significantly increased the probability that the physician would remain to practice in the state.

37. The locational attachment effects of medical school and graduate medical education are discussed in Chapters 4 and 5. It has been reported by Heald et al. (1974), Longnecker (1975), and Coleman (1976) that sizable proportions of physicians either decide on a practice location during military service or claim to have been influenced by military locations in choosing a place of practice. The effects of military service, undergraduate education, and other types of area contact on practice location decisions have not been studied further.

38. The likelihood that physicians will practice in areas where they have had prior contact seems to have declined roughly 20 percent to 25 percent over the period 1935–65. Depending on the type of contact, they are about one-third to one-half as likely to practice in cities of prior contact as in states, and perhaps 75 percent to 80 percent as likely to practice in states of prior contact as in regions. The sources of the figures cited here are Weiskotten et al. (1960), Wiggins et al. (1970), and Held (1972).

39. Lacking data on the physician's residence before medical school, they defined birth as the first type of state contact. They found that, depending on specialty, approximately 85 percent of the physicians whose contacts were confined to a single state entered practice in the same state; 70 percent with only one out-of-state contact remained to practice in the state of most contact; and only 6 percent to 14 percent entered practice in states where they had only one type of previous contact. They also found that, given the number of contacts, the proportion of physicians remaining to practice in the state was generally significantly higher the more recent were the contacts (e.g., residency training rather than medical school).

40. The variables were defined as proxies for physician income opportunities, the quality of living conditions in the state, and so on. They were similar to predictors used to measure area attractiveness in other practice location studies such as those discussed in Chapter 7.

41. According to tabulations by Held, 24 percent of all 1955–65 medical graduates chose states where they had no prior contact, and 50 percent chose states where they had at most one type of prior contact. All the same, it should be mentioned that these figures probably understate the actual amount of contact because Held (like all other investigators) excluded military and government service, undergraduate education, nonmedical employment, and places of family ties as types of prior contact. It is, of course, not difficult to conjecture why geographic attachments occur among physicians. They could be due to preferences for living near family or friends, to special opportunities for beginning practice (e.g., arising out of personal or professional contacts in the area), and to averseness to the uncertainties of living or practicing in new and unfamiliar places.

42. For example, rural general practitioners are highly likely to have been raised in rural areas. Naively, this suggests that rural upbringing might be a strong predictor of the selection of rural general practice. In actuality, however, it is a relatively weak predictor because of the large volume of physician out-migration from rural places of upbringing to urban and suburban practice locations.

FOUR

The Medical School and Physicians' Career Choices

The present structure of undergraduate medical education and the types of physicians it produces are the outgrowth of a complex and ongoing interplay of institutional, technological, and economic forces. Although a full treatment of the medical educational system is beyond the scope of this study, some discussion of background and trends in medical education is essential for understanding physicians' specialty and practice location choices. Accordingly, this chapter first considers the implications of three major historical events which have profoundly affected the character of the modern medical school: the 1910 Flexner Report on medical education, the federal biomedical research program begun after World War II, and efforts by the federal government since the late 1960s to increase the supply of physicians, promote the primary care fields, and encourage physicians to establish practices in medically underserved areas. The federal (and other) policies to alter the specialty and locational distributions of new physicians will be taken up in more detail in Chapter 8.

THE FLEXNERIAN ERA

At the close of the nineteenth century, the great majority of American physicians were poorly trained and controlled by loosely maintained licensure regulations. Partly to raise the reputation of the profession and partly to reduce the number of incompetent or unqualified practitioners, the American Medical Association (AMA) embarked on two basic types of remedial action. One was aimed at strengthening state licensure regulations, the other at improving the quality of medical education.

In 1904, the AMA established the Council on Medical Education to investigate conditions in medical schools, and to recommend any changes deemed necessary. Four years later, the council entered into an arrangement with the Carnegie Foundation for the Advancement of Teaching to conduct a survey of medical schools. A report on the survey, prepared under the supervision of Abraham Flexner, was published in 1910. Singling out medical schools by name, the Flexner Report denounced all but a handful for gross failures of their teaching programs. The report found proprietary institutions so appallingly inadequate that it urged they be closed outright; and, claiming that many nonproprietary schools were little better, it advocated sweeping changes in the medical education establishment as a whole.[1]

Basing its recommendations on innovations undertaken at the newly formed School of Medicine at Johns Hopkins University, the Flexner Report proposed a model medical school embodying five fundamental principles. In particular, it held that: (1) undergraduate medical education is a public service which should be conducted by a university and not a proprietary organization; (2) the medical school's teaching function should be closely integrated with biomedical research; (3) the school should accept only the most highly qualified applicants; (4) it should offer a four-year program, a significant portion of which should be devoted to the biomedical sciences; and (5) the clinical phase of the program should be provided in a major hospital affiliated with the university.[2]

Several forces contributed to the acceptance of the Flexnerian recommendations. First, educational reform was seen as affording important social benefits insofar as it would raise the level of medical technology and the competence of practicing physicians. Thus, from all indications, it was supported by the public at large. Second, universities were receptive toward the recommendation that they assume responsibility for medical education. Third, technological progress in medicine had already begun to create market opportunities for specialization, and demands for the sophisticated type of education advocated in the report had begun to increase.[3] Fourth, the recommended restrictions on the supply of medical education amounted to a substantial barrier to entry in the then crowded medical profession and conferred important economic benefits on established practitioners.[4] Taken together, these forces constituted a powerful array of pressures for reshaping medical schools in the Flexnerian mold.

The two decades following publication of the Flexner Report saw a dramatic restructuring of undergraduate medical education. The number of medical schools declined by one-half to 76, and the number of graduates fell from approximately 4,500 in 1910 to 3,000 in 1920, and did not reach the previous number again until the early 1930s (Fein 1967). Universities rose to a position of dominance and proprietary schools were eliminated.[5] The changes came about primarily through modification of state licensure regulations to make graduation from an accredited school mandatory, and by the withdrawal (or threat of withdrawal) of accreditation from schools failing to meet the new standards.[6] According to Stevens (1971), foundation support awarded to the prestigious private medical schools was another important factor which promoted educational change. The support served both as a source of investment funds for enlarging those institutions, and as an incentive to other schools to adopt the Flexnerian image.[7].

By the 1930s, the shift of undergraduate medical education into the Flexnerian form was completed, and the Flexnerian model has remained the criterion of educational excellence to the present day.[8] Many of the characteristics of the modern medical center can be traced directly to it. Much like its Johns Hopkins prototype, the medical center today is typically a vertically and horizontally integrated producer of undergraduate and graduate medical education, biomedical research and education, education in the allied health professions, and patient care. One obvious implication is that the large medical school has a diverse array of goals competing with the importance it attaches to the undergraduate education of physicians. And, even in terms of their teaching services, medical schools train fewer medical students than undergraduate and graduate students in the biomedical sciences and other health professions (e.g., Crowley 1975b). However, the major historical conflict has occurred between the priorities given teaching and research. In the aftermath of the Flexner Report, biomedical research in medical schools became an important institutional product in its own right and a principal source of technological progress in medicine. But it also created a value system in which skill in specialized research became a measure of both faculty competence and the quality of the school. By many accounts, this research-oriented value system reduced the supply of and demand for primary care training, and was a pivotal factor in the trend toward physician specialization from the 1930s to the 1960s.

According to this argument, research activity caused medical schools to introduce increasingly specialized curricula and to recruit talented and scientifically trained students capable of mastering them. It induced faculty and administrators to regard medicine as a compartmental discipline in which the physician's ability was reckoned in terms of his or her understanding of a narrow specialty area. It awarded honor and income to the research scientist, gave little prestige to the generalist, and produced graduates in the image of the faculty. Graduates were imbued with the attitude that medical practice is primarily a technological rather than comprehensive and patient-oriented profession. They learned that general and primary care practitioners held the lowest status of all physicians and that, because of their lack of specialty training, generalists were also considered the least competent of all physicians. From this perspective, research activity contributed to a perception of medical practice in which specialization and the provision of high-quality patient care were virtually equivalent professional goals. As a result, it was claimed, an increasing number of graduates were turning away from primary care and choosing careers in the specialty fields instead.

Strictly speaking, the argument is probably better thought of as a credible and widely believed hypothesis than as a rigorously documented summary of historical fact.[9] Perhaps the best testimony as to its validity is that it was accepted by educators and served as the basis for many of the curricular reforms of the late 1960s and 1970s.[10] It also motivated many of the recent federal health manpower programs directed at medical schools and designed to increase the supplies of primary care and rural and inner-city practitioners. Medical schools have moved to meet the new public demands for physician generalists, but the Flexnerian tradition is still deeply ingrained in the educational system.

THE FEDERAL BIOMEDICAL
RESEARCH PROGRAM

A signal characteristic of medical schools' financial structures since World War II has been a dependence on outside funding support. Reports of financial distress appeared as early as the late 1940s (Fein and Weber 1971), and after that time medical schools sought and received large volumes of funding from outside sources. By 1958, two-thirds of all medical school operating income was derived from outside sources. In the mid-1960s and early 1970s the fraction had risen to four-fifths, although since that time it has fallen slowly to about three-fifths (AMA 1966, 1976, 1980).

Two factors traceable to the Flexnerian tradition appear to underlie this dependence on outside funding: (1) pricing policies that subsidized medical education and patient care and (2) increasing institutional demands for modern, expensive input mixes. These factors forced medical schools to incur deficits, which led them to turn to outside funding sources. In turn, their dependence on outside income has made them both exceptionally vulnerable to changes in funding levels and sensitive to the demands of funding agencies.

In the past two decades, the largest single source of medical schools' operating income has been the federal government, and, until very recently, federal contributions were the largest single source of investment funds as well.[11] The first flow of federal funding was channeled into medical schools by the National Institutes of Health (NIH) in support of biomedical research. The total value of federally sponsored medical school research increased from $8 million in 1947–1948 to $390 million in 1967–1968, and its share in medical school income rose from 11 percent to 36 percent over the same period (Fein and Weber 1971). Even now, it represents nearly 20 percent of total medical school operating income (AMA 1980).

While most of the evidence on the impact of federal research spending on medical school policies is either descriptive or impressionistic, there is widespread agreement that federal funding greatly strengthened the priority of research. Specifically, the federal research programs furnished the means to enlarge facilities, increase faculty sizes, and expand student enrollments.[12] For medical school faculty, the opportunity to obtain research funding was an avenue to promotion, salary increases, and employment security. There seems little doubt that institutional pressures also stimulated faculty research activity.[13]

One author has characterized medical school faculty of the 1950s and 1960s as researchers employed in institutions whose foremost goals were the production of scientists and biomedical knowledge (Funkenstein 1971). This judgment may not apply to all medical schools, but much of the available evidence tends to confirm its accuracy. For instance, in a nationwide survey of medical school faculty in 1958, Cain and Bowen (1961) found that three-quarters of the members of basic science departments and two-thirds of the members of clinical departments were serving as principal investigators under federal research grants. Seventy-five percent of the basic science faculty and 41 percent of the clinical faculty spent half or more of their time on research. And among the roughly one-third of the respondents who said they were dissatisfied with their academic responsibilities, the desire to devote more time to research was unanimous.

To the extent that their faculty were successful in obtaining research grants, individual departments also became less financially dependent on the medical school. The phenomenon had a fragmenting effect on control within the school, increasing the authority of the basic sciences—the chief beneficiaries of research grants—relative to that of clinical departments (Fein and Weber 1971; Stevens 1971). Indeed, in one study of the impact of NIH funding on medical schools in the late 1960s, Williams et al. (1976) described individual departments as entrepreneurial units whose success depended on their ability to attract outside income.[14] This suggests that federal demands for biomedical research not only generated considerable amounts of research activity in medical schools, but altered the composition of outputs and modified managerial structures, or the loci of internal power, as well. However, since there have been no detailed investigations of the influence of research funding on undergraduate educational policies, any assessment of the effects must be conjectural. Nonetheless, it is reasonable to conclude that the federal biomedical research program substantially reinforced the Flexnerian tradition and helped to divert medical schools from training in primary care.

FEDERAL HEALTH MANPOWER LEGISLATION

In the late 1940s—in the face of substantial increases in the demand for medical care—constraints on the supply of new physicians resulting from the Flexnerian standards became a matter of congressional concern. It was at this time that the first proposals for federal aid to medical education appeared. The concern that there was a shortage of physicians drew increasing attention in the 1950s, and an extended debate took place over what, if anything, the government should do about it. Finally, beginning in 1963, a series of federal statutes was passed giving financial assistance to medical schools and other institutions involved in educating health professionals. Under this legislation, federal support has taken three forms:[15] (1) general operating support tied to enrollment increases and paid on a capitation (per student) basis; (2) funding for the construction of new medical schools and capacity expansion in existing schools; and (3) start-up and operating support for teaching programs in the primary care specialties.

Until 1976, the major objective of the legislation was to stimulate increases in the total enrollment of medical students. The Health Professions Educational Assistance Act of 1963 introduced a program of matching grants for medical schools' investment in new teaching capacity. A 1965 amendment to the act added two types of operating support, "basic improvement" and "special improvement" grants. The former provided general income assistance to medical schools conditional on their meeting certain minimal requirements for enrollment increases. The latter were for the purpose of upgrading curricula and facilities, and were awarded chiefly to the schools whose financial difficulties threatened loss of accreditation. The Health Manpower Act of 1968 changed the name of the special improvement grants to "special project" grants and raised the ceiling on individual awards. By fiscal 1971, 62 of the 108 medical schools then in existence were receiving special project—or so-called financial distress—grants, and they accounted for nearly 40 percent of federal operating support for undergraduate medical education (Carter et al. 1974).

The Comprehensive Health Manpower Training Act of 1971 greatly revised the structure of federal support for medical schools. Basic improvement grants were replaced by a new capitation program which substantially increased the size of awards but made them subject to stringent eligibility conditions.[16] A second capitation system was established which paid medical schools $3,000 for each graduate trainee enrolled in a three-year primary care residency, and support for primary care residency training was extended to all public and nonprofit teaching hospitals. The 1971 statute also increased the federal contribution for construction financing from 66⅔ percent to a maximum of 80 percent of the costs of a new school or a major expansion of an established school, and to a maximum of 70 percent of the costs of building other teaching facilities.[17] Funding authorization for financial distress grants was sharply reduced. Instead, the act identified several other areas where preference would be given for special projects grants. These included efforts by medical schools to increase total enrollment and shorten the M.D. curriculum; to recruit minority, low-income, and rural students; and to initiate teaching in family medicine, particularly where it involved preceptorship training.

The Health Professions Educational Assistance Act of 1976 largely continued the programs initiated by the 1971 legislation. However, it did reflect an end to concern over the general shortage of physicians, and an intensified desire to reallocate physician labor among specialties and geographic locations. It maintained undergraduate capitation grants at reduced payment rates, lowered eligibility requirements regarding enrollment increases, and installed two new conditions for participation. Enrollments had only to be kept at 1976–1977 levels, or at the levels in the years preceding grant awards. The new eligibility conditions stated that the medical school must: (1) offer minimum percentages of first-year residency positions in the primary care specialties (defined as family practice, general internal medicine, and general pediatrics) and (2) reserve an "equitable" number of third-year positions for U.S.-born students who had completed two years of study in foreign medical schools and had achieved passing scores on Part I of the examination given by the National Board of Medical Examiners. The second condition was rescinded in 1977 after 15 medical schools refused to apply for capitation support because of it.

Construction assistance was broadened to cover investment in ambulatory care facilities for primary care training, and one-half of the total appropriation for construction funding was authorized for this purpose. In addition, new special project funding was authorized to start and operate departments of family medicine, to support residency programs in general internal medicine and pediatrics, and to establish Area Health Education Centers.

The federal government's health manpower program has been accompanied by substantial changes in undergraduate medical education, most of them in the directions sought by the legislation. Only 11 medical schools were started from 1935 to 1965, but 19 new schools were established between 1965 and 1976, and another 11 schools became operational between 1976 and 1980.[18] From 1965 to 1974, the annual number of medical graduates rose by 45 percent, the number of first-year students grew by 70 percent, and the average first-year class size increased from 100 to 130 students. In the late 1960s, women represented only 9 percent of all entering medical students, but in 1970 the percentage rose to 11, and in 1979 it was 25. Similarly, minority enrollment increased from 3 percent of all students in 1969 to more than 12 percent of all students in 1979.

By 1974, one-third of all medical schools had accelerated curricula allowing students to graduate in three calendar years, and 12 were experimenting with programs granting the M.D. degree within five to seven years after high school graduation. Most schools revised their curricula to increase the exposure of students to patient care. And, in 1975, 92 schools—as opposed to only 49 in 1973—offered undergraduate courses in family medicine. After 1971, medical schools also devoted a large and rapidly growing share of their new investment to patient care facilities, and many were involved in local programs for providing community medical services.

By outward appearances, the majority of these changes can be traced to incentives created by the federal health manpower legislation. However, except for early reports of their impact on enrollment, the overall effects of these laws on medical schools have not yet been systematically studied.[19] Moreover, their influence on medical schools' behavior would be hard to isolate. Some of the changes were begun by medical educators in the 1960s in response to both self-criticism and outside social pressures—notably the rise in public demands for primary care practitioners and the civil rights movement.[20] Thus, it seems clear that the federal initiatives came at a time when medical schools were receptive to their goals and urgently seeking new sources of operating and investment funds. Moreover, in view of the decline in federal biomedical research spending and the scarcity of private funding over the past decade, it seems likely that medical schools will remain responsive to government manpower policies as long as they are linked with payment incentives.

Whether, as some observers have suggested, the innovations of the 1970s herald a revolution in medical education is another, and as yet unanswered, question. By the mid-1970s some of them were being rescinded—e.g., the three-year M.D. programs—largely, it appears, because of faculty dissatisfaction with the quality of teaching (Berman 1979; Beran 1979; Kettel et al. 1979; Trzebiatowski and Peterson 1979). In other instances—e.g., the implementation of new admissions and curricular policies to increase the outputs of primary care and rural or inner-city practitioners—medical schools' efforts seem to have peaked in the early and mid-1970s, and there has been little movement since that time (Schroeder et al. 1974; Giacalone and Hudson 1977). Within medical schools themselves, there continues to be a strong conviction that professional competence and specialization are closely intertwined. As a result, signs of resistance to the introduction or expansion of general and family medicine programs have been reported for the past decade (see, e.g., Stead 1969; Graves 1973; Mechanic 1974; Lyman 1976; Petersdorf 1975; Egger 1978; and Funkenstein 1978).

Perhaps more importantly, research expenditures constitute 60 percent of all federal operating support provided to medical schools. Influential organizations—even those advocating a larger role for medical education in solving health manpower problems—have argued on behalf of solid institutional commitments to research (AMA 1976; Carnegie Council on Policy Studies in Higher Education 1976), and research activity by medical school faculties may be rising rather than falling. For example, Giacalone and Hudson (1977) indicated that three-quarters of all medical schools employed some faculty who were exclusively or predominantly engaged in research in 1976, as opposed to less than 60 percent of the schools in 1973. Moreover, much of this research was carried on in departments of community or preventive medicine, raising the possibility that they, like specialty departments, are becoming increasingly research-oriented. Some authors have argued that the future of family practice programs hinges as much on the volume and stability of government funding as on any other single factor (e.g., Egger 1978; Geyman 1979). Without such support, they contend, the importance of teaching family medicine is likely to diminish greatly in medical schools' institutional policies. Thus, the actions of the government significantly determine the directions and scope of medical education. But neither the government nor the medical education system has yet reconciled its research goals with its priorities for training medical generalists.

DIVERSITY AMONG MEDICAL SCHOOLS AND PHYSICIANS' CAREER CHOICES

Directly or indirectly, the Flexnerian tradition and the federal biomedical research and health manpower programs have influenced the development of all medical schools. Yet the structure of medical schools, the visible aspects of their institutional policies, and the career-choice behavior of their graduates exhibit great diversity. For example, it is well known that there are systematic differences among the graduates of different types of medical schools in terms of their state locations and propensities to specialize (Theodore et al. 1967; Martin 1975). Consequently, research on physicians' specialty and location decisions has frequently sought to link them with the characteristics of medical schools.

In the absence of useful theoretical models,[21] most studies of the effects of medical schools on their graduates' career choices tend to be descriptive.[22] Their approach consists of identifying the structure of the institution, specifying (or conjecturing) its objectives and policies, and linking those objectives and policies with graduates' career choices. Implicit are the assumptions that the structure of the school limits the range of policies open to its administrators, and that the school's policies influence the career-choice behavior of graduates.

The principal types of institutional policies thought to affect the distributions of medical school graduates among specialties and practice locations relate to admissions, teaching, and research. Since policies are not typically observable, a common procedure is to correlate graduates' career choices with policy proxies. Basically, the proxies employed are structural characteristics of the school and such visible *outcomes* of policy decisions as student and faculty attributes, research expenditures, and school size. Inevitably, of course, this procedure leads to disagreement over the interpretation of findings because one cannot be entirely sure that the proxies are accurate or that the associations between them and career choices reflect causal patterns of medical school behavior.[23]

Two major hypotheses—one having to do with structure and one bearing on school policy—have emerged from studies of the effect of the medical school attended on physicians' career choices. The first is that public schools graduate larger percentages of physician generalists and in-state practitioners than do privately owned schools. The second is that the level of the school's research orientation is inversely related to its output of physician generalists. The ownership hypothesis—which is supported by a variety of descriptive evidence[24]—is based on the notion that state legislatures use legal and budgetary controls on public schools to promote policies for maintaining or enlarging in-state supplies of primary care physicians. Conversely, private ownership is taken to imply weaker institutional motivations for producing either primary care or in-state physicians. The second, and less well specified, hypothesis is based on the belief that research activity and specialized teaching are complementary medical school outputs.

Both hypotheses have proved to be difficult to verify. The research orientation of a medical school's educational program is at best hard to quantify, and the ownership hypothesis is complicated by the diversity of other external and internal controls on institutional behavior.

Fein and Weber (1971) have reported wide variations in the amounts and forms of state support for public schools. Accordingly, if the ownership hypothesis is correct, their findings imply a good deal of variability in the degree of state control. Moreover, a number of states provide operating or special-program support to private schools (Fein and Weber 1971; AAMC 1975; Crowley 1975a, 1975b), so that legislative controls affect private as well as public institutions. And some schools participate in regional programs to train students from other states.

Even the ownership characteristics of private medical schools are by no means uniform. A handful of private institutions are unaffiliated with universities and freestanding. Some have religious affiliations, the implications of which have not been adequately studied. Historically, the prestigious private medical schools have been the wealthiest. Many of the freestanding or religious private schools have ranked among the poorest, and have been most dependent on revenue from student tuition (Fein and Weber 1971).

A few private schools were organized with special educational missions. Two, Howard and Meharry, were established to train black physicians, and as late as 1970 they admitted one-half of all black medical students in the U.S. (Johnson et al. 1975). The Medical College of Pennsylvania was organized specifically to train women physicians, and has admitted male applicants only since 1970. Loma Linda, the only medical school owned by the Seventh-day Adventist Church, produces one of the largest percentages of general practitioners of all U.S. institutions (Martin 1975).

Medical schools regard themselves as organizations whose first responsibilities are to the public, but it is not always clear how they perceive their social obligations or how those perceptions affect their educational policies. The market conditions facing medical schools further complicate analyses of their behavior. For example, we know little about how the effects of the Flexnerian tradition and the federal biomedical research and health manpower programs have been distributed among institutions. Nor do we know the degree to which competition among schools influences tuition, admissions, faculty recruitment, and other educational policies.

As is true of education in general, medical schools are constrained by a number of rules—chiefly those associated with accreditation of undergraduate and graduate teaching programs by the Liaison Committee on Medical Education (LCME).[25] The undergraduate review committees have considerable potential power, since the denial of accreditation can force closure of the school. They compel schools to meet minimum standards with respect to the quality and scope of their teaching, and to incur the concomitant costs. But it is not clear how often or how strongly they have exerted their power over educational policies. Thus, we do not know what role they may have played in the financial difficulties of the poorer schools.

Several attempts have been made to develop a medical school typology. In one, Fein and Weber (1971) constructed cross-tabulations of mid-1960s data on a number of medical school attributes. Their findings indicated that: (1) private schools tended to be somewhat wealthier and more research-oriented than public schools, (2) they admitted students with higher MCAT scores,[26] and (3) they produced considerably smaller percentages of general practitioners. However, the tabulations also showed wide variations among schools in terms of affluence, faculty research activity, student ability, and the percentage of graduates entering general practice within each ownership class. Furthermore, they showed that research orientation, student ability, and the percentage of graduates choosing specialty practice all increase with school affluence regardless of the type of ownership. Thus, ownership, affluence, faculty research activity, and student ability were interrelated characteristics, and each could be used as an independent predictor of graduates' specialty choices.

Morgan and Jones (1976) constructed a measure of institutional research orientation,[27] and cross-tabulated it against budgetary, enrollment, and faculty-size data on 86 medical schools for 1964–74. Many of their results are similar to those reported by Fein and Weber. Specifically, they found that schools with the highest research orientation had much the highest operating budgets, were the most dependent on federal research income, and were the least dependent on state and local government income. Their tabulations showed no strong association between research orientation and the number of students, but they did indicate that the numbers of faculty, basic science faculty, and interns and residents were all largest in the most research-oriented schools.[28]

Morgan and Jones found no discernible relationship between school research orientation and the percentage of graduates entering patient care practice, but they did not examine the distribution of graduates among patient care specialties. They did find, predictably, that the most research-oriented schools produced the largest percentages of academic physicians.

Four other studies (Richards et al. 1968; Rodgers and Elton 1974; Otis et al. 1975; McShane 1977) factor-analyzed large numbers of medical school variables including student or graduate characteristics (e.g., MCAT scores and specialty board certification rates, ownership indicators, admissions criteria, curricula, the volumes and sources of income, and the sizes of undergraduate and graduate programs). Richards et al. and Rodgers and Elton both obtained three factors they described as representing private and public ownership traits, undergraduate class size, and the size of graduate programs.[29]

Using a much larger set of variables than either of these studies, Otis et al. found five factors which they interpreted as the school's "eminence," size, curricular orientation toward clerkship or basic science training, emphasis on course electives, and dependence on service or research funding. Applying a cluster analysis to the factor scores, they then derived 10 different groupings of schools which appeared to fall into three distinct classes: one consisting of new institutions, another composed of two groupings of older institutions with high eminence scores, and a third made up of older institutions with average or below-average eminence scores.

Matching their classification of older schools against the 1960–64 specialty distributions of graduates, Otis et al. showed that the two groups of "eminent" schools produced by far the smallest percentages of general practitioners and the largest percentages of internists, pediatricians, general surgeons, faculty, and researchers. School size, curricular variation, clerkship orientation, and funding sources were weakly or negligibly related to the specialty distribution of graduates.

Most of the variables that Otis et al. found to be strongly correlated with their eminence factor were described by Fein and Weber as correlated with the school's affluence. Among the variables positively correlated with that factor were student scores on the science portion of the MCAT, the specialty board certification rates of graduates, total expenditures and training support per student, research income per faculty member, the faculty-student ratio, and a measure of school affluence. In addition Otis et al. noted that 18 of the 24 schools in the two eminent groups were privately owned. Finally, although their eminence factor does not seem to be a pure surrogate for research orientation, one of the two eminent groups contained all five of the most research-oriented medical schools according to an index published in the mid-1970s by the AAMC (1975b).[30]

McShane's study was very similar to that by Otis et al. He derived eight clusters of medical schools which, in general, reflect the dimensions of institutional structure found by other authors. McShane made no attempt to relate his dimensions of institutional structure to the specialty distributions of the schools' graduates, but he did indicate that the smallest percentages of general practitioners were produced by schools with large graduate education programs, by new schools, and by those with large volumes of sponsored research.

The results of these various studies suggest certain generalizations. First, the medical school characteristics most strongly associated with variation in the specialty distributions of graduates are prestige, affluence, ownership, research orientation, and funding sources. Second, it is evident that these institutional characteristics are highly interdependent, so that it is difficult to select any particular one of them and claim that it alone best "explains" the specialty distribution of graduates.[31] Third, there are some indications that the schools that produce large percentages of specialists admit disproportionately many students whose abilities (as measured by high MCAT scores, for example) make them likely to become specialists, while the reverse is true for schools which produce small percentages of specialists.

These results are consistent with the two major hypotheses that underlie studies of the relationships between physicians' specialty choices and their medical school backgrounds. The first holds that medical schools influence the specialty distributions of their graduates through the process of admissions filtering. That is, even though a particular school may have little formal interest in the specialties its graduates choose, it tends to attract and admit students with certain configurations of abilities and personality traits. These, in turn, tend to be associated with actual or latent specialty preferences, with the result that the school heavily influences—albeit indirectly—the specialty distribution of its graduates. The second major hypothesis holds that the teaching environment shapes students' specialty preferences through its value system, the role models it provides, and other direct or indirect effects that it exercises on students. The two hypotheses are perhaps more complementary than competitive, but most authorities stress one or the other. We consider them in more detail in the next two sections.

THE INFLUENCE OF ADMISSIONS POLICIES ON SPECIALTY CHOICE

Because medical schools typically set their tuition rates well below market-clearing levels, each school faces a large excess demand for its first-year positions.[32] First-year places are then rationed to applicants according to five basic admissions criteria: (1) performance on the MCAT;

(2) undergraduate overall and science grade-point averages (GPAs); (3) performance in a personal interview with the admissions committee; (4) age; and (5) state of residence. Nearly all schools employ the first four, but the last is used almost exclusively by public institutions.[33]

Admitted applicants are typically those with the highest MCAT scores and GPAs, and most schools either discourage or refuse applications from candidates older than their late twenties.[34] Nearly all private schools charge the same tuition to in-state and out-of-state students, and in most cases there is little reason to believe that their admissions policies discriminate against out-of-state applicants.[35] Conversely, public schools' tuition rates and residency requirements are usually set by state legislatures and discriminate strongly against out-of-state applicants. Public schools' tuition rates for out-of-state residents are typically two to three times higher than those for in-state students, and only a small percentage of first-year places are allocated to nonresident entrants.[36]

The overt implication of the academic admissions criteria is that medical schools prefer and accept the most capable, academically proven, and competitive applicants.[37] The growth of the total applicant pool has almost certainly accentuated the trend, and—although longitudinal comparisons of test scores and grade-point averages may be misleading—the average MCAT scores and undergraduate GPAs of entering medical students have risen steadily over the past two decades.[38] Most entrants are educated in the more prestigious undergraduate colleges and universities, and the vast majority take undergraduate majors in the biological or physical sciences (AMA 1967, 1974; Crowley 1975a).

Descriptive evidence as to the impact of admissions screening on the distribution of students' other background traits is ambiguous. For example, Johnson et al. (1975) found that students admitted to medical schools in 1972 were more likely than the average applicant to come from the highest-income and best-educated families. However, they reported that the distributions of parental income, educational attainment, and occupational status were nearly identical for admitted students and applicants as a whole. In a study of applicants and admitted students in 1976, Waldman (1977) showed that applicants from high-income families (above $10,000 per year) had higher MCAT scores and undergraduate GPAs than those from low-income families. Although family income is not known to have a direct influence on admission, this suggests that the weight given to MCAT scores and GPAs discriminates against low-income applicants, and Waldman indicated that this is probably so. His data show that 41 percent of the white applicants from high-income families, but only 31 percent of the white applicants from low-income families, were admitted into medical schools in 1976.

Cullison et al. (1976b) also reported that medical school admissions policies do not appreciably alter the overall rural-urban distribution of applicants' hometown locations. Specifically, they divided hometown locations into three county groupings—large metropolitan, small metropolitan, and nonmetropolitan—and found essentially the same percentages of 1973 applicants and admitted students residing in each grouping.[39]

On the basis of historical enrollment patterns, a prima facie case can be made that medical schools formerly discriminated against women and nonwhite minorities. The objections to women are said to have arisen from antifeminist attitudes and the belief that women were more likely than men to end their academic or professional careers after marriage and childbirth (see, e.g., Bowers 1968; Lopate 1968; Kaplan 1971; Morgan 1971; and Notman and Nadelson 1973). Nevertheless, the indications since 1970 are that medical schools have not discriminated against women (Fruen et al. 1974) and have actively recruited minority students.[40]

No study has shown whether admissions criteria discriminate according to applicants' personality characteristics. However, it has been reasonably well documented that student performance in medical school is correlated with certain personality traits. The most able students tend to score high on psychological tests of the need for achievement and social recognition, self-reliance, and self-discipline.[41] In short, the profile of the "best" medical student—competitive, forceful, and self-assured—conforms roughly with the personality stereotype admissions committees have been said to prefer. Even so, it is not clear that admissions committees are capable of identifying preferred personality traits.[42] Indeed, most of the evidence indicates that admissions committees are not strikingly successful in selecting high academic performers.[43]

A number of studies have found systematic and apparently stable differences between the background traits of students in public and private schools. We have already observed that average MCAT scores are lower in public than in private schools, and other differences in students' traits appear as well. Lyden et al. (1968), Smith and Crocker (1970), and the U.S. Department of Health, Education, and Welfare (1974) have shown that relative to private medical school students, public school students are: (1) somewhat more likely to be married; (2) more likely to be married with children; (3) less likely to come from the highest-income and best-educated families; (4) slightly more likely to have lived in small, rural communities; and (5) much less likely to have lived in large cities. In addition, public school students incur lower average annual expenses than private school students of the same marital status.

The different student mixes of private and public schools could have at least two explanations. One is that the applicant pools differ substantially—i.e., demands for positions in the two types of schools are not homogeneous. As shown above, for example, school attributes such as prestige and research orientation vary with ownership. Since such attributes are related to the school's attractiveness to medical students, they may lead to systematic differences in applicant pools. On the other hand, it is also possible that differences in admissions policies account for the observed differences in student background traits. Unfortunately, the relative importance of student self-selection and admissions screening cannot be determined on the basis of existing evidence.[44] There are, however, several reasons for believing that observed patterns of student traits are more the result of admissions policies—if not necessarily admissions screening—than a systematic segmentation of applicant demands.

First, the chronic excess demand for positions gives medical schools a large range of choice as to which students to accept. Second, the discriminatory policies of public schools toward out-of-state applicants restrict the sizes of their applicant pools relative to those of private schools. In 1974, for example, the mean number of applicants per first-year place was 15.5 in public schools and 32.7 in private schools (Dube and Johnson 1975). Public schools' admissions policies consequently limit the number of academically superior applicants.[45] Third, since public medical schools are less concentrated in urban states than private schools, the preferential treatment they give in-state applicants may explain why they have proportionately fewer applicants with urban backgrounds. Finally, the comparatively low in-state tuitions charged by public schools may indicate why lower-income and married applicants are more attracted to them than to private schools.

Several other hypotheses are suggested by the relations between physicians' background traits and career choices described in Chapter 3. One is that admissions policies have had the effect of discriminating against potential general practitioners, and perhaps against other primary care generalists as well. In particular, the characteristics of general practitioners—average or below-average MCAT scores and college GPAs, and especially their relatively high age—are not favored by admissions committees.

Whether they are the result of admissions discrimination or not, the historically low enrollment rates of women have depressed the supply of pediatricians, but have probably enlarged the supplies of general practitioners. Likewise, the historically low enrollments of blacks and other minority applicants have restricted the supplies of physicians to the black and minority populations. Recent increases in admissions of women and minority applicants should reverse both of these trends. In the same vein, the recent growth of public medical schools—which tend to admit larger percentages of the less academically qualified, older, and nonmetropolitan applicants than private schools—should mean an increase in both the absolute and relative numbers of potential primary care and nonmetropolitan practitioners.

The MCAT and its predecessor tests were designed to identify applicants with high risks of dropping out of school or repeating classes (Sanazaro and Hutchins 1963).[47] Indeed, a case can be made that all of the basic admissions criteria except for state residency requirements are for the same purpose. Medical schools' desires to control the risk of dropouts and repeaters stem from two interrelated factors: (1) the conviction that precious social resources are wasted on students who fail to graduate on time,[48] and (2) the high, quasi-fixed costs of medical school training. By far the largest part of total training costs is the combination of salary and capital expenses. As a result, short-run marginal costs are probably close to zero over large ranges of output below maximum student capacity.[49] This means the loss of each student in the first or second year—the years in which the great majority of dropouts occur—reduces school revenue by the amount of the student's forgone tuition over the remaining two to three years with little if any reduction in total training costs. Given the financial difficulties medical schools have faced in the past 30 years, the expected costs of dropouts must provide substantial incentive to control attrition rates. And the federal capitation grants paid to medical schools since 1971 have reinforced this incentive.

A few studies of individual medical schools have cast doubt on the ability of the academic criteria—especially MCAT scores—to distinguish between graduates and dropouts (Garfield and Wolpin 1961; Geertsma and Chapman 1966; Bartlett 1967). But the most comprehensive analysis of student attrition yet conducted (Johnson and Hutchins 1966) concluded that all of the common standards do discriminate between them with a reasonably high degree of accuracy. In that analysis, Johnson and Hutchins reviewed data on 28 medical schools from 1949 to 1958 and found that: (1) academic and nonacademic dropouts had significantly lower MCAT Scores and college GPAs than graduates;[50] (2) the likelihood of dropping out increased with the student's age at matriculation, and markedly so at ages over 30; (3) the rates of attrition were two to three times higher among students from the lower-rated undergraduate colleges than among students from the major universities; and (4) the dropout rates for women were approximately twice as high as the rates for men.

In a study of 10 classes at the Colorado School of Medicine, Conger and Fitz (1963) showed that MCAT scores, undergraduate GPAs, and interview ratings were more reliable predictors of dropout probabilities when used in combination than when employed individually. Hence, their results support the hypothesis that medical schools historically preferred young, high-performing, male applicants who displayed "dedication," emotional stability, and good health because they were most likely to complete the medical curriculum.

The points raised in this section can be briefly summarized. First, most of the basic admissions criteria were devised—and are probably still used—to control the costs of dropouts. Little evidence indicates that they are meant to select high medical school performers as such or to regulate the specialty composition of graduates. Second, in the aggregate, admissions policies favor young applicants, possibly those from the upper income classes (insofar as family income is positively related to MCAT scores and GPAs), and, in the past decade, women and minorities as well. There are also substantial differences between the student mixes of public and private schools due, at least in part, to differing admissions policies toward in-state and out-of-state applicants. Third, there is reason to believe that academic and age standards discriminate against certain types of potential primary care practitioners. Thus, however incidental their effects are to their purpose, admissions policies bring into medical schools students with background traits known to be related to specialty choices.

THE INFLUENCE OF THE MEDICAL SCHOOL ENVIRONMENT ON SPECIALTY CHOICE

Sanazaro (1965) has described undergraduate medical education as a "black box" which transforms inputs of students into outputs of graduates. In the course of this poorly understood process, many influences may act on the students' specialty-choice decisions—from faculty attitudes and the charisma of certain teachers to the information students acquire about the choice of alternatives. Researchers have taken two somewhat different approaches in exploring them. One group has concentrated on the development of student attitudes and preferences during medical school, implicitly assuming that medical education affects physicians' perceptions of the profession in certain systematic ways. The second has sought to correlate observed specialty choices with medical school characteristics, postulating that different types of medical schools affect the decisions in different ways.

Numerous investigators have reported that students' cynicism increases markedly during medical school.[51] Typically, students begin medical school eager for patient contact and believing they will be trained for humanitarian service. But the educational process involves two years of initial course work in the sciences, which students view as having minimal connections with patient care. Moreover, this work demands long hours of study, stresses memorization, defines success chiefly in terms of grades and faculty approval, and is often a profound source of disillusionment.[52] Not atypically, students describe themselves as overwhelmed by how much there is to know about medicine and how little of it they can reasonably expect to grasp. As a consequence of this kind of experience, students' humanitarian motives, their perceptions of medicine as a patient-oriented profession,[53] and their self-confidence in treating patients all decline during medical school. Thus, the educational process itself may be an important factor accounting for the shifts in preferences toward specialization that were discussed in Chapter 1.[54]

Among the institutional forces acting on medical students' specialty preferences, three—curricula, faculty influence, and medical student culture—have received the most attention. Several studies indicate that such curricular features as all-elective years, clerkships, and courses in family medicine do influence students' immediate specialty preferences. Even so, there is considerable doubt as to whether the changes are permanent.[55] The results, although mixed, generally support the conclusion by Otis et al. (1975) that curriculum content is not a major determinant of specialty selection.

Medical school faculty influence students' career choices by providing subjective or objective information on alternative specialties, counseling, and serving as specialty role models. But medical schools themselves seldom make substantial efforts to influence or assist in students' specialty decisions. For example, Zimny and Senturia (1974) found that only 24 of the 76 schools they surveyed in 1971–72 had organized counseling procedures. The remaining schools relied on informal devices such as elective course work, meetings describing internship and residency alternatives, and student-initiated contact with faculty members. Many of the respondents questioned the effectiveness of formal career counseling and the ability of the school to provide it. They cited such problems as the difficulties of finding suitable advisors, lack of faculty time, and the belief that most students have no need for specialty counseling.

The low priority that most medical schools give to specialty counseling contrasts with the importance of faculty influence as reported by students. In an early study by Coker et al. (1960), 54 percent of a sample of nearly 2,700 students at eight medical schools claimed that the faculty had influenced their specialty plans to some degree. Faculty members who were rated as having the most influence were also regarded as the best teachers, and were most often consulted by students for advice on personal problems. Interestingly, the findings also raise doubts about the validity of role modeling as a critical factor in specialty decisions. For example, Coker et al. found little tendency for students to share the professional attitudes of influential faculty. In addition, they observed that sizable percentages of students did not plan to enter the specialties of the faculty for whom they had the highest regard.

Some more recent results also tend to undermine the role-model theory, and, more generally, the notion that faculty have a crucial effect on students' specialty preferences. Funkenstein (1978) reported that only 10 percent of the medical students at Harvard in the mid-1970s professed to have faculty role models. He observed that students' specialty choices were mostly determined by social and economic conditions outside the university environment. According to Eagleson and Tobolic (1978), 1976 graduates of Wayne State University who went on to family practice residencies rated faculty influence as the least important factor in their specialty decisions. Similarly, Cauthen et al. (1980) found that only 10 percent of the 1977 graduates of the University of Texas Health Center at San Antonio described faculty influence as a major factor in their specialty choices. Curiously, Cauthen et al. indicated that experience in clinical courses was the most influential factor shaping students' choices, while Eagleson and Tobolic found that it was of only minor importance.

These results conflict with the remaining evidence on the role-model hypothesis. Indeed, it is possible that the significance of role modeling in specialty decisions varies both between schools and over time. Becker et al. (1961) and Bloom (1971) reported that medical students at the University of Kansas and the State University of New York at Brooklyn tended to assume the same attitudes as their faculties toward patient care and research, even though they felt that the faculty treated them as outsiders and a burden. According to Becker et al., students at Kansas selected rotating internships—the traditional path into general practice—primarily because the faculty placed high value on a well-rounded background for patient care. Likewise, Lyden et al. (1968) found that public medical school graduates were much less likely than private school graduates to take residency training and to be encouraged by faculty to do so.

The effects of faculty role models were also examined by Weil et al. (1981) and Weil and Schleiter (1981) in their work on residents in internal medicine. Both found that having a medical school faculty role model was a highly important predictor of the residents' interests in a subspecialty career as opposed to general medicine. However, Weil et al., like Funkenstein (1978), reported that the substantive content of the field was the most important factor in the choice of a career path. Weil and Schleiter drew no conclusions at all. Thus, the results may show that an expression of faculty interest in a student contributes to the student's interest in specializing, but they could also indicate that students with specialty interests are those who are most likely to choose role models from the medical school faculty.

Several studies have sought to correlate medical school graduates' specialty or internship choices with proxies for faculty influence. For example, Perlstadt (1972) regressed the percentage of 1966 graduates entering rotating internships from each school in his sample on five "influence" variables. The strongest predictor was a dummy variable indicating school affiliation with a private, nonsectarian hospital.[56] Perlstadt found a negative coefficient on the variable and suggested that the result was due to the heavy staffing of such hospitals by specialists who influence medical students to choose specialized graduate training. Whether his inference is valid is, of course, conjectural.

Sociological case studies (e.g., Becker et al. 1961) have implied that student cultures in medical school may also affect specialty choices. However, the only statistical investigation of this was done by Anderson (1975). Using stepwise discriminant analysis, he estimated a six-way classification of graduates' specialty choices at an unnamed southern medical school, and concluded that measures of social behavior in medical school were the strongest predictor variables. Among the 58 variables that entered into the discriminant function, three of the first four were the amount of the graduate's leisure time in medical school, a measure of his or her difficulty in making friends, and an indicator of the importance he or she attached to student interpersonal contact. The first of these variables tended to group general practitioners and academic physicians apart from other graduates. The second separated out general practitioners, and the third tended to identify internists.[57] It seems evident, though, that Anderson's proxies for "social behavior" are also proxies for personality traits. As a consequence, it is questionable whether his results really show that student culture exercises a significant influence over specialty choice, since the relationships he observed may have been due to personality traits.

Other efforts to estimate the effects of the medical school on specialty choice fall largely into the "black-box" category. That is, they seek to establish correlations between graduates' specialty choices and a variety of structural and policy characteristics of medical schools (e.g., ownership and research orientation) without developing hypotheses regarding the causes of specialty choices.

For example, Yett et al. (1973) regressed the percentages of 1960-64 graduates entering each of four specialty fields (general practice, medical specialties, surgical specialties, and other specialties) on the percentage of women among graduates and dummy indicators of school ownership, religious affiliation, university affiliation, rural location, and a predominantly black student body. They found that the only significant predictor of specialty choice was ownership, with public schools producing larger percentages of general practitioners than private schools.[58]

Using data on 1960 graduates, Hadley (1975, 1977, 1979) estimated a group of linear regressions in which the dependent variables were the probabilities of individuals' choosing each of five to nine specialty fields.[59] He reported that all variables describing the structure and policies of the medical school—including ownership, mean student MCAT scores, percentage of out-of-state students, faculty-student ratios, and research expenditures per faculty member—were either statistically non-significant or else entered the regressions with implausible signs.

Williams et al. (1976) employed stepwise discriminant analysis on a sample of 1965, 1969, and 1972 graduates of 10 medical schools to derive a four-way classification. of specialty choices (internal medicine, other primary care specialties, surgical specialties, and all other specialties). Their predictor variables included individual background traits such as age and sex, MCAT scores, medical school GPAs, a selectivity index for undergraduate college, and a group of federal funding variables. According to their findings, the most significant predictors were sex and class ranking. The amounts of total federal funding for internal medicine and primary care departments were also sigificant, but research funding variables were not.

Hay (1980, 1981) used a logit probability model to predict the specialty choices of a large sample of physicians who were in active practice during 1970. He defined three specialty categories—general practice, internal medicine, and other specialties—and specified two medical school characteristics—type of ownership and a measure of the school's research orientation—as predictors of the choice probabilities. Essentially, his results showed that general practitioners were significantly more likely than other physicians to have graduated from publicly owned and non-research-oriented schools, and that internists were significantly more likely than other physicians to have graduated from private schools.

It is not easy to draw firm conclusions from these disparate sets of findings. On the one hand, the theory of professional socialization argues that physicians' attitudes and preferences toward specialties are strongly conditioned by the medical school environment. The theory is plausible, and a great deal of case study evidence shows that physicians' attitudes toward *medicine and medical care* are greatly influenced by their experiences during medical school.[60] However, little research has been performed on the relationships between specialty choices and aspects of the medical school environment when other factors such as students' personality and background traits are held constant. Consequently, there is no large or consistent body of evidence demonstrating that the medical school environment per se has any significant impact on students' specialty preferences. This is not to say that no such evidence can be adduced, but to date it has not been brought forward.

Another type of anomaly arises from the findings of the "blackbox" studies, where specialty choices are merely correlated with medical school characteristics. Studies that use the medical school as the analytic unit typically find associations between the specialty distributions of graduates and certain institutional characteristics. For the most part, these results indicate that the percentage of general practitioners falls as the school's research orientation rises, and that the percentage is lower in private schools than in public schools. Yet the few studies which use the individual physician as the analytic unit report that specialty choices are at best weakly related to institutional characteristics after the individual's background traits are taken into account.

These findings suggest three tentative conclusions regarding the observed associations between medical school attributes and physicians' specialty choices. First, it is arguable that learning environments have a far less important impact on specialty preferences than admissions filtering and admissions policies. A school's research orientation, prestige, wealth, size, and ownership undoubtedly describe its learning environment. But these same attributes also define the types of students the school attracts, and those whom it prefers and admits. In Chapters 2 and 3 we showed that many individual background and personality traits appear to be significantly related to specialty choices. Insofar as these traits are linked, directly or indirectly, with students' choices of medical schools and the schools' choices of students, we can infer that the admissions process tends to select applicants with latent or preestablished specialty preferences. This alone may be sufficient to explain why the specialty distribution of graduates differs across medical schools. Conversely, the evidence we now have on the influence of the learning environment consists chiefly of reasonable hypotheses rather than operational mechanisms by which specialty choices can be predicted. Until specialty choices can be reliably forecasted given a knowledge of the learning environment, we must have reservations about the utility of the environmental theories.

Second, there has been a distinct historical tendency for graduates of medical schools that are clinically oriented to enter general practice. On the basis of what has just been said, this tendency is probably due largely to admissions filtering and self-selection. Applicants have some prior knowledge of medical schools' teaching policies, if only through the schools' reputations. Hence, it is reasonable to believe that potential generalists prefer institutions whose teaching structures are relatively non-research-oriented. Similarly, admissions policies in clinically oriented schools ordinarily place less emphasis on applicants' scholastic abilities than do those of the more research-oriented schools. This has also undoubtedly favored the matriculation of future general practitioners in clinically oriented institutions.

Third, there is little evidence that medical school characteristics are correlated with specialty distributions except for the distribution between general practice and the specialties. Therefore, it is not clear whether the schools' admissions and teaching policies systematically favor or oppose choices of the primary care specialties other than in this one respect. To the extent that potential generalists are attracted to less research-oriented schools, these schools may produce disproportionately large numbers of primary care physicians. But, in the absence of better supporting evidence, this conclusion must be viewed as a speculation.

THE INFLUENCE OF THE MEDICAL SCHOOL ON PRACTICE LOCATION CHOICE

Research on the influence of medical schools on their graduates' practice locations has centered on two interrelated factors: (1) school ownership and (2) the school as a source of prior contact with the area of practice. It has long been known that larger percentages of public school graduates than private school graduates become in-state practitioners (Weiskotten et al. 1960; Theodore et al. 1967; Martin 1975). However, this quite likely reflects the fact that public schools admit considerably larger percentages of in-state students than private schools. That is, on the average public school graduates have more in-state contact than private school graduates, are initially less mobile geographically, or both, and these characteristics lead them to settle in the state. This hypothesis is supported by existing evidence.

For example, Fein and Weber (1971) estimated that in-state medical school entrants in the 1950s were more than three times as likely as out-of-state entrants to become practitioners in the state where they attended medical school. On this basis, they concluded that the graduate's state of origin is a much more important predictor of the state of practice than is the state location of the medical school.

Even more persuasive findings were reported by Yett and Sloan (1974). Their tabulations showed that only 11 percent of general practitioners and 2 percent of all other physicians who entered practice in 1966 did so in states where their previous contact had been confined to attending medical school. Conversely, 60 percent of general practitioners and 29 percent of other physicians began practice in states where their previous contact consisted of birth and medical school. Taken together, these results strongly suggest that the differential retention rates of public and private medical schools are explained by the admissions policies of the former, which favor in-state applicants.

The same issue was also addressed by Hadley (1975) in his analysis of the practice location choices of 1960 medical school graduates. Using regression methods, Hadley estimated the conditional probability of a physician's locating in a state given that his or her prior educational contact with the state consisted only of attending medical school there. Along with predictors standardizing for the effects of other locational influences, including state of birth and upbringing, he specified three medical school variables in the regressions: an ownership dummy, the average school MCAT score, and the percentage of out-of-state students admitted. As a group, the medical school variables were not significantly correlated with the retention probability. But, like the results of Yett and Sloan, Hadley's regressions indicate that birth or upbringing in a state significantly increases the likelihood of retention.[61]

The relationships between medical school location and the urban-rural aspect of the physician's practice location decision have been explored in a number of studies, all of which used variants of the prior-contact hypothesis. Breisch (1970) reported a significant tendency for graduates of "high-quality" and urban schools to practice in urban areas. He regressed the percentage of a school's graduates up to 1966 who practiced in Standard Metropolitan Statistical Areas (SMSAs) on the school's expenditures per student (a proxy for quality) and the population of the county in which the school was located. Both variables were significantly positively correlated with the percentage of graduates who located in SMSAs. Breisch attributed these findings to: (1) the propensity of physicians from high-quality schools to locate in urban areas where sophisticated medical facilities and support are available; and (2) the propensity of all physicians to locate in communities like those in which their medical schools are located. Although his results are consistent with these interpretations, they are weakened by the failure to standardize for certain key characteristics—notably specialty composition and individual background traits (e.g., the location of upbringing).[62]

Most medical schools also provide another type of area contact to students through their preceptorship programs. Under these programs, students spend two weeks or more working as apprentices to physicians practicing outside the medical school. The first such programs were begun in the 1920s, but most were established in the 1970s with funding provided by the Comprehensive Health Manpower Training Act of 1971. Many programs either allow or require the student to serve in a rural community, the thesis being that contact with a rural practice or community favorably disposes the student to select a rural practice location. The evidence as to the effects of this brief form of prior contact on practice location decisions is mixed, but most results indicate that the preceptorship has only a minor influence on location choices. We discuss the specific findings concerning preceptorships and location decisions in Chapter 8.

On balance, the state of knowledge concerning undergraduate medical education and physicians' practice location choices is still tentative. The major implication is that the medical school affects the geographic distribution of physicians through its admissions policies. Publicly owned schools that admit large percentages of in-state applicants typically exhibit much higher graduate retention rates than privately owned schools that admit large percentages of out-of-state applicants. The school itself is a source of state contact for future practitioners, but the pattern suggests that the combination of in-state upbringing and medical school contact has a considerably stronger attachment effect than medical school contact alone.[63]

It is not clear whether medical school environments significantly shape physicians' preferences for urban or rural practice communities. Many researchers have inferred that an educational system that teaches the sophisticated medical management of patients in an urban hospital setting is likely to increase graduates' preferences for urban practice. But it can also be argued that the medical school environment is not a critical factor in locational decision making since it represents only part of the physician's total educational experience. These competing hypotheses remain to be rigorously tested.

SUMMARY

The current structure of undergraduate medical education contains elements militating both for and against the supply of primary care training. One is the Flexnerian tradition, in which the foremost educational objective is the production of physicians of high quality, where quality is defined as the depth of the physician's knowledge of a specialty field. The other is the mixture of federal programs and public pressures introduced in the 1970s to increase the production of primary care practitioners. Through its support of research, larger enrollments, and primary care training, the federal government has been the largest overall source of medical schools' incomes. In that capacity, it has been both a major force perpetuating the Flexnerian tradition and the principal agent promoting physician manpower policies that are in fundamental conflict with that tradition. Throughout most of the 1970s, critics charged that the medical education system failed to supply physician generalists in the numbers society needed. If that claim is true, then a significant cause of the failure is the volume of federal support for medical school research over the past generation. Medical schools themselves have competing institutional goals of producing generalists and specialists, and these were matched by the competing payment incentives of federal funding programs.

Two hypotheses have been advanced to account for the influence of medical schools on the specialty and practice location distributions of their graduates. The first is that admissions policies and self-selection of medical schools by students generate distributions of student attributes which cause the observed patterns. The second is that medical school learning environments cause these patterns. The evidence on the first is indirect, consisting chiefly of findings that: (1) physicians' career choices are linked with their background and personality traits, and (2) configurations of these traits appear to vary with medical school characteristics. The evidence on the second, which has been applied mostly to specialty preferences, is mixed, and little of it has been oriented toward predicting physicians' career choices. Both hypotheses are probably true to some extent, but it is our feeling that the first provides the more powerful instrument for prediction. We believe that its policy implications—namely, the possibility of influencing specialty and location distributions by modifying admissions criteria—are stronger as well.

The principal admissions criteria are academic achievement, age, and residency status. The ostensible purpose of the academic and age standards is to control the risk of dropouts and accompanying institutional losses, but their probable indirect effect has been to limit the numbers of potential physician generalists in the medical education system. Residency requirements imposed by public schools lead to the production of graduates with relatively high levels of in-state contact, and it appears that they are largely responsible for the high rates of in-state retention of public school graduates. There are indications that public schools may admit larger proportions of rural students than private schools, so that admissions filtering or applicant self-selection may also affect the urban-rural distribution of public and private school graduates.

Because many of the underlying issues have not yet been resolved, it is prudent to regard these conclusions with caution. At least three different areas merit further investigation before the effects of undergraduate medical education on physicians' career choices can be considered well understood.

The first is the relationship between the medical school's characteristics and its output of primary care practitioners. The prevailing view that emphasizing research and specialty training reduces outputs of primary care physicians is based chiefly on statistical results concerning the percentages of general practitioners among graduates. However, the number of graduates in general (or family) practice may not be an accurate proxy for a school's output of primary care physicians, and there are few indications that a school's emphasis on research and specialty training is a successful predictor of specialty composition among the remaining fields. Beyond that, recent evidence suggests that a considerable amount of primary care is provided by physicians who are nominally referral specialists (Wechsler et al. 1978; Aiken et al. 1979). Thus, the observed specialty composition of a school's graduates is not necessarily an accurate indicator of its output of physicians who do, in fact, provide primary (or referral) care. Although it is clearly a difficult undertaking, studies of career choices based on actual patterns of patient care provided, rather than on nominal specialties, would improve our understanding of the ways that medical schools affect the content of their graduates' medical practices.

Second, we lack empirically tested models of how admissions filtering alters the distribution of latent career preferences in applicant pools, and how the career preferences of admitted students are further changed by the educational process. Here, the major question is whether quantitative measures can be developed which would show the extent to which the specialty and location distributions of graduates might be changed by altering admissions or teaching policies in prescribed directions. Without such measures, we must be cautious about attempting to change specialty and location distributions by altering medical school policies.

Finally—and more generally—what is needed is a more detailed look inside the "black box" of medical education, an identification of the various important types of learning experiences, and a rigorous determination of how these experiences bear on physicians' career choices. A large literature exists on the socializing effects of medical schools, and many hypotheses have been advanced to explain how medical students develop attitudes toward professional practice.[64] However, much of the evidence from statistical studies indicates that medical school experiences are not a dominant influence on physicians' specialty or location choices. These results may be accurate, but they could also be due to the failure to specify the socializing factors correctly. Until rigorous, large-sample studies of these socializing factors are carried out, we cannot be confident that changing the medical school environment will significantly alter the patterns of physicians' career choices.

NOTES

1. The Flexner Report recommended closing 124 of the 155 medical schools then in existence and reducing class sizes in the remaining schools to approximately 70 students each. Twenty schools allegedly shut down rather than be exposed by the report, and Flexner himself was threatened with bodily harm after the report was published. See, e.g., Stevens (1971).
2. Much the same vision of the ideal medical school had already been expressed by the Council on Medical Education. See, e.g., Stevens (1971).
3. For example, the first specialty board (in ophthalmology) was established in 1917.
4. The economic implications of the Flexner Report have been stressed by several authors, notably Kessel (1958, 1970, 1974), who claimed that it marked the capture of medical schools by organized medicine. However, the report did not simply call for reductions in the supplies of medical education and practitioners; it argued for the rationing of education among the most highly qualified institutions and the rationing of positions among the most highly qualified applicants. In this sense, it was not simply a device for erecting barriers to entry and raising the incomes of established practitioners.
5. One apparently incidental consequence of the elimination of proprietary schools was a sizable reduction in the supply of medical education for blacks. Most of the black medical schools were proprietary, and only two university-based institutions, Howard and Meharry, survived the transition (Stevens 1971; Kessel 1974).
6. While the AMA had no direct control over state boards' licensure policies, its Council on Medical Education was the sole medical school accrediting authority from 1906 to 1942. In 1942, the authority was passed to the Liaison Committee on Medical Education, which included members from the Association of American Medical Colleges as well as those from the Council. The committee has since added representatives of federal government and the public (AMA 1973).
7. A different view of the role of foundation support—particularly that of the first Rockefeller Foundation—has been advanced by Brown (1979, 1980), who argued that corporate philanthropy forced the reforms in medical education in order to reshape the medical profession according to its own special interests. However, he failed to explain why these interests were better served by schools with a greater emphasis on biomedical research than by the pre-Flexnerian clinical model.
8. For instance, the Carnegie Commission on Higher Education (1970, pp. 3–4) stated that: "The Flexner model has been the sole fully-accepted model in the United States since 1910. Some schools have fulfilled its promise brilliantly; others have been pale imitations; but all have tried to follow it."
9. For representative evidence and opinion on the issue, see Kendall (1971), Jason (1970), Mumford (1970), Funkenstein (1971, 1978), Stevens (1971), Sheps and Seipp (1972), and Mechanic (1974).

10. See, e.g., the Carnegie Commission on Higher Education (1970). The commission took the position that, despite its contributions, the Flexnerian medical school model was no longer adequate to meet society's needs for practitioners and professional health education. The establishment of family practice as a new specialty in 1969 was one of the efforts by educators (albeit at the graduate level) to counteract the growth of specialization in the demands for and supply of medical education.

11. In 1958–59, federal spending accounted for 30 percent of total medical school operating revenue. By the mid-1960s the figure had increased to roughly 55 percent; and, while it has recently declined, it stood at 30 percent in 1977–78 (AMA 1966, 1980). Since 1968, the federal share of funding for medical schools' purchases of plant and equipment has ranged from 27 to 42 percent of the total (AMA 1971, 1980; Crowley 1975a, 1975b).

12. See, e.g., Stevens (1971) and Fein and Weber (1971) on this point. From 1951 to 1960, the number of full-time-equivalent faculty per medical school doubled, and the number of full-time-equivalent faculty per 100 medical students grew from 24 to 45 (Powers et al. 1962). The increase in the faculty-student ratio is misleading, however, for most of the additional faculty seem to have been used to expand graduate programs. Between 1950 and 1961, the numbers of interns and residents supervised by medical school faculties doubled and tripled, respectively, while enrollments in all other programs except continuing physician education increased by less than 20 percent (Powers et al. 1962).

13. For a discussion of the value of faculty research productivity to the medical school, see Comroe (1962).

14. The Williams et al. study is the only rigorous effort to examine the effect of federal research and training grants on medical school behavior. Their principal findings were that federal expenditures significantly increased department sizes, basic science (non-M.D.) enrollments, and average faculty salaries, but had no important influence on the size of internship and residency programs. The results concerning basic science and graduate enrollments do not agree with those noted in the text above, but they apply to a somewhat later time period. Moreover, some of the methodology used in the study may be questionable. For instance, to determine the effects of research awards on faculty sizes, Williams et al. regressed the current-year number of faculty on the current-year numbers of medical students and graduate trainees, NIH research and training grants, and, in one equation, patient load. Since it is likely that all of the explanatory variables are dependent on the number of faculty, the estimates of the regression coefficients may have been biased.

15. Also see Chapter 8.

16. To receive a capitation grant, the medical school had to increase its first-year enrollment by 10 percent over its fall 1970 figure if the class size was less than 100, and by the larger of 5 or 10 students if the class size was 100 or more. The total award for each graduate of a four-year curriculum was $11,500; but to provide incentives for shortening degree programs, the award was set at $13,500 for each graduate of a three-year school.

17. The Veterans Administration Medical School Assistance and Health Manpower Training Act of 1972 authorized construction funding for eight new medical schools. In 1975, six schools in the developmental phase were receiving support from this source (AMA 1976).

18. For the figures cited here and below, see AMA (1973, 1976, 1980), AAMC (1975a), Crowley (1975a, 1975b), and Carnegie Council on Policy Studies in Higher Education (1976).

19. The Council on Medical Education (AMA 1970) credited the first round of enrollment increases in 1969 to funding incentives under the Health Manpower Act of 1968. And Carter et al. (1974) concluded that the 1971 capitation grant program produced substantial further increases, noting that 23 schools showing negligible changes in enrollment up to 1970 enlarged their first-year class sizes by an average of 14 percent from 1970 to 1972.

20. For example, the AAMC and the AMA both endorsed the principle of expanding medical school capacity after 1960, and the AAMC actively supported the 1963 statute and all later health manpower legislation. State legislatures have also played a vital role in medical school construction since the 1950s. One indication of their importance is the fact that 9 of the 13 new medical schools which became operational after 1970 were public institutions.

   Federal antidiscrimination conditions may have had something to do with the liberalization of admissions policies. By 1970, however, following a recommendation by the AAMC in 1968, medical schools had already begun to recruit women, blacks, and other minority students. Debate over curricular reform—both shortening the time to graduation and raising the emphasis on patient care—also started in the mid-1960s. See Coggeshall (1965), Funkenstein (1966, 1971), Matlack (1972), Johnson et al. (1975), and Carnegie Council on Policy Studies in Higher Education (1976).

21. Hall (1976) proposed an interesting model in which the medical school is assumed to maximize a utility function defined in terms of the number of graduates, the quality of educational services produced, and a composite "other" good denoting outputs of research, etc., subject to a budget constraint. He specified medical students as inputs in the production of both graduates and institutional quality. Whether this type of "consumer" model will prove more useful than those in which the school is viewed as a seller remains to be determined empirically. For instance, product differentiation of medical schools along the lines of quality can be thought of either as the result of some complex utility-maximizing (or utility-satisficing) process, or as a device for attracting buyers of educational services, research, and other outputs. In turn, the sale of, and income generated by, such outputs may well enter into a utility function by producing reputational capital, assuring survival and stability of the institution and its employees, or otherwise satisfying the controlling interests. Obviously, many theoretical models can be conceived of, but it is difficult to choose among them in the absence of knowledge about institutional goals.

22. For some descriptive evidence on medical school behavior, see, e.g., Fein and Weber (1971), Carter et al. (1974), and Williams et al. (1976).

23. To illustrate the problems, suppose that a given school admits students of average ability, offers an all-elective fourth year, derives a negligible fraction of its income from research support, and produces a small percentage of primary care practitioners. Intuitively, the first three characteristics might suggest that the school provides a non-research-oriented and unspecialized teaching environment, a description which is difficult to reconcile with its tendency to produce a small percentage of primary care physicians. In fact, the school may have preferred and sought both applicants of higher ability and a higher level of research funding than it attracted. And, in keeping with these goals, its curriculum and teaching policies may have been strongly specialty-oriented. Thus, it is difficult to say whether teaching environment or factors external to the medical school led to the observed propensity of its graduates to specialize.

24. See, e.g., the tabulations in Theodore et al. (1976), Lyden et al. (1968), and Martin (1975).

25. These are by no means the only cooperative mechanisms in medical education. For example, the American Association of Medical Colleges (AAMC) frequently serves as the industry's public spokesman, and it influences some aspects of educational policy. In this regard, the liberalization of admissions policies in 1970 followed a study by the AAMC which advocated increased enrollments of women and minority applicants. Medical schools also maintain a clearinghouse for applicants, participate in a centralized procedure for placing graduates in hospital training positions, and engage in many collaborative programs for disseminating information and improving the quality of medical education.

26. The same tendency was also reported in a descriptive study of 1950 and 1954 medical graduates by Lyden et al. (1968).

27. Their measure was derived from a factor analysis of school research expenditures per faculty member, per basic-science faculty member, and per dollar of total school expenditures.

28. They also remarked on a feature of the medical schools which has received inadequate attention—namely, that the distribution of school characteristics is by no means homogeneous across regions of the country. For instance, they reported that: (1) the most research-oriented schools were located in the Northeast and on the Pacific Coast; (2) the Northeast had the smallest proportion of public schools of all regions; and (3) southern schools tended to be the most service-oriented (in terms of their dependence on professional fee income) and to have the smallest graduate programs. Insofar as graduates' specialty and practice location choices are correlated with medical school characteristics, these results suggest that the pattern of choices should display differences across geographic regions.

29. Richards et al. (1968) added Canadian schools to their sample and obtained a fourth factor, which distinguished between the admissions requirements of U.S. and Canadian institutions.

30. The five were Columbia, Harvard, Johns Hopkins, Pritzker (Chicago), and Yale. The AAMC index defined a six-level classification of research orientation which, as might be expected, "explains" a large part of the variation in the percentages of graduates entering general practice. For example, using data from Martin (1975) on the specialty distributions of graduates, we ranked schools from most to least research-oriented, and found that the mean percentages of their 1960–64 graduates choosing general practice were 1.4, 3.2, 9.0, 13.8, 19.6, and 20.4, respectively. The AAMC index also appears to "explain" a large part of the variation in the MCAT scores of medical students. For 35 schools that reported the MCAT scores of their first-year classes in 1974 (AAMC 1975a), the mean MCAT scores of students in the most to least research-oriented institutions were 630, 614, 597, 588, 569, and 550. This suggests that both MCAT scores and propensity of students to specialize strongly increase with institutional research orientation.

31. Although private ownership and a high research orientation accompany the tendency of graduates to specialize, on statistical grounds the same tendency can also be attributed to school prestige, affluence, or even federal funding.

32. Currently, the ratio of applicants to positions for individual schools ranges from about 5 to more than 90, and the ratio of all applicants to all positions is about 2.5 to 1. The ratios for individual schools are higher than the overall ratio because of multiple applications. On the average, applicants apply to more than nine different schools (AMA 1980).

33. See, e.g., Gough (1971) and AAMC (1975a). The role of the personal interview in the admissions process is not well understood, but its ostensible purpose is to furnish the admissions committee with an impression of the applicant's motivation and dedication to medicine, emotional stability, health, and social attractiveness (Gough 1967, 1971).

    Other criteria, such as the quality of personal recommendations, are used in preliminary screening. Most schools require undergraduate course work in the sciences, and the quality of the applicant's undergraduate college is commonly taken into consideration in evaluating GPAs. For descriptions of current admissions procedures, see Rosenberg (1973), Carter et al. (1974), and Cuca et al. (1976).

34. For descriptive and case-study evidence on these points, see Hutchins and Gee (1961), Littlemeyer (1969), Page and Herron (1969), Dube et al. (1971), AMA (1972, 1973), Carter et al. (1974), Dube and Johnson (1974, 1975), Fruen et al. (1974), Rothman et al. (1974), AAMC (1975a), Crowley (1975b), Cuca et al. (1976), and Olmstead and Sheffrin (1981).

35. Private schools receiving state support may, and in some instances are known to, reserve explicit numbers of positions for in-state applicants (Crowley 1975a).

36. In two representative entering classes (1970 and 1978) 45 percent and 53 percent, respectively, of the students in private medical schools were residents of the state in which their school was located; the percentages for public schools were 87 and 91 (AMA 1971, 1980).

37. Some observers have emphasized the role of student selectivity as a means of producing high-quality physicians in the Flexnerian tradition. For example, Hall (1976) argued that medical schools deliberately set low tuition rates in order to create large applicant pools and thus maximize their admissions selectivity.

38. For example, 12 percent of the entering students in 1963 had overall undergraduate GPAs of 3.6 or higher on a 4-point scale, but in 1974 the percentage was 39 (Crowley 1975b), and in 1977 and 1978 it had risen to 50 (AMA 1980).

39. They did show that the average MCAT scores of nonmetropolitan applicants were substantially lower than those of metropolitan applicants. If this difference applies to past applicant populations as well, it suggests that medical schools may have discriminated against rural applicants on the basis of MCAT scores.

40. For instance, many schools established remedial preadmission programs for blacks and other minority students. And the average MCAT scores and premedical academic credentials of minority students in 1971 and 1976 were considerably lower than those of white students. See Johnson et al. (1975) and Waldman (1977).

41. See Beiser and Allender (1964); Gough and Hall (1964, 1975a, 1975b); Ingersoll and Graves (1965); Lief et al. (1965); Schofield and Merwin (1966); Korman et al. (1968); Rothman and Flowers (1970); Gough (1971); and Rothman (1973). For reviews of the literature on medical students' personality traits, see Lief (1971) and Webster (1975).

42. Little information exists on how admissions policies select individuals with preferred personality traits. Levitt (1966) and others have argued that admissions procedures favor "healthy obsessive-compulsive" applicants. In one study at the University of Toronto in 1972, Rothman et al. (1974) showed that admitted students scored lower than rejected applicants on measures of dominance, exhibition, nurturance, and order, but higher on measures of harm avoidance. At least superficially, these results seem to conflict with the belief that admissions committees seek out the traits ascribed to the "best" students.

    The AAMC expressed concern over the tendency of the MCAT to discriminate against minority applicants without superior academic and scientific backgrounds, and it redesigned the test to reduce its emphasis on science. The new version was given for the first time in 1977. The AAMC has also explored the possibility of using personality tests as part of the admissions procedure, but such tests are unlikely to become standard in the immediate future because of the obvious difficulties in interpreting and applying the results (Petty 1976).

43. Almost unanimously, the large number of studies of MCAT scores, college GPAs, and interview ratings have reported that they are at best weak predictors of medical school grades and other performance measures such as National Board scores. Achievement on the various admissions tests is most strongly correlated with medical school performance in the first two years

when dropout probabilities are highest. It seems to be weakly (or even inversely) correlated with clinical performance in the final two years. See Gough (1971, 1978) for summaries of the large literature on these points.

Most of the early studies of admissions standards employed fairly crude statistical methods such as pairwise correlations or comparisons of means of admissions ratings and medical school performance. More recently, efforts have been made to predict academic performance from multiple regressions in which admissions performance variables are combined with measures of student background and personality traits (Schofield 1970; Best et al. 1971; Gough and Hall 1975a, 1975b; Schofield and Garrard 1975; Hall 1976), but they have not been especially successful. In studies where R^2s have been reported, the equations predicted at most about a third of the variation in academic performance measures.

Whatever its exact goals and effectiveness, the admissions procedure is by no means inexpensive. Rosenberg's (1973) estimates of admissions costs at four schools in 1972 ranged from $544 to $1,755 per admitted student.

44. An attitudinal study of medical students at Case Western Reserve by Aronson et al. (1965) indicated that the school's reputation and curriculum were the most frequently mentioned reasons for attending the school, but whether the same is true for other medical schools is not known. Perlstadt (1975) argued in favor of the admissions screening hypothesis, citing the unpublished results of a study by the National Opinion Research Center. According to Perlstadt, high college academic performers were about equally distributed among three groups of medical schools classified by their research orientation. But 80 percent of the students in the most research-oriented schools were high performers, compared with 62 percent of the students in schools with an average research rating and only 29 percent of the students in schools with a low research orientation. The results, he contended, show that bright students do not necessarily single out research-oriented schools, but that research-oriented schools prefer bright applicants.

45. This would especially be the case in states producing few college graduates. Clearly, if applicant MCAT scores were identically distributed among medical schools, then the probability that a given number of applicants had MCAT scores above any fixed level would increase with the size of the applicant pool.

46. In 1973, for instance, nearly 40 percent of all entering private school students attended institutions in three heavily urbanized northeastern states: Massachusetts, New York, and Pennsylvania. But the northeastern states as a group accounted for only 11 percent of the students entering public schools (Crowley 1975a).

47. This is not to say that the only objective of admissions screening is to eliminate potential dropouts. Individual candidates may be accepted because they show promise as researchers or for other special reasons, and the application of admissions standards varies among schools (Carter et al. 1974). There are no indications that the process is used to predetermine the specialty distributions of graduates. Any impact on the specialty choice appears to be indirect,

resulting from the design of curricula and the selection of students capable of completing them.

48. Currently, the dropout rate is about 2 percent, but in the late 1950s it was as high as 11 percent (Johnson and Hutchins 1966; AMA 1980), and educators expressed considerable concern over student attrition. Johnson and Hutchins estimated that the number of dropouts during the 1950s represented a loss in the supply of new physicians equivalent to the closing of eight medical schools.

49. We use the word "capacity" in the loose sense, since the enrollment experience of the early 1970s demonstrates that the physical capacity of medical schools is by no means inflexible.

Unfortunately, it is impossible to be very precise about the structure of medical school costs because little empirical research has been devoted to the subject. Only two relatively recent efforts have been made to estimate undergraduate training costs, and they employed somewhat different samples and accounting methodologies (Institute of Medicine 1974; U.S. Department of Health, Education, and Welfare 1974). One attempt has been made to estimate cost functions for medical schools (Wing and Blumberg 1971), but it has been challenged on methodological grounds (Latham 1973).

50. Academic dropouts are students who are dismissed because of low grades; nonacademic dropouts are students who voluntarily withdraw from school for reasons unrelated to their academic performance. In the Johnson and Hutchins study, nonacademic dropouts had somewhat higher MCAT scores and college GPAs than academic dropouts.

Little et al. (1960) also showed that the rate of attrition increases as the school's average MCAT score declines. But because they used the school as the unit of analysis, differences in institutional characteristics may have accounted for the pattern they observed.

Roughly half of all those who drop out do so for nonacademic reasons (e.g., study pressures, loss of interest in medicine, or personal or financial problems). There is some evidence that the personality traits of nonacademic dropouts differ from those of graduates (Johnson and Hutchins 1966; Gough and Hall 1975a), and the academic environment may affect the withdrawal decision as well. For instance, in the sample studied by Johnson and Hutchins, the medical school with the highest attrition rate was wealthy and research-oriented. According to Hutchins (1965), its faculty believed that research took precedence over teaching, treated students contemptuously, and imposed great pressures on them to succeed. By contrast, in a school having one of the lowest attrition rates, Hutchins claimed that the environment provided an intellectually stimulating and nonstressful relationship between students and faculty.

51. The original findings are by Eron (1955) and Becker and Geer (1975). For a summary of the literature, see Rezler (1974).

52. See, e.g., Coombes and Boyle (1971) for a discussion of students' opinions on this point.

53. In one case study, for example, Snyder (1967) found that one-third of the fourth-year students had difficulty in establishing their professional priorities with respect to service to patients, concern for their colleagues, and adhering to impersonal principles of good medicine. Recent findings also tend to show that students become more conservative in their social, political, and medical views as they progress through medical school (e.g., Leserman 1980).

54. Actually, little is known about how medical students develop and revise their perceptions of specialties, although some evidence indicates that views of specialties do change during medical school. For example, at the University of New Mexico, Otis and Weiss (1972) found that freshman medical students regarded internal medicine as a primary care specialty, while seniors regarded it as a referral field.

55. See, e.g., Chyatte and Slater (1971); Herrmann (1972); Levine and Bonito (1974); Maurice et al. (1975); Preiss and Jackson (1978); and Burke et al. (1979). Also see Rezler (1974) for a summary of the literature on students' attitudinal responses to experimental curricula.

   In a study of 1960 graduates of 26 medical schools, Hutchins (1962) examined the tendency of research-oriented medical schools to produce larger percentages of academicians and smaller percentages of general practitioners than non-research-oriented schools. He argued that the difference was due to differences in learning environments—and especially to the curricula in research-oriented schools requiring or encouraging student research. However, students who attend research-oriented schools presumably expect to participate in research, and self-selection rather than participation in research may have accounted for the observed career-choice pattern.

56. The other explanatory variables were the class mean MCAT score, the percentage of basic science faculty supported by federal grants, the ratio of first- and second-year students to basic science faculty, and sponsored research expenditures. The coefficients on all variables but the last were negative.

57. The six specialty fields defined by Anderson were general practice, internal medicine, general surgery, academic medicine, other specialties, and an "undecided" category. The discriminant function containing all 58 explanatory variables correctly classified 85 percent of actual specialty choices. A function containing the first 10 variables correctly classified nearly 50 percent of the choices.

   Although Anderson made no explicit attempt to identify specialty characteristics, his results concerning general practitioners resembled those of other researchers. In particular, he found that on the average general practitioners were older, had lower grades, and were more sociable than other physicians. Interestingly—and unlike other findings—MCAT scores and background traits (e.g., sex, father's occupation, and size of hometown) contributed little incremental explanatory power to the discriminant function.

58. For similar studies using simple rather than multiple regression methods, see Hutchins (1964) and Sanazaro (1965).

59. See Chapter 6 for a fuller discussion of Hadley's model and the one by Hay cited in the text below.

60. For a review of the literature, see Bloom (1979).
61. Three studies of single states or single medical schools have also shown that a physician's probability of remaining to practice in a state is relatively small when his or her prior contact with a state is restricted to undergraduate medical education (Gough and Hall 1978; Wilensky 1979; and Watson 1980b).
62. Weiskotten et al. (1960) also reported that physicians tend to remain in cities where they attended medical school. They showed that, nine years after graduation, nearly 20 percent of the graduating classes of 1945 and 1950 were practicing in cities where they had attended medical school. However, less than 1 percent of each class practiced in cities where their only previous contact was medical school. Like other results, this indicates that medical school contact by itself produces weak attachments to areas.
63. Certain prominent exceptions exist to the general rule that percentages of public school graduates staying to practice in their medical school states are higher than the percentages of private school graduates. For example, public schools in Vermont have low retention rates, while private schools in California have exceptionally high retention rates. In these cases, the locational distributions of graduates seem to be better explained by taste or economic hypotheses than by prior contact. Still, they tend to indicate that medical school attachments are weak—either because medical school contact has an inherently weak effect on practice location, or because the choice of a medical school can depend on preestablished locational preferences.
64. For a review of the literature, see Bloom (1979).

FIVE

Graduate Medical Education and Physicians' Career Choices

Unlike undergraduate medical education, the graduate training of physicians takes place in a labor market for physicians' services. The teaching hospital[1] provides educational services to its graduate trainees, and trainees are an important source of skilled labor to the hospital.

Since the demand for graduate labor is derived from the hospital's production policies, the number and specialty composition of the training positions it offers depends, in general, on the volume and mix of its patient services, input prices, and managerial objectives. The demands for positions—or supplies of graduate labor—arise from the emerging specialty and location preferences of graduates, licensure requirements,[2] and market signals. Market signals consist of three types of payment made to graduates in exchange for their labor services: salary, remuneration in kind (such as room and board), and educational services which are transformed into increases in the graduates' stocks of human capital.

Like medical schools, teaching hospitals produce a differentiated educational service based on the perceived quality and ultimate investment value to physicians of their training programs. Most indications are that the supply side of the educational market is strongly segmented by the perceived quality of training services,[3] and the demand side is segmented as well, chiefly by hospitals' perceptions of the quality of trainees. Foreign medical graduates (FMGs), who enter the educational system at the graduate level and comprised approximately one-fifth to one-third of the graduate labor force in the 1970s, are typically ranked below U.S. medical graduates (USMGs) in hospitals' preferences for trainees.[4]

Teaching hospitals and trainees are unevenly distributed geographically, with the highest concentrations occurring in the Middle Atlantic and East North Central states. From 1975 through 1978, about 62,000 interns and residents served in U.S. teaching hospitals, but 10 states each had fewer than 150 and 3 had none (AMA 1976, 1980).

Most teaching hospitals are nonprofit, but otherwise hospital ownership takes a variety of different forms which influence the nature of the learning environment. In addition, external controls on the content and quality of teaching programs are exercised by a host of different professional organizations. It is within this complex and little studied background that physicians finally make their specialty and practice location choices.

THE STRUCTURE OF GRADUATE MEDICAL EDUCATION

Graduate medical education has traditionally consisted of one year of internship followed, if the physician wished to specialize, by one or more years of residency training in a specialty.[5] Internships and residencies were usually separate and self-contained programs, often taken in different hospitals under different teaching staffs.

Internships were divided into three types: rotating, mixed, and straight. The first involved short periods of training in all or most of the major specialties, and was the form of service commonly chosen by general practitioners. The second involved an intensive period of training in one specialty with shorter periods in one or more others. The third was essentially the first year of a residency program.

In 1975, the American Medical Association (AMA) listed 34 different residency specialties, for which the standard lengths of training ranged from one to six years beyond internship (Crowley 1975b). The lengths of residency training are determined, in effect, by the 22 specialty boards,[6] which set minimum periods of specialty education as eligibility conditions for board certification. The boards exercise indirect control over the length of graduate training, in part through their conditions for specialty certification.

A specialty board confers certification on a physician only if he or she meets its requirements for length and scope of residency training, and demonstrates medical competence by passing its tests. Although board certification has no legal status, it is a professional device for differentiating physicians by specialty and, more importantly, by the depth and quality of their specialty training. As such, it is a means for physicians to shift their demand function outward (i.e., to attract patients and referrals from other physicians), secure hospital admission and practice privileges, obtain staff appointments, and increase their professional status. Specialty certification consequently enlarges physicians' lifetime earnings and psychic income opportunities, and creates demands for extended residency training sufficient to meet the boards' requirements.[7]

The control of graduate medical education is distributed among a large number of hospital ownership and control categories. In 1974, 7 percent of the nearly 44,000 USMG interns and residents served in federal hospitals, 19 percent served in state and local governmental hospitals, 33 percent were in private nonprofit hospitals, and 41 percent served in two or more hospitals giving joint programs (AMA 1976).[8] Ninety-five percent of all USMG interns and residents served in hospitals affiliated with medical schools, and 94 percent served in hospitals having 200 or more beds.

Graduate programs are also subject to external approval by review committees. The review committees hold considerable power over the structure of programs because of the incentives for physicians to take approved training. Hospitals which fail to meet the committees' standards stand to lose access to their graduate labor supplies as well as their prestige and their attractiveness to patients and private physicians.

Until 1975, internship review committees were composed of representatives of the AMA's Council on Medical Education, the Association of American Medical Colleges (AAMC), the American Hospital Association (AHA), and the Federation of State Medical (licensing) Boards. Residency review committees were composed solely of representatives of the AMA and the specialty boards. In 1975, the committees were merged into a single authority, the Liaison Committee on Graduate Medical Education (LCGME), but the conduct of field reviews has evidently remained unchanged (Crowley 1975a).

By outward appearances, the principal sources of program control are medical schools and the specialty boards. At least one authority has contended that the present structure of graduate medical education was erected by the specialty boards, which, in the absence of competing interest groups, took on the responsibility for determining the scope, content, and length of residency training (Holden 1969).[9] It is difficult to judge how different the graduate labor markets would be in the absence of external program review. However, it seems clear that the specialty boards have been a critical factor promoting the growth of specialized residency training.

Another, and largely unanswered, question is the extent to which hospitals' market power influences the supply of training positions. Historically, teaching hospitals have been described as behaving like a loose cartel, with their apparent main interest being the preservation of a low-cost supply of physician labor.[10] The basic cartel-like device used in the graduate labor markets has been the National Intern and Resident Matching Program (NIRMP), now the National Resident Matching Program (NRMP), which was established by hospital and educational institutions in 1951.

Excess supplies of graduate positions began to appear in the 1930s and 1940s. As a result of the rapid expansion of hospital capacity and sharp decline in the number of new graduates after World War II, the aggregate vacancy rate for positions rose to 25 percent in 1950 (AMA 1968). The recruitment of graduates became chaotic, and there were reports that hospitals had begun to contract with junior and even sophomore medical students to fill their open internship positions (Curran 1959). The NIRMP was formed ostensibly to relieve the pressures on students—a purpose it definitely fulfills[11]—but probably also to forestall potentially costly price competition among hospitals for graduates.

First applied to internships, and then to residencies in 1968, the NIRMP is a centralized mechanism for allocating applicants to hospitals on the basis of the ranked preferences of both. It does not prevent price bidding, but it restricts large-scale price competition by limiting the number of contacts between applicants and hospitals. However, since the program exerted no control on the supply of positions, it did not materially lower vacancy rates, which averaged approximately 20 percent up to 1970 (AMA 1973).[12]

The NIRMP and the chronic excess supply of positions have been cited as examples of the forms and effects of collusive behavior by teaching hospitals,[13] but there have been no detailed studies of the labor market itself. One consequence of the period during which there was little price competition for graduates is that hospitals probably sought to attract graduates via the quality or range of their teaching programs, and by offering amenities such as a desirable location or pleasant working conditions, as well as other nonpecuniary devices. Hence, their pricing behavior may have led them to broaden the variety of human investment options available to graduates.

The principal type of differentiation in educational programs occurred between those given by hospitals with medical school affiliations and those given by unaffiliated hospitals.[14] Traditionally, unaffiliated— or "community"—hospitals have been much more service-oriented than hospitals affiliated with medical schools, and their graduate programs have reflected that fact. That is, they were much more likely than affiliated hospitals to offer rotating internships, internships without residencies, and residency programs in the primary care specialties.[15]

Two reasons seem to account for the differences. First, because community hospitals were primarily service-oriented, their labor demands tended to be of a generalized nature. Second, community hospitals were largely unable or unwilling to provide the large and diversified teaching staffs necessary to supervise internship or residency programs in the referral specialties. As a result, the conventional view is that community hospitals were the training grounds for physician generalists. Affiliated hospitals, where programs were maintained by medical schools under the Flexnerian educational standards, were the base for academic physicians and trainees planning to enter the specialty fields. Inasmuch as the degree of medical school control varies among affiliated hospitals, this contrast is probably an oversimplification, but it has persisted as a fundamental characterization of the graduate training environment.

Like undergraduate medical education, the overall structure of the graduate environment has undergone substantial changes since 1960. One of these changes has been the rapid growth of control by medical schools, accompanied by the equally rapid decline of the role of community hospitals and the abolition of the rotating internship.

Partly owing to the then limited teaching capacity of affiliated hospitals, the number of community hospital teaching programs increased considerably after World War II. By 1960 three-quarters of all teaching hospitals were unaffiliated with medical schools. In the late 1950s, however, medical educators began a two-sided attack on this trend. One—the less public of the two—was aimed at the allegedly poor quality of the community hospitals' teaching programs. The other, and more vigorous, criticism was directed at the rotating internship—the core of most community hospitals' graduate programs. Community hospitals, it was charged, were unable to provide adequate training because their educational functions were dominated by service commitments, and because they lacked the full-time teaching resources available to affiliated hospitals.[16] Moreover, educators contended, graduate medical education was a university responsibility under the Flexnerian tradition, and did not belong in unaffiliated hospitals.

The attack on the rotating internship was much more catholic in nature, centering on programs in both affiliated and community hospitals. Medical educators argued that the first graduate year had lost its historical function as a preparation for medical practice and had become instead a precursor to residency training. They claimed that the rotating internship was poorly taught, superficial, and commonly offered by community hospitals as a means of acquiring inexpensive physician labor.[17] Graduates who went on into residencies were penalized by having to repeat their first-year training in order to qualify for board certification. Citing these criticisms, the influential report of the Citizens Commission on Graduate Medical Education (AMA 1966) proposed (1) that the university be the provider of graduate education and (2) that internship and residency training be combined into single programs.

The second recommendation was adopted by the AMA's House of Delegates in 1970 and became effective in mid-1975. Under the new regulations—which applied to all graduate teaching programs approved by the LCGME—internships were replaced by first-year residencies called "GME-1." These, in turn, were designated as "flexible" or "categorical," and were meant to satisfy part of the training time requirements for specialty board certification. Flexible and categorical residencies replaced mixed and straight internships, respectively. The rotating internship was eliminated. In effect, this new system prevents community hospitals from employing unspecialized intern labor, and forces them to offer full multiyear residencies. Thus, short of abandoning their graduate programs altogether, most community hospitals have the option of seeking medical school affiliations or entering into joint arrangements with other (not necessarily affiliated) hospitals to provide the required programs on a shared basis.[18]

It is tempting to view the events of the 1970s as the final phase of the competition between medical schools and community hospitals for the graduate labor supply.[19] But it is probably just as reasonable to interpret the medical schools' motives as reflecting their growing concern over the quality and content of graduate medical education. Moreover, both the number of rotating internships and the share of the graduate labor market held by community hospitals had fallen dramatically even before the announcement of the merger of internships and residencies in 1970. To be specific, in 1960, 74 percent of all teaching hospitals were not affiliated with medical schools, but by 1970 the percentage had declined to 41, and by 1975—on the eve of the merger of internships and residencies—it had fallen still further, to 30. In 1960, rotating internships represented 70 percent of all internships offered, but by 1970 they represented only 17 percent, and in 1975 they accounted for nearly the same percentage (19). In the six-year period 1964–70, the total number of rotating internships fell by 47 percent, from 9,057 to 4,760, with 85 percent of the positions eliminated being in community hospitals.[20]

In spite of the declining number of positions, vacancy rates for rotating internships remained high throughout the 1960s, particularly in community hospitals. In the late 1960s, for example, the vacancy rates for rotating internships averaged about 35 percent in unaffiliated hospitals and 20 percent in affiliated hospitals. Furthermore, by 1970, the vacancy rate for all graduate positions was 30 percent in unaffiliated hospitals but only 15 percent in affiliated hospitals. In the same year, more than 90 percent of USMGs served in affiliated hospitals. Community hospitals were left to rely on FMGs, who represented 65 percent of their interns and 59 percent of their residents. Without access to the large and growing supply of foreign physicians during the late 1960s, community hospitals' market position would almost certainly have deteriorated even more quickly than it did. Thus, while the expansion of medical school control is certainly part of the explanation for the increasing specialization of graduate medical education since 1960, an equally important factor has been the shift in the types of graduate training positions demanded by USMGs.[21]

On the other hand, the supply of graduate medical education has also been affected by despecializing influences arising, in part, from within the university-based system. One factor was the establishment of the specialty board in family practice in 1969. The result of a 10-year effort by educators in comprehensive care, the new specialty board established a three-year family practice residency. The goal was both to upgrade the professional status of general practitioners and to provide primary care training outside of the traditional inpatient environment (Lienke 1970).[22] Motives similar to those reflected in the development of family practice residencies also led in the early 1970s to the increased involvement of medical schools with health maintenance organizations (HMOs), neighborhood health centers, regional health programs, and the expansion in their production of patient services in general.

Although many of these new activities were heavily subsidized by the federal legislation, it would be an oversimplification to ascribe them solely to the government's policy initiatives. In this respect, it is important to recognize that medical educators do not constitute a single homogeneous interest group. Indeed, it has long been apparent that they differ widely in terms of their professional values and judgments. In this sense, the push to develop primary care residencies and to broaden participation in related programs had important ideological roots. It reflected, in part, growing opposition within the ranks of medical educators to the traditional emphasis placed on competence in a narrow specialty field (see, e.g., Knowles 1965; Wingert 1966; Wise et al. 1966; and Deuschle 1969).

Although federal funding for residency positions in primary care was available before 1970, it was explicitly extended to all nonprofit teaching hospitals by the Comprehensive Health Manpower Training Act of 1971. In 1976, support was authorized for residency positions in general internal medicine and general pediatrics as well. As an additional and potentially powerful stimulus to medical schools to increase the number of residents in primary care, the 1976 act also made the award of undergraduate capitation grants contingent on a school's meeting minimum requirements with respect to the percentage of its filled residency positions that were in family practice, general internal medicine, and general pediatrics.[23] Clearly, Congress sought to create incentives not just for increasing the supply of positions in primary care, but for undertaking policies to assure that the positions were in fact filled.

The increase in the number of family practice residencies offered by teaching hospitals has been remarkable—from 467 in 1970 to 7,328 in 1980 (AMA 1971, 1980)—and it is reasonable to credit much of this growth to federal subsidy programs. However, it is not known how permanent a trend this growth represents. For example, although the vacancy rate for family practice residencies is now about equal to those for the other major fields, and 10 to 13 percent of all GME-1 residents are selecting family practice positions (Graettinger 1979; AMA 1980), it is not known how many of these potential family practitioners would otherwise have chosen to enter general practice or another primary care field.

Some experts are of the opinion that the popularity of family practice may have peaked (e.g., Egger 1978). However, it is probably fairer to say that medical schools' attitudes toward the field are still in a state of transition. A survey conducted in early 1973 by Schroeder et al. (1974) showed that 22 of the 105 then existing medical schools neither operated nor planned to establish family practice residencies. In addition, the survey revealed a somewhat more receptive attitude to family practice by public than by private medical schools. At that time, 67 percent of the state-supported schools, but only 36 percent of the privately owned schools, had operational family practice residency programs. Likewise, certain other well-publicized medical school activities, such as their involvement with HMOs, also seemed to be off to a slow start. Among the 34 schools with functioning or planned HMO affiliations in 1973, only four actually engaged the majority of their graduate trainees in providing primary care to HMO subscribers, and only 14 involved 5 percent or more of their trainees in primary care.

Another survey of medical schools carried out in 1976 by Giacalone and Hudson (1977) indicated a mixed pattern of progress toward providing graduate training in family practice. The number of schools not contemplating the introduction of family practice residencies fell from 22 to 10, but 8 of the 10 were privately owned institutions. Most of the schools reported that they had either established new departments of family medicine or expanded those already in existence, and they appeared to have made significant efforts to recruit family practice faculty. On the other hand, there was a decline in medical schools' involvement with HMOs and no movement toward developing clinical locations for family practice training. Giacalone and Hudson also found that generalist residency programs in pediatrics and internal medicine accounted for less than half the total number of programs offered in each field.

These fragments of evidence are obviously inconclusive, and they may indicate nothing more than the normal lag between the introduction and implementation of new educational technologies. Even so, they raise the possibility that medical schools' perceptions of their social obligations include a somewhat limited commitment to supply primary care training. Because of this, some authorities argue that the future supply of graduate training in the primary care specialties is strongly dependent upon the directions and the vigor of related federal subsidy policies.[24]

GRADUATE TRAINING AND PHYSICIANS' SPECIALTY CHOICES

Although federal policy has increasingly focused on graduate training as the avenue for influencing physicians' specialty choices, exceptionally little evidence has been produced on the outcome. Chapter 1 described a number of studies which show that a significant percentage of physicians—perhaps even the majority—delay their *final* specialty choices until entry into graduate training. These findings suggest that the graduate training environment is an influential decision factor for a large number of physicians. Nevertheless, if physicians either determine their specialty choices or at least reduce them to a few alternatives before medical school graduation, it follows that they will tend to choose training hospitals and residency programs that feature their specialty preferences. To the extent this is the case, the observed patterns of hospital and program selection represent the effects rather than the causes of specialty choices. Thus, analyses of specialty choices and the graduate training environment must address an important methodological question: is the type of graduate training environment self-selected, or does it have a material causal impact on physicians' specialty choices?

The view that the medical school affiliation and research orientation of the graduate training hospital are important determinants of a trainee's perceptions of medical practice was documented in a case study by Mumford (1970). Mumford examined the development of interns' attitudes toward medicine and specialization in two unnamed midwestern hospitals during the late 1950s. One hospital held a major affiliation with a prestigious and research-oriented university medical school, while the other was a small, unaffiliated hospital located in the suburbs of the same city. In most respects the two hospitals mirrored the description of affiliated and community hospitals given above.[25] According to Mumford, a primary goal of the university hospital was the production of specialized research, and the foremost goal of the community hospital was the production of patient services. In each case, the hospital's objectives were communicated to its interns in a variety of formal and informal ways. By the end of the training year many of the interns came to adopt the hospitals' value systems as their own.

In the university hospital, interns were continuously reminded of the reputation of the medical school and the faculty, and were encouraged to attend the many research lectures given. The hospital was organized into self-contained specialty departments among which there was little professional or social contact. The faculty maintained a formal structure of consultive support, and interns were systematically discouraged from making medical judgments without first consulting their seniors in the hierarchy. Patients were admitted to the hospital only if they represented useful opportunities for teaching or research, and attending physicians and other medical personnel were accorded low professional status. Interns were given direct control only over ward patients, and their activities, particularly record keeping—on which the faculty placed great emphasis—were closely monitored by the senior staff. At the end of the year, Mumford contended, interns had accepted the hospital's procedures as essentials for the competent practice of medicine. They tended to consider patients principally as "interesting" or "uninteresting" cases, to be reluctant to diagnose or prescribe treatment without consultation, and to be little aware of the hospital environment outside their specialty departments.

By contrast, the interns in the community hospital were repeatedly informed that their first obligations were to patients, and that they were training to become practicing physicians. At the very beginning of their service they were assigned major responsibilities for patient care, which they appeared to enjoy. They even found satisfaction in emergency-room service because of the responsibility for patient welfare that it conferred on them—unlike their counterparts in the university hospital, who regarded the duty as tedious and unrewarding. The interns were encouraged to model their behavior after that of attending physicians,[26] and to look upon nurses as allies who might have superior medical judgment by virtue of their experience. The hospital admitted all patients regardless of their teaching potential—a policy the interns took pride in—and quartered the interns together. Out of their social contacts and rotation through the hospital's major clinical departments, the interns acquired familiarity with a range of different specialty practices. At the end of the year, Mumford argued, they had developed the attitude that medicine was a generalized experimental art centered on the individual's responsibility for providing patient care.[27]

Mumford gave no direct evidence of the effect of the different hospital environments on interns' specialty choices, so in this respect her results are merely suggestive of the "specializing" or "despecializing" impact of graduate training. She implied, however, that the environment has a causal effect on specialty decisions. To support this view, she cited results from a 1968 national survey by Columbia University showing that 11 percent of the interns in small unaffiliated hospitals but only 1 percent of those in large affiliated hospitals did not plan to take residency training.

At least two other hypotheses are also consistent with this finding— namely, that it was caused by either graduate self-selection or hospital recruitment policies. That is, graduates who had already chosen, or were inclined to choose, general practice may have selected unaffiliated hospitals because of the characteristics of their training programs; or unaffiliated and affiliated hospitals may have chosen graduates with disproportionately high and low propensities, respectively, to enter general practice. In either case, of course, the training environment may have had little immediate influence on specialty preferences. Mumford noted that the university hospital sought and attracted graduates who ranked in the upper third of their medical school class, but that the community hospital neither sought nor attracted unusually capable trainees. In light of the evidence (presented in Chapter 3) that the highest scholastic achievers are ordinarily the least likely to choose general practice, the difference in observed intern characteristics suggests that the university hospital did, in fact, recruit trainees with weaker preferences for the primary care specialties.

Because of the lack of empirical models of hospital choice by interns and residents, it is difficult to separate the effects of self-selection, recruitment, and the training environment in the reported associations between hospital affiliation and the choice of general practice. For example, in a study of the 1950 and 1954 graduating classes of 12 medical schools, Lyden et al. (1968) found that public school graduates were markedly more likely than private school graduates to serve internships in unaffiliated hospitals, to take rotating internships, and to enter general practice. In addition, they showed that, even among private school graduates, those with the highest MCAT scores were much more likely than those with low MCAT scores to intern in major teaching hospitals and to take straight internships. The implication is that physicians' choices of training hospitals, length of training, and specialty are all substantially predetermined by their background or the characteristics of the medical school they attended.[28]

An attitudinal study of internship hospital choice by 1970 and 1971 graduates of seven medical schools (Paiva et al. 1974) further narrowed the range of possible interpretations. Dividing training hospitals into three types—university, municipal, and private—they found that the types that graduates selected were *not* related to most measured personality traits or to such data as MCAT scores and undergraduate college GPAs. By contrast, the choice of training hospital was strongly associated with characteristics of the respondents' undergraduate medical education and planned specialty fields. Interns choosing university hospitals attributed far more influence to medical school faculty and advisers than either of the other two groups, and reported far more (and more enjoyable) participation in research during medical school. They were also least likely to be planning to enter general practice and most likely to be planning careers in a specialty or in research and teaching.[29] Interns choosing municipal or private hospitals were disproportionately oriented toward primary care practice. These findings, Paiva et al. argued, indicate that preferences for internship hospitals were primarily shaped by medical school experiences and already developed specialty plans.

However, a third study of physicians' career paths by Zuckerman (1978) reached somewhat different conclusions. Zuckerman used a three-way classification of career outcomes—general practice, specialty practice, and teaching/research. He proposed six different educational pathways leading to these outcomes, each of which was defined in terms of physicians' academic abilities, the academic or clinical orientation of their medical school, the degree of affiliation of their internship and residency hospitals, and the types of internships they had taken (rotating or straight).

Zuckerman's major hypothesis was that the medical education system evaluates students and graduates and, on the basis of these evaluations, places them in training tracks leading toward specific career outcomes. Using data from the AAMC's longitudinal study of 1960 medical graduates, he sought to test this hypothesis by matching career outcomes with the six educational pathways. The attempt largely failed. The most successful match occurred for general practice, but only 12 percent of the general practitioners in his sample actually chose the pathway Zuckerman predicted.[30] Moreover, he reported that the 2,500 sample members had, in fact, followed more than 1,100 different pathways. Thus, if it is the case that physicians do select particular fields early in their training, these results suggest that they do not choose a particular sequence of learning environments in which to prepare themselves for those fields. Nevertheless, like Paiva et al., Zuckerman found significant correlations between physicians' internship hospital choices and the orientations of their medical schools. He also found significantly positive associations between the affiliation levels of their internship and residency hospitals. He took this as evidence supporting his "track" hypothesis. A corollary of this hypothesis is that physicians follow particular routes through the graduate educational system partly because they have already decided on their practice specialties.

On the other hand, it is known that an important degree of specialty switching takes place even after physicians begin their residency training. For example, Ernst et al. (1978) examined the first and last residency specialties of approximately 4,500 physicians who entered practice in 1970. They reported that the numbers of physicians in 12 specialties changed from −50 percent to +96 percent between first and last residency programs. The numbers of persons in general practice, internal medicine, and pediatrics fell by 11 percent, 18 percent, and 4 percent, respectively, but the largest numerical losses occurred in internal medicine and general surgery. In the latter two fields, nearly all of the losses were to other medical and surgical specialties, indicating that residency training is commonly accompanied by switches from more general to less general programs.

Two other studies also suggest that a considerable degree of specialization occurs after physicians begin their residency training. Wechsler et al. (1978) surveyed physicians who had been residents in internal medicine, pediatrics, or obstetrics-gynecology in Massachusetts during 1967–72. Fourteen percent of the respondents reported that they had changed fields during their residency service. Even more significantly, 17 percent had changed specialties after they began practice. In addition, there was a marked tendency among those who did not change specialties to subspecialize within their primary fields. Indeed, Wechsler et al. calculated that, on a full-time-equivalent physician basis, only 27 percent of the former residents in internal medicine, 42 percent of the former residents in pediatrics, and 39 percent of the former residents in obstetrics-gynecology were providing primary care. These findings are especially striking in view of the fact that when the survey was conducted in 1976, the respondents had been in practice less than 10 years—some for as little as 4.

A similar pattern was observed in a more recent study by Jacoby (1981), which also indicated that specialty switches and subspecialization continue to occur after entry into practice. Jacoby outlined a simple forecasting model which he used to predict the practice specialties of physicians from a knowledge of their first residency fields. To implement the model, he examined the specialty histories of 160,000 U.S. medical graduates from the classes of 1960–77. Although he did not present a complete set of figures, his illustrative data showed that subspecialization takes place both before and after entry into practice. Of particular importance here is his finding that only 57 percent of the physicians who begin their residencies in primary care fields will actually function as primary care practitioners. The remainder, he predicted, will either switch into referral specialties or take up subspecialties within the primary care fields.

These results demonstrate that: (1) first residency specialties are only moderately good predictors of practice specialties; (2) far more physicians enroll in a first-year primary care program than ultimately become full-time primary care practitioners; and (3) during their residency training, physicians are much more likely to switch from generalized to specialized fields than the reverse.

In terms of the issue at hand, the paramount question is why these patterns appear. Are they the result of the emphasis and prestige given to specialization by the medical education system? Do they simply reflect the specialty plans of physicians that were decided before the start of residency training? Or are they part of a normal process in which physicians gain clinical experience and discover that they prefer sub- or referral specialties to more generalized fields?

Unfortunately, the existing evidence does not provide clear-cut answers. The observed patterns are obviously consistent with the thesis that, in a variety of ways, the medical educational system encourages specialization. But the trend toward specialization after entry into practice can be read as either supporting or refuting this thesis. Presumably, physicians in practice are immune to the direct influence of the graduate training environment. To the extent that they continue to specialize, their behavior can be interpreted as a natural response to their practice experience and inherent specialty preferences. Nevertheless, if the learning environment exercises a pervasive and long-lasting effect on physicians' attitudes, any tendency of practicing physicians to further specialize can be viewed as the indirect consequence of values inculcated by a medical educational system biased in favor of specialization. Beyond that, many specialty boards—including those in the medical fields—encourage or require a generalized first year of residency training.[31] As a result, graduates may enroll in a general first-year program such as internal medicine with the intention of switching later to a sub- or referral specialty. On balance, it is not possible to conclude at this time the extent to which residency and practice specialization is due to the nature of the graduate training environment versus the extent to which it is due to self-selection by physicians themselves.

Few studies investigating the effects of graduate training on physicians' specialty choices have controlled for other factors that may influence specialty decisions. One that did (Hadley 1975, 1977, 1979) used a number of predictor variables—including internship hospital characteristics—to estimate the probabilities that 1960 medical school graduates would choose one of five to nine different specialties. His hospital variables included a dummy indicator of a major teaching affiliation, the autopsy rate, and the percentage of straight internships offered. All were considered to be proxies for the hospital's prestige, with the most prestigious (or research-oriented) institutions being distinguished by a major teaching affiliation, a high autopsy rate, and a high percentage of straight internships.

Hadley's findings indicated that internship hospital characteristics were the most significant predictors of physicians' specialty choice probabilities (in comparison with background and personality traits, medical school characteristics, etc.). In particular, he found that (holding the other factors constant) service in a prestigious hospital greatly reduced the probability that a physician would select either general practice or anesthesiology. On the other hand, hospital prestige did not successfully distinguish other primary care practitioners from referral specialists. Having an internship in a prestigious hospital appeared to raise the probabilities of choosing internal medicine and pediatrics, but it also raised the probabilities of choosing the referral specialties other than anesthesiology.

Hadley's results with respect to general practitioners are consistent with the evidence from the other studies we have reviewed. However, inasmuch as correlations between specialty choice probabilities and other variables do not establish the direction of causation, they do not prove that internship environments materially affect specialty choices.

The same problem clouds another study. Pozen et al. (1979) investigated the stability of specialty choices by residents in pediatrics and internal medicine programs at the Boston City Hospital. The residents were trained in two "pathways," one traditional (which allowed individuals to subspecialize) and one devoted to primary care. Pozen et al. found that there was little change in their subjects' career plans (in terms of subspecialty orientation and intention to provide direct patient care) regardless of which pathway they had chosen. They concluded that both pathways "stabilized" their subjects' career preferences, and, ipso facto, that these preferences are affected by residency training. However, their findings can also be interpreted as being the product of individual self-selection. That is, if the residents had already determined their career plans, it is reasonable to suppose that they would choose the pathways most compatible with their plans. Thus, it is not particularly surprising that most of them exhibited no changes in career preferences. Indeed, changes in preferences—an issue that Pozen et al. did not examine—might well be considered stronger evidence of the effects of the training environment than the absence of such changes.

A third study by Weil and Schleiter (1981) reached rather different conclusions. As will be recalled from our earlier discussion of it, this study concerned the effects of personal and educational background characteristics on resident internists' interest in entering primary care as opposed to subspecializing. Another aspect of the study dealt with the relationships between the same characteristics and the residents' interest in medical practice versus academic careers. Weil and Schleiter classified residency programs according to their size, complexity, differentiation, and research orientation. The type of program chosen was found to be significantly associated with the type of medical school the resident had attended, but not with his or her interest in primary care or in an academic career. On this basis, Weil and Schleiter concluded that postgraduate training has little direct effect on physicians' career preferences. Instead, they contended that it "enhances" the influence of prior conditioning factors more than it "counteracts" them.

Taken together, these last three studies illustrate how difficult it is to interpret evidence on the hypothesis that graduate medical teaching environments affect specialty preferences. Two of the studies concluded that there is such an effect, but they can be questioned on methodological grounds. The third found that the effect is minor, but it did not consider residents' choices among greatly different fields. All in all, these findings can best be viewed as weak. Although it is apparent that graduate specialties are useful predictors of final specialty choices (since many of the latter are made at the beginning of graduate training), it is far less clear that the type of initial graduate program or teaching hospital has an important causal impact on most physicians' selection of field.

THE RELATIONSHIP BETWEEN GRADUATE TRAINING AND PRACTICE LOCATION

The relationships between graduate training and practice location have been studied mostly in the context of the prior-contact hypotheses of location behavior (described in Chapter 3). Graduate training provides an important source of contact with a potential practice area, and numerous analyses have shown a strong tendency for physicians to choose practice communities in the same states as their graduate training. Moreover, physicians are more likely to remain in the states where they have taken graduate training than in the states of their undergraduate medical education. Weiskotten et al. (1960) reported that 59 percent and 63 percent, respectively, of large samples of 1945 and 1950 medical graduates still practiced in their states of residency training nine years after graduation. By contrast, only 42 percent of each sample chose practice locations in their states of medical school graduation. Mason (1975) found that 52 percent of the population of 1960 graduates were practicing in the same states as their internship or residency hospitals in 1975, as opposed to 43 percent who were practicing in the same states as their medical schools. Similar patterns have been described in studies of Texas physicians by Brandt et al. (1979), Stefanu and Pate (1978), and Stefanu et al. (1979), and in a study of Michigan physicians by Wilensky (1979).

Even more striking indications of the differential retention effects of medical schools and graduate training appear when the recency of state contact is taken into account. Tabulations by Held (1972) of 1955–65 medical graduates showed that 20 percent remained to practice in states where their only prior contact was graduate training, but only 3 percent remained in states where their only contact was attending medical school. Among physicians entering practice in 1966, Yett and Sloan (1974) found that 11 percent of the general practitioners chose states where their only previous contact was medical school, and 20 percent chose states where their only previous contact was graduate training.[32] However, the percentages for specialists were only 2 and 15, respectively, suggesting that specialists as a group are more mobile than general practitioners.

While it is clear that a correlation exists between the state location of graduate training and choice of practice location, there is—as was stressed in Chapter 3—considerable disagreement with respect to its cause. Weiskotten et al. (1960) argued that graduate training locations are a causal influence on practice location choices. In contrast, on the basis of their regression analysis, Fein and Weber (1971) concluded that interns and residents are attracted to a state by the state's desirability as a future practice site. Yett and Sloan (1974) estimated a modified form of the Fein-Weber regression equation and reported results contrary to those of Fein and Weber.[33]

Thus, it is an open issue whether the state of graduate training influences or is influenced by the choice of a state of practice. This ambiguity is especially unfortunate in view of the important policy implications of the issue. In particular, policies to modify the geographic distribution of physicians by altering the state locational patterns of graduate training will be ineffective if the choice of training location is dependent on selection of a state in which to practice.[34]

Little is known of how the characteristics of graduate training hospitals affect practice location patterns. Indeed, no substantive hypotheses that might account for a relationship have been advanced. Hadley (1975) suggested that graduates may migrate between states in order to serve in especially desirable hospitals. But unless some states possess a disproportionate number of desirable hospitals and succeed in retaining their trainees, his speculation is of limited value in helping to understand the interstate distribution of physicians.[35]

Relatively little is known of the links between graduate training and practice locations at the intrastate level. In their study of 1945 and 1950 medical graduates, Weiskotten et al. (1960) found that approximately 35 percent of each class entered practice in cities where they had taken graduate training, and that 13 percent of each class entered practice in cities where their only previous contact was graduate training. Similarly, Ernst et al. (1978) found that 29 percent of a large sample of USMGs who entered practice in 1970 chose to practice in the counties where they had taken their last graduate training.

Despite the evidence that contact with a local area may have a strong influence on intrastate practice location choices, the factors that might account for such an influence have been explored in only two studies. Watson (1980a) used discriminant analysis to identify the characteristics of urban and rural practitioners among graduates of the University of Utah College of Medicine. Among other results, Watson reported that physicians practicing in urban locations were significantly more likely than rural practitioners to have settled in cities where they had taken their internships. While this finding may be only tautological (since most teaching hospitals are located in metropolitan areas), it raises the possibility that the attachment effects of training in a city may inhibit physicians from selecting rural practice locations.

The other study by Lee (1980) was discussed in Chapter 3. Lee's evidence did not support the hypothesis that prior contact with a community during residency service leads physicians to locate their practices in that community. Instead, he concluded that physicians tend to select residency communities where they plan to establish their practices. The results on which he based his conclusion should be regarded as tentative. Nevertheless, they do indicate that the matter deserves further investigation.

Thus, while correlations exist between graduate training locations and practice locations within as well as among states, we do not yet understand what causes them. They could be due to attachments developed during physicians' graduate training experiences. Alternatively, they could be due to attachments formed at earlier career stages, or they could be brought about by physicians' prior practice location choices independent of previous contact with the area.

As part of the general proposition that graduate training discourages physicians' interests in primary care, it has also been asserted that the graduate training environment discourages preferences for rural practice locations. According to this argument, graduate service is normally performed in an urban inpatient setting where the most modern medical technologies and a broad spectrum of consulting and support personnel are available to the physician. Consequently, physicians come to perceive these resources as essential to "good" medical practice. And, inasmuch as such resources are scarce in rural areas, this means that the same type of learning environment that undervalues primary and ambulatory care leads physicians to prefer metropolitan over rural practice communities.

Despite its intuitive appeal, the foregoing hypothesis has not been systematically tested.[36] It is not really known to what extent graduate training would, by itself, induce physicians to settle in rural areas if it deemphasized the roles of urban-based hospitals, technology, and support systems. A final resolution of the issue awaits further investigation.

SUMMARY

According to the prevailing theories, graduate medical training exercises a causal impact on physicians' specialty and practice location choices. First, it is contended that the learning environment actively promotes specialization because of the high value placed on it by the majority of teaching hospitals. Second, it is argued, graduate training locations give physicians attachments to areas which prompt them to establish practices in those areas.

By and large, the evidence to this point is consistent with both theories. Although we do not know the exact volume of specialty switching that takes place during graduate training, it appears to involve roughly 10 to 20 percent of all physicians. In addition, several studies have indicated that the switching occurs from more generalized to less generalized fields. This seems to be particularly true for physicians who begin their residencies in the primary care specialties. Currently, 55 to 60 percent of all first-year residents are entering the primary care fields, but these figures are much larger than the percentages of new physicians who ultimately become primary care practitioners. The best estimates now available indicate that at most three-fifths—and perhaps many fewer—first-year residents will practice in primary care, with the rest becoming sub- or referral specialists.[37]

Similarly, the existing evidence on location patterns shows a marked tendency for physicians to enter practice in states, counties, and cities where they received their graduate training. For example, we can predict up to 30 percent of all physicians' county-of-practice locations, and a somewhat larger percentage of their state locations, simply by knowing the counties and states of their last graduate training.

However, the importance of these results for policy hinges on their causal implications. Altering the graduate learning environment and the location of graduate training will affect the specialty and locational distributions of physicians only insofar as each has a causal impact on specialty and location decisions. And on this point the evidence is, at best, ambiguous.

Regarding the trend toward specialization during graduate training, it is not yet clear how much of this tendency is the result of customary pregraduate career planning. Historically, major teaching hospitals have produced a disproportionate number of specialists while unaffiliated hospitals have produced a disproportionate number of generalists. But this may have been the result of hospital recruitment policies or self-selection by graduates seeking preferred training settings. The tendencies of physicians to subspecialize even after they have begun practice also suggest that specialization has a momentum beyond whatever impetus it may be given by graduate medical education.

Likewise, the hypothesis that graduate hospital locations influence physicians' practice location choices has been challenged. According to the counterargument, relationships between hospital and practice locations are caused by physicians' self-selection of hospital locations. Although the findings on this point too are inconclusive, the possibility that the line of causation varies with individual physicians cannot be ruled out.

The structure of graduate medical education has altered markedly since 1960. The four most significant changes have been: (1) the enlargement of medical schools' control over the graduate training environment, (2) the abolition of rotating internships in favor of earlier specialty training, (3) the introduction of the family practice residency, and (4) the expansion of primary care programs in response to federal subsidies initiated in the early 1970s. Depending on how one regards the theories and evidence concerning graduate medical education and physicians' career choices, these changes may or may not have important long-term effects on the functional distribution of new physicians.

If one accepts the prevailing theories, the first two trends militate for continuing physician specialization and a continuing scarcity of practitioners in rural areas. The third, which has enhanced the status of general primary care practice, should stimulate physicians to select a primary care field if they are otherwise marginally undecided between the primary care and referral specialties. The fourth tends to assure an adequate supply of residency positions for physicians preferring the primary care fields.[38] The problem is that the evidence to date does not permit us to predict reliably whether these trends will, in toto, increase, reduce, or not change, the percentage of primary care practitioners currently being produced by the medical education system. Their ultimate impact depends on their relative strengths. The educational system's resolve to produce primary care practitioners may therefore be contingent on the government's—and the public's—commitments to primary care training. Whether, for instance, medical schools would continue to offer large-scale primary care training programs without government funding—especially in light of their current financial problems—must be considered to be an open question.

If one rejects the prevailing theories, the implication then is that all changes in the graduate medical educational system are unlikely to affect the functional distribution of physicians except insofar as they limit training opportunities. What might be called the "skeptical position" holds that physicians' specialty preferences—and, to a lesser degree, their practice location choices—are determined before residency service. Thus, graduate medical training cannot significantly influence residents' career choices in favor of particular specialties or practice locations. Nonetheless, even in this view, it could have a constraining effect on them—e.g., if the supply of primary care positions were sharply cut back or the number of hospital locations were drastically reduced.

Regrettably—given the importance of the issue—tests to date of the prevailing theories have not been sufficiently rigorous to determine whether they accurately portray the influence of graduate medical education on physicians' career decisions. The challengers of the prevailing theories are a minority, but they have raised issues that need further investigation.

NOTES

1. We use the expression *teaching hospital* to denote any hospital that offers formal training programs to medical school graduates. The training is carried out under the supervision of a teaching staff, and, unless the graduates are licensed, they are forbidden by law from giving unsupervised patient care.
2. In the 1970s, 39 of the 55 state and territorial licensing boards required at least one year of approved graduate training of candidates for licensure (AMA 1971; Goodman and Mason 1976; Wunderman 1979), and all boards required candidates to demonstrate their clinical competence. In general, proof of competence could be established either by passage of the board's own licensure examination—which had become uniform by the mid-1970s —or by passage of the three-part examination of the National Board of Medical Examiners (NBME). Each test is based in part on the candidate's internship experience, so that internship training was a de facto condition for licensure in all states and territories. In the past, some medical schools required a year of postgraduate clinical training for the M.D. degree, but the practice was largely abandoned in the 1930s and the last of the major medical schools to maintain it, Northwestern, eliminated it in 1949. For discussions of the history of internships, see Curan (1959), Campbell (1964), and Stevens (1971, 1978).
3. Actually, the evidence on this point is neither recent nor precise. In a study of 1,200 interns serving in hospitals that were affiliated with medical schools, Saunders (1961) reported that more than 90 percent had rated the medical reputation of the hospital as a major consideration in their choice of training institutions. Other factors such as the hospital's location and caseload were

listed as important selection criteria by two-thirds or less of the study group. Collectively, teaching hospitals have had excess supplies of positions for more than three decades, but prestigious hospitals evidently have little difficulty in recruiting trainees. Malt and Grillo (1969) stated that in one recent year, Massachusetts General Hospital had 96 candidates for 12 surgical internship positions even after a preliminary screening. Mumford (1970) found a similar situation at a prestigious (unnamed) hospital in the Midwest. There have been no studies of the choices of training hospitals, but other findings, discussed in the text, imply that the quality of programs is a significant factor in the selection process. Also see Heine (1960) and Hutchins (1961).

4. See Stevens and Vermeulen (1972) and Lockett and Williams (1974) for discussions of the issues concerning FMGs. The demands for FMGs also appear to be segmented between Asian and other graduates. The former, who made up two-thirds of the foreign physician supply, are generally regarded by hospitals as the least desirable trainees.

5. At various times in the past, a few medical schools have offered two-year internships through their affiliated hospitals. Originally, internships were intended to provide a year of clinical training before entry into practice, and residencies, designed for physicians planning to specialize, are a relatively recent innovation. General practitioners ordinarily ended their graduate training with internship service. Physicians who dropped out of residency training might identify themselves either as general practitioners or as specialists in their residency fields. Except for specialty board certification, a matter we will return to below, the medical profession has no legal or private system of specialty classification, and physicians are free to list their specialties in whatever fields they choose.

6. The boards are private agencies operated by the various specialty societies. Most were formed during the 1930s, but the two newest, those for allergy and immunology and for nuclear medicine, were created in 1971.

7. Board certification is frequently used by the public and the medical profession as an indicator of physician quality, but its effect on lifetime earnings has received little research attention. However, tabulations of data on all U.S. practicing physicians in 1965 by Dyckman (1976, pp. 75–76) showed that the average net incomes of board-certified practitioners were 50 to 100 percent higher than those of noncertified practitioners, depending on specialty. The figures were not standardized for physician age, workyear, location, or other characteristics that influence net income levels, but it would be surprising if the differences were explained by these other factors alone. In 1973, 53 percent of all pre-1966 graduates of U.S. medical schools were board-certified, and the percentages for 1955–59 and 1960–64 graduates were 64 and 60, respectively (Martin 1975).

8. The figures include a small number of Canadian graduates who are not ordinarily distinguished from American graduates in published data. In 1973, teaching hospitals represented 24 percent of all U.S. hospitals but 52 percent of total bed capacity (Crowley 1975a).

9. The boards and the medical schools appear to have parallel interests in maintaining the length of residency programs. However, the Council on Medical Education has expressed concern about the time required for specialty certification (AMA 1972, p. 1017). It has been suggested that the state licensing boards also have different conceptions of the amount of training necessary to establish professional competence (Holden 1970). Thus, despite the seeming mutuality of viewpoints of these various controlling organizations, there are indications that they represent something less than a unified front.

10. See, e.g., the discussion in Adams (1962).

11. See, e.g., the favorable comments on NIRMP by the Student American Medical Association (1972).

12. Hospitals' collusive pricing behavior was partly broken in the 1960s, and from 1960 to 1970 the average annual graduate salary rose from approximately $2,500 to $7,500 (AMA 1968, 1972). Whether this was brought about by the excess supply of positions or by other factors is not known. The decade was one of vigorous competition between university and unaffiliated hospitals for graduates, but it was also marked by the growth of private health insurance and the passage of Medicare-Medicaid, which enabled hospitals to pass along their increased costs to private insurers and the federal government. The large inflows of FMGs during the middle and late 1960s were, of course, a depressing influence on graduate salary rates.

13. See Adams (1962). Adams also remarked on instances of tacit or express collusion on pricing in local markets during the 1950s. For a discussion of oligopsonistic and other interpretations of excess demands for hospital labor in a somewhat similar situation, see the analysis of nurse markets by Yett (1975).

14. Since 1965, the AMA has defined three levels of hospital affiliation with medical schools: major, limited, and graduate. Hospitals having major or limited affiliations provide clerkships to medical undergraduates. A major affiliation means that the hospital is also a major teaching site for the medical school's undergraduate program, while a limited affiliation means that it is a minor site. A hospital having a graduate affiliation provides graduate training only. To establish a graduate affiliation, the hospital must have one or more of the following relationships with a medical school: the school must formally assist in the organization and supervision of the graduate program, provide regular faculty teaching services, help the hospital select its trainees, or use the hospital as a training site in conjunction with its major teaching hospital. Accordingly, the type and degree of medical school control over hospitals with graduate (or even limited) affiliations varies greatly. In fact, in some instances hospitals are not even located in the same counties or states as the medical schools with which they are affiliated.

15. For example, in 1970—albeit after a general decline in popularity of the rotating internship—53 percent of the internship positions offered by unaffiliated hospitals, but only 15 percent of the positions offered by affiliated hospitals, were of the rotating type. In the same year, 9 percent of the first-year residency positions in unaffiliated hospitals, and only 2 percent of those in affiliated hospitals, were in general and family practice (AMA 1971).

16. See, e.g., Child (1964) and Renner (1964) for discussions of the archetypal university and community hospitals described above. Especially see Child for an illustrative statement of universities' viewpoints about community hospitals. On the same point, also see Millis (1969) and Peterson and Bendixen (1969). Interestingly, there is little independent evidence of the supposed low quality of community hospitals' graduate programs. The issue was studied by Levit et al. (1963, 1964), who used the performance of interns on Parts II and III of the NBME examination to assess the effects of programs in affiliated hospitals. Interns in affiliated hospitals had the highest scores on both parts of the examination, a result Levit et al. attributed to the greater ability of affiliated hospitals to attract able graduates. But improvement in the test scores (taken before and after internship service) was not significantly different between the two groups of hospitals.

17. See, e.g., Gee and Schumacher (1961), Saunders (1961, 1964), Clute (1963, Chapter 23), and Willard (1964) for statements of and evidence on these points. The negative opinions of Saunders (1961) concerning rotating internships were based on a survey of programs conducted in university hospitals, which indicated that they were not immune from the criticisms leveled at community hospitals. There seems little doubt that hospitals' demands for trainees were strongly conditioned by economic motives. Remarking on the results of a 1962 hospital survey, Campbell (1964) claimed that hospitals sought interns largely to staff their accident floors. (He also reported that interns were desired because graduate programs added to the prestige of the hospital.) The demands for trainees have been an important factor in attracting FMGs into the U.S. (Stevens and Vermeulen 1972; Lockett and Williams 1974), and there are reports that hospitals actively recruited FMGs from abroad (Evans 1970). At the empirical level, only one effort has been made to estimate demand functions for graduate labor, but it suggests that the number of residency positions offered is related to service commitments. Sloan (1970a) estimated an illustrative demand function for residents (in ophthalmology) in which he regressed the number of positions on the resident salary rate, a dummy for medical school affiliation, average daily census, and the number of outpatient visits. Both output measures were significantly positively correlated with the number of positions offered, while the salary rate and affiliation dummy both entered the equation with significantly negative coefficients. The last result tends to support the view that affiliated hospitals were less likely than community hospitals to employ residents for their labor services alone.

18. In 1972, the AAMC issued a statement saying that all graduate medical education should eventually come under the control of medical schools through their affiliated hospitals. Apparently to disassociate itself from that position, the AMA advised community hospitals that they might be able to meet the new program approval conditions by providing training in combination with other institutions. See AMA (1973, p. 954).

19. No firm evidence on this point exists, but there were some indications of such competition even in the 1950s. Curran (1959) reported complaints from

community hospitals that universities held an unfair advantage in graduate recruitment because they were able to influence students' choices during medical school.

20. The figures cited here and in the next paragraph were taken from AMA (1966, 1968, 1971, 1976).

21. It is not known to what degree the shift in USMGs' demands led to the closing of community hospitals' teaching programs before 1970. There are, however, indications that the contraction was accompanied by efforts on the part of such hospitals to obtain medical school affiliations. In 1973, the AMA reported that medical schools were favorably disposed toward these efforts since their own hospital capacity was not adequate to absorb the growing supply of graduates (AMA 1973, p. 954). This supports the view that the integration of internship and residency training was more a device for extending medical schools' control over the quality of graduate training than a market exclusionary tactic. In this respect, the number of teaching hospitals grew from about 1,400 in 1960 to 1,700 in 1970, and the number of hospitals with graduate affiliations only—the weakest form of medical school association—increased from 0 to 141 during the same period.

22. A similar program leading to board certification in internal medicine was also established (e.g., Taylor and Johnson 1973). The program is one year longer than the family practice residency and requires two initial years of clinical training.

23. The specified percentages for fiscal years 1978, 1979, and 1980 were 35, 40, and 50, respectively. If the national average percentage in a given year fell below the target percentage, the requirement was reduced to the target for the preceding year.

24. See, e.g., the comments by Maloney (1970), Perlstadt (1972), and Mechanic (1974).

25. For instance, the university hospital's teaching staff consisted of full-time members of the medical school faculty; the hospital offered only straight internships, routinely filled its internship positions, and accepted few FMGs. The community hospital's teaching staff was composed of part-time attending physicians (i.e., private practitioners); it offered only rotating internships, usually failed to fill all of its positions, and employed a much larger percentage of FMGs than the university hospital. However, the university hospital was probably an extreme example of its type, even in the 1950s. Not all medical schools were as research-oriented as Mumford's, nor did all affiliated hospitals offer only straight internships or successfully fill their internship positions. See, e.g., Saunders (1961) for a somewhat different, and probably more representative, portrait of internship programs in affiliated hospitals during the late 1950s. In the past decade, the range of affiliations has also broadened, so that it would be misleading to regard Mumford's university hospital as characteristic of the majority of affiliated hospitals today.

26. That is, attending physicians were presented as exemplifying the roles the interns were expected to assume. Mumford noted that the staff suggested that interns who planned to start practice in the hospital's community should de-

velop good relationships with attending physicians as a matter of investment. She also noted that a number of physicians in the community had
done their internships or residencies in the hospital.

27. Some of the effects of the environment were less visible. Mumford observed
that interns in the community hospital became careless about record keeping
by the end of their service, abbreviating it whenever possible in the belief
that it was desirable but not essential for good patient care. At the university
hospital, where performance was measured by the accuracy and detail of patient records, interns grew to regard the precision of record keeping as an
important measure of physician competence. Mumford went on to argue
that patient records were the main form of communication between consulting physicians and were used for that purpose in the university hospital. In
the community hospital, where consultation was given a much lower priority, interns failed to learn the specialist's "language." Without it, they presumably became less able, as well as less willing, to communicate professionally with specialists after they entered practice.

28. Glaser (1959) presented a similar argument in an earlier and chiefly nonem-
pirical paper. The chronic excess capacity of graduate training programs,
which tends to increase graduates' range of hospital choices, also favors the
self-selection hypothesis. Knobel (1973) argued that the supply of FMGs is
an additional factor increasing USMGs' bargaining power vis-à-vis the
choice of both hospital and residency specialty. Using a national sample of
data from 1967, he found that FMGs from the least developed countries—
putatively those having the most inferior medical schools—were disproportionately likely to serve in primary care residencies. He contended that the
pattern resulted from the placement of USMGs and FMGs from developed
countries in the preferred referral specialties, with "low-quality" FMGs rele-
gated to the least desirable primary care positions in unaffiliated hospitals.

29. Among respondents intending to enter general practice, 12 percent chose university hospitals, 46 percent chose municipal hospitals, and 42 percent chose
private hospitals. Among respondents intending to enter a specialty, the percentages were 57, 24, and 19, respectively. For prospective academicians and
researchers, the percentages were 76, 15, and 9, respectively.

30. The pathway was similar to the training background that other authors have
described for general practitioners. It was characterized by the physician's
low academic standing, graduation from a clinically oriented medical school,
rotating internship service in an unaffiliated teaching hospital, and no residency training.

31. According to Graettinger (1978), this practice is becoming more prevalent.

32. The small-sample study by Wilensky (1979) cited above reported the same
type of result.

33. Fein and Weber (1971) regressed the fraction of state residency positions
filled by USMGs in 1966 on the percentage of positions offered by unaffiliated hospitals, the average residency salary rate, and the total number of
positions offered divided by the number of 1950–59 graduates practicing in
the state. They argued that the last variable declined as the state's desirability

as a practice site increased, and they found that the regression coefficient on the variable was significantly negative. From those results they inferred that the number of USMG residents increased with the desirability of the state.

Yett and Sloan replaced the "desirability" proxy with four specific measures of the state's attractiveness to physicians: the percentage of population growth due to in-migration, the mean net income of specialists, the percentage of the population living in metropolitan areas, and the mean annual number of degree-days. Individually, the four variables were weakly related to the fraction of residency positions filled by USMGs, and, except in the case of in-migration, the estimated regression coefficients had implausible signs. Yett and Sloan (1974) concluded that physicians do not select their graduate training sites on the basis of their planned practice locations.

34. As was discussed in Chapter 3, the lateness of practice location decisions tends to imply that training location influences the choice of a practice location rather than vice versa. On the other hand, it is evident that practice location decisions are made (and sometimes revised) throughout the entire training process, from preentry into medical school to graduate service. Thus, the site of graduate service may have little effect (and may even depend) on the practice location choices of those physicians who make early decisions, while it may be a critical factor for those who make late decisions.

35. For example, Hadley (1975) found that a physician's choice of state in which to practice was essentially unaffected by characteristics of his or her internship hospital. Thus, even if physicians migrate between states to serve in desirable hospitals, such migration does not appear to materially influence their practice location decisions.

36. Empirical results with respect to special programs to promote decentralized graduate medical training are discussed in Chapter 8.

37. One study has even indicated that the fraction of the physician population entering primary care may be falling (Langwell 1980a).

38. This matter is the subject of some disagreement. See Chapter 8.

SIX

Econometric Studies of Specialty Choice

In preceding chapters we alluded to certain aspects of specialty choice behavior which are compatible with a priori expectations. In many ways, however, that discussion overstated the contribution of theory to an understanding of observed behavior. This is because of the lack of comprehensive theoretical models of occupational choice—comparable, say, with economic models of consumer choice or firm behavior —which can be translated into a working empirical framework.

The early sociological work by Ginzberg et al. (1951), Blau et al. (1956), and Super (1957)—which is still the foundation of noneconomic research in the field—held that occupational choice is a developmental process which may take place over many years. During this process individuals acquire a growing knowledge of their self-image and desired professional role, their capabilities and limitations, and information about the choice alternatives and the means of achieving them. Blau et al. emphasized that social attitudes affect the process as well. More particularly, they contended that social structures condition the individual's self-image, provide or deny training opportunities, and ultimately admit the individual into an occupation.

Although sociological theory has advanced a general model of occupational choice, it has never rigorously hypothesized the precise mechanism of selection. As a result, empirical research based on this framework has sought chiefly to identify variables (e.g., family background, intelligence, sex, race, personal attitudes, training opportunities, and barriers to entry) which may account for differences in choices.[1]

Economic theories of occupational choice ordinarily do not treat role selection as a fundamental element of the decision process. A common hypothesis in the economics literature two decades or so ago is that occupations are chosen to maximize the individual's anticipated lifetime earnings (e.g., Becker 1963). More recently, the income-maximization hypothesis has been replaced by a general utility-maximizing hypothesis in which the choice is assumed to reflect tastes and preferences regarding income, leisure, and borrowing (e.g., Thurow 1970; Freeman 1971; Lindsay 1973; Becker 1975). Training costs, initial wealth, and interest rates (or access to borrowing) are absorbed into the constraints on the decision. Insofar as they are recognized at all, role preferences are subsumed under the individual's tastes. Yet economists, unlike sociologists, have not attempted to model the longitudinal character or other details of occupational selection.

Econometric research on occupational choice has followed two approaches. The first takes the individual as the unit of analysis, and the researcher estimates the probabilities of a person's choosing among a discrete number of occupational alternatives. The variables used to predict the probabilities include individual attributes such as sex and race, and characteristics of the alternatives such as income and training costs (Boskin 1974; Schmidt and Strauss 1975b). The second approach employs the market as the unit of analysis. Using time-series data, the researcher estimates a long-run labor supply curve for the occupation—i.e., the number of persons entering it—as a function of lifetime earnings (or a proxy) and other relevant variables (Freeman 1975a, 1975b).

Only four econometric studies of physicians' specialty choices have been undertaken, one following the market approach and the other three employing an individual or micro model. Since they represent the current "state of the art," these four econometric models of specialty selection will be considered in some detail. But first, by way of background, we will discuss the general influences on specialty choice that all such models should address.

THE ELEMENTS OF SPECIALTY CHOICE

One reason that no general economic model of occupational choice exists is that modeling efforts to date have been designed for a variety of specific purposes. For example, some models of occupational choice have been constructed to give a broad conceptual account of behavior, while others were intended to provide a realistic and detailed understanding of some particular aspect of the process. Some were meant to predict the outcomes of career decisions without explaining them. Others were tailored for a given set of data or a particular estimation technique. Still others were designed to highlight special features of behavior such as those amenable to policy influence. More often than not, objectives such as these involve the use of specific types of choice models in which certain—but differing—variables or dimensions of behavior are stressed.

Another reason for the lack of a general economic model of occupational choice is that some aspects of career decisions are inherently difficult to model. In the case at hand, for example, most physicians choose their specialties well before entry into practice, in greater or lesser ignorance of income opportunities and practice working conditions. Hence, the researcher must decide whether to introduce uncertainty regarding these factors into the model or to treat specialty choices as though they occur with perfect knowledge and foresight. Those who elect the first approach must devise methods for dealing with: (1) the amount and reliability of information the physician receives, (2) the physician's perceptions of the information and attitudes toward risk, and (3) the mathematical formulation of uncertainty.

These difficulties notwithstanding, it is important to adopt a general framework for examining physician specialty decisions. The one that we feel is best suited is adapted from a model proposed by Freeman (1971). In this model there are l different occupations (specialties) indexed by i ($= 1, \ldots, l$). In the present context, a physician can be regarded as choosing the specialty i and number of work hours which yield the highest level of utility:

$$U[w_i x_i sh + W, (1 - s)L + n_i x_i sh], i = 1, \ldots, l, \qquad (1)$$

where U is the physician's utility function and

> w_i = the pecuniary rate of earnings in specialty i,
>
> x_i = 1 if the physician selects specialty i, and 0 otherwise,
>
> s = the proportion of time spent working ($0 \leqq s \leqq 1$),
>
> h = the maximum number of hours available for work or leisure,
>
> W = net nonlabor income,
>
> L = the rate of nonpecuniary or "psychic" income derived from leisure,
>
> n_i = the rate of nonpecuniary or "psychic" income from practicing in specialty i.

A plausible hypothesis[2] is that the physician selects values of i and s that maximize a utility function depending on pecuniary income $w_i x_i sh + W$ and nonpecuniary income $(1 - s)L + n_i x_i sh$. Provided the utility function and underlying decision process satisfy the usual assumptions,[3] the model also extends to other types of optimizing behavior. For example, the physician might normally be expected to make trade-offs between pecuniary and nonpecuniary income. However, if the marginal utility of nonpecuniary income is zero, the choice becomes a pecuniary-income-maximizing decision. Conversely, if the marginal utility of pecuniary income is zero, the choice becomes a nonpecuniary-income-maximizing decision compatible with role-model or similar noneconomic theories. If both marginal utilities are zero, the choice can be thought of as a satisficing decision in which two or more specialties satisfy the physician's minimum desires for pecuniary and nonpecuniary income.

Consider next the major components of the model and their implications for empirical analysis of specialty choice.

The Present Value of Lifetime Earnings

Suppose the physician decides on a specialty in a given year (designated as 1). Since a first year of graduate training is ordinarily required for licensure, year 1 is likely to be the beginning of the second or any later residency year.[4] Suppose further that the physician expects to work T years before retiring. Let y_{it} denote the net income he or she expects to receive in the i'th specialty for the t'th year following his or her decision. Then the present value (PV) of anticipated lifetime earnings in specialty i is:

$$PV(w_i x_i sh) = \sum_{t=1}^{T} [1/(1 + r)]^t y_{it}, \quad i = 1, \ldots, l, \qquad (2)$$

where r is an interest or discount rate. The expression can be estimated by applying reasonable values of r to sample data on annual net income in the i'th specialty. The latter (e.g., compiled as averages or medians) must come from figures for practitioners at different stages (years) spanned by their earnings, including the period of residency training (e.g., Sloan 1970b).

Clearly, the actual lifetime earnings for a specific physician depend on a number of discretionary and nondiscretionary variables. The expected productive lifespan T and the appropriate discount rate r may vary from individual to individual. Up to a point, physicians can affect their hourly rates of income by their choices of pricing policy, location, patients, practice setting, scale of practice, outputs of laboratory or x-ray services, etc. Furthermore, physicians' perceptions of their income opportunities may vary from individual to individual even though the actual income opportunities are the same.[5] As a practical matter, these qualifications imply that virtually any estimates of lifetime earnings or hourly income rates are likely to be, at best, rough approximations of actual earnings expectations.[6]

Yet despite these (essentially empirical) problems, certain theoretical propositions can be derived from the role that lifetime earnings expectations play in the utility-maximizing apparatus sketched above. One concerns the interrelationships between the physician's age, earnings expectations, and specialty choice. Specifically, income considerations should lead physicians to select a length of training that varies with their age at the beginning of their productive life. The older physicians are at the start of their training, the shorter, ceteris paribus, should be the length of training planned. Since specialization ordinarily requires a longer rather than shorter period of graduate training, physicians who are relatively older at the time they make the choice should tend to choose general practice or a generalized (e.g., primary care) field at higher rates than those who are younger.

Consider, for example, two career options open to every physician. Let option 1 denote the alternative of ending training and beginning practice in year $t = 1$ (i.e., at the end of the first graduate year). This can be called the general practice option. Let option 2 denote the alternative of taking another year or more of graduate training starting in year $t = 1$, with entry into practice deferred until a later date. Assuming that this option involves at least some specialty training for the physician, it can be called the specialty practice option. Let y_{1t} stand for the physician's expected annual income in year t if he or she chooses option 1, and let y_{2t} stand for expected annual income in year t if he or she selects option 2. Ordinarily, y_{1t} should be larger than y_{2t} for t close to 1; but since annual incomes are usually higher for specialists than for general practitioners, the reverse should be true as t grows beyond 1. The difference between total discounted lifetime earnings for career options 1 and 2 is

$$\sum_{t=1}^{T}[1/(1 + r)]^t(y_{1t} - y_{2t}), \tag{3}$$

where the annual income differences $y_{1t} - y_{2t}$ are discounted much more heavily for large t than for small t.[7]

Assuming that the physician plans to retire at a given age, the length of his or her productive life varies inversely with his or her age at the beginning of it. Hence, if the physician is sufficiently old at $t = 1$, the difference in lifetime earnings is positive, and career option 1 yields the higher income. Only if the physician is young enough to anticipate having a long productive life in which to recover income forgone in the early years of training will career option 2 prove to be the more remunerative choice.

Since option 2 can be regarded as specialty training or training leading to board certification, the comparison of lifetime earnings in equation (3) implies, ceteris paribus, that: (1) the older physicians are at the end of internship, the more likely they are to choose general practice; and (2) the older physicians are in any year of graduate training, the less likely they are to become board-certified. It is also evident that: (3) the sooner physicians plan to retire, the more likely they are to choose general practice; and (4) any increase in physicians' income as residents (e.g., in the form of salary, grant, gift, or fellowship) reduces their likelihood of choosing general practice and increases their likelihood of seeking board certification. Hypotheses 2 through 4 have not been adequately tested but existing evidence supports the validity of hypothesis 1.[8]

Ability

As a rule, specialties require a variety of intellectual, physical, social, and emotional skills, each of which contributes to the value of a physician's output. Since all specialties do not demand the same types or amounts of skills, the value of a given ability presumably varies from field to field. For example, the "shadow price"—i.e., the implicit or imputed value—of skill in interpersonal relationships is probably high in primary care practice, but low in specialties such as radiology and pathology where there is less physician-patient contact.

Using Freeman's approach, the role of ability in the physician's specialty choice decision can be represented as follows:

$$w_i = \sum_{k=1}^{K} p_{ik} a_k + B, i = 1, \ldots, l.$$

As before, w_i stands for the expected hourly net income rate. K is the total number of relevant abilities; a_k is the individual's endowment (in units) of the k'th ability; p_{ik} is the shadow price of the k'th ability in the i'th specialty; and B denotes the effects of other decisions such as the choice of practice setting, etc.[9]

Because units of ability and their shadow prices are not observable, the expression has limited empirical applications. Nevertheless, it does imply that individual endowments of abilities affect specialty choices through their impact on expected incomes. In particular—other things being equal—physicians are not likely to choose specialties which place high shadow prices on skills they lack. Unfortunately, this raises still another problem with respect to using *observed* lifetime earnings differentials (or annual net incomes) to predict specialty choices. If physicians do select specialties where their skills are most highly valued, sample data on annual net incomes will overstate their forgone net income opportunities in the specialties *they did not choose*. For instance, a physician may well select a specialty where observed lifetime earnings are lower than in other fields. Yet the decision may still be income-motivated because that physician's particular endowment of skills provides *him or her* with a higher expected earnings stream in the first specialty than the others. We will return to this matter below. The point we want to stress here is that observed annual net incomes may not be reliable measures of the earnings opportunities that *individual* physicians face when they choose their specialties.

Little empirical evidence regarding the effects of ability on specialty choices exists. In Chapter 3 it was shown that such measures of ability as MCAT scores, medical school GPAs, and National Board scores are related to specialty choices. But it is not clear what skill dimensions these measures capture. Moreover, the effects of manual dexterity, insightfulness, skill in patient management, and other abilities have not been studied.

A further complicating factor is that endowments of abilities themselves may be related to physicians' tastes. That is, individuals may sharpen the skills required for an activity because they enjoy the activity, or they may prefer activities in which they are especially skillful. In either case, the "psychic income" individuals derive from a specialty will be positively related to their skill level in performing the specialty's activities. Accordingly, the effects of preferences may reinforce those of income opportunities in specialty decisions. This, of course, complicates the problem of determining the extent to which preferences and income expectations, respectively, account for the observed associations between specialty choices and dimensions of physician ability.

The Present Value of Net Lifetime Nonlabor Income

Ordinarily, the value of physicians' lifetime nonlabor income (W) can be expected to be higher the greater their initial wealth. Assuming that the marginal utility of pecuniary income diminishes as total lifetime earnings increase (i.e., that the marginal utility of income falls as income increases), several empirical hypotheses follow. In particular, physicians from the wealthiest families should be the least sensitive to lifetime earnings differentials when they choose specialties. Conversely, they should be the most sensitive to perceived psychic income differentials. In addition, since any unrestricted grant, gift, or scholarship preserves or enhances a medical student's initial wealth, it should weaken his or her responsiveness to income differentials in deciding on a specialty. Large expenditures during medical school should have the opposite effect, but their impact should be greatest on the least wealthy students.

If perfectly functioning markets for human capital services existed, borrowing to finance a medical education or to augment current income during training would not affect specialty decisions. Physicians who borrow for such purposes would have to forgo future income by the amount of interest payments required. Physicians who are self-financing in effect borrow from their families or themselves. They forgo future income by the amount of interest payments they could have received from lending funds to someone else. Thus, if the relevant borrowing and lending rates were the same, the physician who borrows and the physician who is self-financing would forgo the same amounts of future income (given the size and the payback provisions of the loan). Consequently, each would face the same structure of expected income opportunities, and, if they were otherwise identical, their specialty choices should be the same.

There are, however, many imperfections in the markets for human capital. Accordingly, for any of several reasons, physicians who borrow to finance their medical education have greater incentives than those who are self-financing to curtail their graduate training. In particular, lacking collateral to pledge as security for the loan, they may be unable to borrow beyond a certain amount at any interest rate. Or, if they can borrow, they must typically pay interest rates higher than those they would impute to themselves if they were self-financing.[10] Or they may be averse to the risks inherent in accumulating large debts. In each of these cases, physicians who borrow may be constrained by the amount of financing they can secure, or else faced with large (or psychically onerous) payment obligations if they decide to extend their graduate training.

Because those who borrow most extensively during medical training are likely to be the least wealthy students, the foregoing considerations suggest, ceteris paribus, that they are the ones who will tend to take the shortest periods of graduate training. Hence, they are disproportionately likely to enter general practice or, if they choose other fields, not to become board-certified or to subspecialize. Although it is fragmentary at best, the empirical evidence described in Chapter 3 is compatible with these hypotheses.

The Present Value of Lifetime Nonpecuniary Income

The second argument of the utility function 1 represents the effects on specialty decisions of the psychic incomes derived from leisure $(1 - s)L$ and specialty-related working conditions $n_i x_i sh$. Most of these effects are immediately evident. For example, physicians who place the highest shadow prices on their leisure time (i.e., on time not spent in practicing medicine) will tend to work the fewest hours and to select specialties whose hours and other working conditions interfere least with their nonprofessional activities. As shown in Chapter 3, women physicians who marry and bear children display these tendencies. Indeed, their behavior is possibly the clearest testimony to the impact of high-priced leisure time (due to marital roles) on physician career decisions.[11]

The expected nonpecuniary income derived from practicing in the i'th specialty can be recast formally in a manner consistent with the noneconomic interpretations of specialty choice. First, assume that the various specialties embody J different characteristics or activities which generate different amounts of utility to the physician. Next, let z_{ij} and N_j denote the average number of units per hour in the i'th specialty and the shadow price of the j'th such attribute ($j = 1, \ldots, J$).

Then the average nonpecuniary income rate in the i'th specialty can be written

$$n_i = \sum_{j=1}^{J} N_j z_{ij}, \quad i = 1, \ldots, I.$$

That is, the psychic income rate (n_i) the physician attaches to the i'th specialty depends on its attributes (the z_{ij}) and the unit values the physician assigns to these attributes (the N_j). The attributes might include such things as patient contact, the intellectual demands of the field, regularity of working hours, control over the outcomes of patient care, or any group of factors that physicians perceive as defining specialties.

However, since neither attribute levels nor the values that physicians attach to them are directly observable, the applications of this formal expression are chiefly qualitative. In particular, it is useful as a theoretical framework for depicting the roles of the variables stressed in the noneconomic studies of specialty choice (discussed in Chapters 2 and 3). In those studies, specialty choices are typically correlated with physicians' personality or background traits under the hypothesis that physicians choose fields which best enable them to fulfill their preferred professional roles. This approach can be cast in the context of the economic specification that a physician assigns a psychic income rate to each alternative specialty.

First, assume that each specialty is reasonably well characterized by a set of attribute levels. Hence, its utility-generating properties will vary among physicians according to the different shadow prices that they attach to its attributes. Physicians should tend, other things being equal, to choose the field whose attributes they value most highly because by doing so they are likely to derive the greatest utility.

Since it is reasonable to suppose that individuals with different personality and/or background traits place different values on the same attributes, the economic approach, in effect, argues that these traits ought to be correlated with specialty choices. The traits themselves can be viewed as proxies for the shadow prices of the various specialty attributes.

The use of the psychic income rate expression can be extended a step further to suggest how medical education affects specialty choices. Thus far it has been implicitly assumed that the values physicians give to specialty attributes are predetermined, and that the attributes are also fixed. Obviously, the nature of physicians' educational experiences can influence both their perceptions of the attributes and their evaluations of them. One type of experience may convince the physician that specialty i has low levels of attributes he or she values highly (for example, professional status), while another might suggest that the same field has high levels of the desired attributes. Similarly, such factors as the types of curricula physicians are exposed to, faculty role models, and experience with research or patient management may all affect the value they implicitly assign to each attribute. In either case, the medical educational environment may alter the structure of psychic incomes physicians expect to receive from alternative specialties. Hence, by directly affecting he amounts of utility physicians anticipate from alternative career choices, medical training programs have the potential to significantly influence the choice of a specialty.

The foregoing argument provides a useful way of interpreting the environmental theories of specialty choice reviewed in Chapters 4 and 5. This approach also highlights the empirical testing issues considered in those chapters. Namely, it is intrinsically very difficult to disentangle the effects of predetermined specialty preferences from those attributable to the influence of the educational environment in empirically implementing models of specialty choice. Taken alone, either innate preferences or educational experiences could explain how physicians come to perceive the psychic incomes they anticipate from their specialty choices. Ideally, a general theory of specialty choice should provide a means of assessing the relative magnitudes of the impacts of preestablished preferences and preferences induced by medical education. The development and testing of such a general theory constitutes an important challenge for future research.

EMPIRICAL STUDIES

The foregoing discussion was intended to show that most of the implicit or explicit theories of specialty choice can be accommodated within a framework that postulates utility-maximizing behavior on the part of physicians. However, to date, the empirical work by economists has concentrated on the role of pecuniary income opportunities in specialty decisions. In one sense, this merely reflects the central position that prices—here the price of physicians' time—occupy in economists' thinking. In terms of the proposition that the quantity of any commodity or service supplied depends on price, the choice of specialty becomes one of several factors determining the supply of a particular type of physician manpower. Ceteris paribus, the rate of entry into a field should rise or fall as the rate of lifetime earnings in the field rises or falls relative to earnings in other specialties. If it does not, the economist's typical reaction is to search for evidence of market imperfections and appropriate remedial policies.

Some forms of physician manpower policy involve offering income incentives to physicians to induce them to make desired specialty or practice location choices. (We will consider the findings relating to such policies in Chapter 8.) The important point, with respect to the issue at hand, is that such policies *presume* some noticeable degree of responsiveness by physicians to income opportunities when they make their career decisions. But much of the research we have reviewed so far indicates that specialty choices are not markedly income-motivated. If correct, such findings imply that programs relying on income incentives to promote given types of specialty choices will be ineffective. In this context, it is unfortunately the case that assessing the effects of income motivation on specialty choice is easier said than done. The principal difficulty involves measuring the income opportunities themselves. In the studies we now turn to, different approaches were taken regarding the measurement issue, and different methods were used to derive and interpret the empirical results.

The first of the four econometric studies of specialty choice is by Sloan (1970a), who estimated market-level demands for residency positions (i.e., the supplies of physicians by residency specialty) in nine fields. He specified two alternative demand equations, which were of the forms:

$$R_t = a_0 + a_1 E_{t-1} + a_2 P_t + a_3 F_t \qquad (4a)$$
$$R_t/P_t = b_0 + b_1 E_{t-1} + b_2 F_t, \qquad (4b)$$

where the a's and b's are constants, t denotes the year of observation ($t=$ 1956, 1960, and 1966) and

R_t = number of residents in the specialty,

E_{t-1} = present value of lifetime earnings in the specialty lagged by one year,

P_t = number of residency positions offered in the specialty,

F_t = number of foreign medical graduates in all residency positions.

To construct the lifetime earnings estimates, Sloan assumed that physicians: (1) take four years of residency training beginning at age 27; (2) follow their residency training with two years of military service; and (3) enter practice at age 33 and retire at age 65. He discounted the lifetime earnings estimates at alternate rates of 5 percent and 10 percent.[12]

Sloan's reasoning underlying the demand equations 4a and 4b is straightforward. If specialty choices are sensitive to lifetime earnings differentials, higher values of lifetime earnings should induce larger values of R_t and R_t/P_t. That is, specialties having the highest lifetime earnings should attract the largest numbers of residents and the highest proportions of filled positions. When Sloan estimated the equations, he found that the coefficients on lagged lifetime earnings were, as his hypothesis predicted, significantly positive. But they were also numerically small. Indeed, they indicated that for most specialties a doubling or tripling of lifetime earnings would increase the number of residents in the field by less than 100 per year. On those grounds, Sloan concluded that lifetime earnings differentials do not have a material impact on specialty choices.

However, owing to weaknesses in the specifications of the regressions, Sloan's conclusion is tenuous. First, it is not consistent with economic theory to specify the quantity of a good or service supplied as a determinant of the quantity demanded, as is the case with respect to his first regression in which the number of positions supplied, P_t, is used to "explain" the number of positions demanded, R_t.[13] Likewise, the second regression cannot be interpreted as being either a demand or a supply function for residency positions. The proportions of specialty positions that are filled depend on the number that are offered as well as on the number demanded. Regardless of how attractive a residency field is, specialty programs in that field could have low percentages of filled positions if hospitals persist in offering many more positions than are demanded. Thus, the implications of Sloan's second regression regarding the demands for specialty training are unclear.

Still another problem with Sloan's regression equations 4a and 4b is that they do not standardize for nonpecuniary differences among specialties. That is, each medical school graduate is assumed to select a type of training (or specialty) solely on the basis of the lifetime earnings associated with it. This is an extremely strong hypothesis which precludes the influence of tastes, skills, and other nonpecuniary factors on specialty decisions.[14] (It also precludes the possibility of substitution effects among choices—i.e., that demands for training in one field change as lifetime earnings in other fields change—since the demand for positions in each specialty depends only on lifetime earnings in that particular specialty.) Although many of the findings discussed in Chapters 2 and 3 were not available at the time of Sloan's study, it is now evident that physicians' tastes play a large part in their specialty choices. Consequently, tastes are important omitted variables in his regression equations. And it is known from econometric theory that the omission of significant variables can bias the estimates of the coefficients on the variables that are included. As a result, it is doubtful whether estimates of equations 4a and 4b would adequately measure physicians' income motivation even if the supply of residency positions were deleted from the regressions.

The second econometric study of specialty choice—and the most comprehensive to date—is by Hadley (1975, 1977, 1979). Using a model of individual choice, Hadley estimated the probabilities of selecting five (1975, 1977) and nine (1979) specialties or groups of specialties. Included among them were general practice, the other primary care fields, and various of the referral specialties. Hadley estimated a separate regression for each specialty or specialty group, with the dependent variable defined as one if the physician chose the field and zero otherwise. His data consisted of a large cross-sectional sample of records from the AAMC's longitudinal study of 1960 medical graduates.

Three sets of explanatory variables were included in the regressions. They represented proxies for various elements of the lifetime earnings expression described above (net annual income by specialty and state, MCAT and National Board scores, age, sex, marital status, parental occupation, etc.), nonpecuniary income (specialty prestige, personality and career preference traits, religious preference, size of hometown, etc.), and educational experience (characteristics of the physician's medical school and internship hospital).

Three of the explanatory variables—net annual specialty income, a measure of specialty prestige (the fraction of filled residency positions in the field),[15] and the modal length of postgraduate training in the field— were specific to the choice alternatives. In order to introduce variation in these variables across the sample members, Hadley employed the following convention. With X_i denoting the value of any of the three variables for the i'th specialty, he respecified each in ratio form X_i/X_j, where j indexes an "alternative" specialty and X_j is the value of the given variable for the alternative specialty. The alternative field was defined as: (1) the specialty actually chosen by the physician if it was not specialty i; or (2) the last previous field preferred by the physician if, in fact, he or she selected specialty i but had once preferred a different field; or (3) the modal specialty choice of the physician's medical school class if he or she chose specialty i and had never stated a preference for another field.

Many of Hadley's findings have been described in the preceding chapters. Consistent with the results of the personality and background studies of specialty choice, the most significant predictors of the choice probabilities were personality-trait measures relating to specialty tastes.

The selection probability for general practice was positively related to the physician's age at graduation, having a large family, and having a rural upbringing, but the probability of choosing another field was generally not significantly associated with any of these background variables. This, too, is compatible with other results.

Measures of the physician's academic performance tended to be poor predictors of the choice probabilities, as did medical school characteristics such as average class MCAT scores. In one version of his study (1977), Hadley indicated that internship hospital attributes were generally not significantly related to the choice probabilities. However, when he used a nine-way specialty classification (1979), he found that, as a group, these attributes were about as significant as the personality-trait proxies. On the average, his regressions accurately predicted from 54 to 58 percent of the specialty choices—a success rate comparable to those reported by the personality studies described in Chapter 2.

Hadley's regressions did, however, produce several anomalous results in terms of occupational choice theory. First, the coefficients on the income variable either were not significantly different from zero or else were significantly negative. This indicates that increases in specialty net incomes vis-à-vis alternatives generally do not affect the choice probabilities, and may even lower them. Second, the coefficients on the length-of-training variable were almost uniformly positive and in many cases significantly so. This pattern conflicts with the theoretical proposition that —other things being equal—lifetime income incentives should lead physicians to select fields with the shortest periods of graduate training. Third, in two-thirds of the equations the coefficients on the specialty prestige variable were negative, implying that a reduction in the prestige of these fields raises the probabilities that physicians will select them. The first two of these three results led Hadley to conclude that specialty choices are insensitive to income differentials across the fields.

Because of their potential policy importance, Hadley's results deserve closer examination. In particular, it could be argued that they are at least partly due to the definitions of the income and length-of-training variables he employed. First, it is questionable whether specialty lifetime earnings differentials are accurately reflected by mean *annual* net income differences across fields, even when the physician's age at graduation and the length of residency training are included in the regressions as standardizing variables.

Second, Hadley's specification of the relative net income, length-of-training, and specialty prestige variables involves "alternative" fields which the physician may not have considered in making his or her specialty choice. Suppose, for example, the i'th field is general practice, and let Y_i and Y_j denote mean annual net incomes in general practice and the "alternative" field, respectively. As described above, relative income opportunities between general practice and other fields were characterized by the variable Y_i/Y_j in the general practice regression. If the physician chose general practice but had earlier preferred another specialty, Y_j was defined as the income in the last such field. In this case, presumably, Y_i/Y_j captures the marginal influence of income differences on the physician's choice between two fields he or she had actively considered. But if the physician selected general practice without expressing a prior preference for another specialty, Y_j was assigned an essentially arbitrary value. And if the physician chose specialty j, Y_i/Y_j was still designated as the relative income attractiveness variable even though the physician may never have preferred general practice. As a result, the definitions of Y_i/Y_j differ conceptually across physicians, and it is at least doubtful whether either of the last two definitions correctly represents relative income opportunities as physicians perceive them.[16]

Third, Hadley's regressions embody the restrictive assumption that the effects of length of training on specialty choices are independent of those of income. This can be seen as follows. Let Z_i and Z_j stand for the modal lengths of graduate training in specialties i and j. Since the equations were linear, the relative income and length-of-training variables appeared in the i'th specialty equation as the expression $a(Y_i/Y_j) + b(Z_i/Z_j)$, where a and b are parameters. The coefficient b is interpreted as the marginal change in the probability of choosing specialty i due to a change in Z_i/Z_j, given that the effects of all other variables *including* Y_i/Y_j are held constant. That is, to interpret the equation, one *assumes* that changing the lengths of training between specialties has no impact on relative specialty incomes. If physicians are income-motivated, this assumption is clearly false. Medical school graduates would avoid specialties with long residencies because they had zero investment values. As the numbers of entrants into these fields declined, ceteris paribus, net incomes in them would rise to new long-run equilibrium values. In effect, Hadley's specifications precluded the possibility of inferring income motivation from the coefficients on Z_i/Z_j. His finding that the coefficients were mostly positive is arguably more the result of his assumption that length of training has no effect on income than it is evidence that specialty choices are insensitive to income.

On balance, Hadley's conclusion that specialty choices are at most weakly income-motivated is, like Sloan's, vulnerable to criticism, and it too should be regarded as tenuous. More recent work on the issue has concentrated on geographic location as a determinant of income differentials across fields and on methodological refinements of specialty choice models.

Using 1975 data and a technique similar to Sloan's (but with adjustments for differences in work hours and years), Langwell (1980b) estimated lifetime earnings for physicians in four specialty groupings (general/family practice, other primary care fields, surgery, and other nonprimary care fields) and three types of geographic areas (rural, semirural/small urban, and urban counties). Although she did not attempt to model specialty choices, she did report a surprising pattern of specialty earnings differentials across fields. According to her estimates, the present values of general/family practitioners' lifetime incomes were uniformly higher than those of specialists in urban counties, and mostly lower than those of specialists in rural counties.

These findings have provocative implications for physicians' specialty choice behavior. If specialty choices are predominantly income-motivated, one would expect physicians planning urban practice locations to select general/family practice, and those planning rural locations to select a specialty. In any event, we should observe a large proportion of physicians entering general/family practice because of its comparative income advantage over the specialties in urban areas where most physicians settle. In fact, the evidence shows neither that general/family practitioners have disproportionately large tendencies to choose urban practice locations nor that specialists are exceptionally likely to choose rural locations. Moreover, general/family practitioners do not constitute a large portion of the physician population. Consequently, Langwell's results are consistent with two alternative interpretations. Either the structure of comparative earnings between general/family practice and the specialties is changing and the structure of physician supply has not yet adapted to it, or—as Sloan and Hadley argued—physicians' career choices are not predominantly income-motivated.

In the past decade, econometricians have employed a variety of statistical models to predict and analyze individuals' choices in situations where there are two or more discrete choice alternatives. The most widely used are known as "logit" models because they utilize the bivariate or multinomial logistic probability distribution.[17] A natural application of logit models is to individuals' occupational choices, and the final two studies of physicians' specialty choices discussed here both used variants of the multinomial logit model.

Using a simultaneous logit model proposed by Schmidt and Strauss (1975a, 1975b), Werner et al. (1978) estimated the probabilities that a physician would select general practice (as opposed to a specialty) and a practice location in a shortage county (as opposed to a nonshortage county). Despite the narrowness of this choice classification, their model —unlike others—explicitly included location as a predictor of specialty and specialty as a predictor of location. Their other explanatory variables consisted of three background traits—indicators of age at entry into practice, sex, and rural upbringing—and four self-reported career attitudes—measures of the individual's desires to locate where there were continuing education facilities and a high medical need, the importance of income as a locational influence, and the importance of a loan-forgiveness program as a locational influence. The data were the same as those used by Heald et al. (1974) and Cooper et al. (1975), which have been discussed in other chapters.

The results with respect to background traits were similar to those obtained in other studies. Older physicians, males, and physicians reared in rural communities were especially likely to select general practice. Those practicing or planning to practice in rural communities were also significantly more likely to choose general practice than a specialty. Physicians desiring proximity to continuing education facilities, those whose location plans had been influenced by loan-forgiveness programs, and those desiring to locate in areas of high medical need were found to be significantly more likely to choose general practice than a specialty.[18]

Of special noteworthiness, however, was the effect of the attitudinal variable—the importance of income opportunities as a locational influence—on specialty choices. The variable itself was significantly positively related to the probability of selecting a specialty rather than a general practice. This suggests that income motivation in some sense affected the choices between fields. Beyond that, it is difficult to know what to make of the finding. It could be interpreted as merely showing that some physicians' career decisions are probably income-motivated. But it tells us nothing about how sensitive physicians are to differences in income opportunities.

The most recent econometric study of specialty selection is by Hay (1980, 1981). It is of particular interest here because of its methodological implications. Earlier we remarked that observed earnings levels among specialties may not accurately represent the alternative income opportunities that individual physicians perceive when they make their career choices. For instance, individuals who chose specialty A might have done so because their particular skills brought greater financial rewards in A than in other specialties. If the physicans who chose specialties B, C, etc., behaved in the same way, actual incomes observed in the latter fields would overstate the earnings that physicians who selected specialty A would have received had they chosen a specialty different from A. Under these circumstances, actual earnings levels are upward-biased estimates of the incomes physicians would have been likely to earn in specialties other than the ones they chose. The resulting measurement bias is likely to distort the findings from econometric efforts to measure the sensitivity of specialty choices to net income differences.

Arguing in this vein, Hay proposed the hypothesis that specialty choices and specialty earnings are jointly dependent. Under his hypothesis, single-equation estimates of specialty choice probabilities—i.e., estimates obtained by assuming that choice probabilities depend on earnings levels but not vice versa—are subject to simultaneous-equations bias. Moreover, it is known that the effect of this type of bias is to give spuriously low estimates of the impact of specialty earnings on choice probabilities. Hay therefore argued that his hypothesis would be confirmed if a single-equation regression of the choice probabilities yielded a smaller coefficient on specialty earnings (treated as exogenous) than a simultaneous-equations model in which the choice probabilities and earnings were treated as jointly dependent.[19]

To test his hypothesis, Hay first formulated a simultaneous logit and ordinary least squares model of specialty choice with the choice probabilities and earnings defined as jointly endogenous. He designated three specialty groups (general practice, internal medicine, and other specialties) and fitted the model to a large sample of 1970 data on physicians in practice. Specialty earnings were defined as physicians' annual net incomes, and the model included exogenous variables denoting physicians' background traits (age, sex, race, and country of medical school graduation) and, for U.S. medical graduates, medical school environments (type of ownership and a measure of the school's research orientation). He next estimated a single-equation model of the choice probabilities using the same data and the same set of background and medical school descriptors, but with specialty net income added as an exogenous variable.

The estimates of the two models strongly supported Hay's hypothesis. In the estimated single-equation model, the specialty choice probabilities were negatively and not significantly related to net income. But in the simultaneous-equations model, the probabilities were positively and significantly correlated with specialty net income.

Inasmuch as his sample consisted partly of foreign medical graduates, Hay's results are not strictly comparable to those of Sloan, Hadley, or Werner et al.[20] Moreover, as has already been noted, one can question the use of annual net incomes as proxies for specialty lifetime earnings. Nevertheless, the findings are important for two reasons. First, they constitute the only *econometric* evidence to date that physicians' specialty choice decisions are income-motivated. Second, they raise serious doubts about the reliability of estimated specialty choice–earnings relationships that are derived from the assumption that earnings are exogenous to the relationship.

In particular, they suggest that Hadley's and Sloan's models—in which specialty earnings were treated as exogenous—underestimated the strength of physicians' pecuniary motivation. In both models earnings were defined as mean values over all the physicians who actually chose a given specialty. To the extent that there is variation among physicians in terms of the types of talents they possess—and among specialties in terms of the rewards each affords different talents—this is an unrealistic assumption. Hay's results indicate that this assumption may have distorted our previous understanding of specialty choice behavior.

SUMMARY

For the most part, the various noneconomic theories of physicians' specialty choices hold that the basic influences are nonpecuniary. In contrast, economic theories hold that—given such factors as tastes, skills, work hours, and barriers to entry—career choices are determined by differences in the net present values of expected lifetime earnings. Although neither type of theory excludes the other, they have different implications regarding appropriate policies to influence physicians' specialty choices. The first type of theory implies that a target distribution of new physicians can be achieved by controlling the types of persons admitted to medical schools and by modifying the learning environment itself. The second type of theory contends that the same result can be achieved by altering the structure of specialty net lifetime earnings through subsidies (or, in principle, taxes) provided during physicians' medical education. Although the prescribed policies in each case are not mutually exclusive, their relative costliness and chances for success are clearly contingent on the actual strength of physicians' income motivation in selecting specialties.

There are several a priori grounds for believing that income motivation has, in fact, only a minor effect on the majority of physicians' specialty choices. Typically, physicians come from families with above-average incomes; make their choices in greater or lesser ignorance of their future earnings; may decide on fields under short-run academic pressures to commit themselves; and can influence their earnings streams by location and managerial decisions made after they enter practice. Each of these factors militates against income motivation as a major force acting on physicians' specialty decisions.

The econometric evidence on the issue can best be described as inconclusive. Two of the studies discussed in this chapter rejected the hypothesis that specialty decisions are income-motivated. A third indicated that—contrary to several personality studies of physicians—general practitioners may have weaker pecuniary incentives than specialists. The fourth supported the income-motivation hypothesis and raised serious questions concerning the validity of the two studies which rejected it. We concur in the latter view, with the proviso that the research needs to be replicated before the hypothesis can be regarded as verified.

Moreover, it should be stressed that even if the income-motivation hypothesis can be proved, it would not follow that earnings are a dominant factor in specialty choices. Each of the three econometric studies of individual choices found that proxies for physicians' tastes were significant predictors of the choice probabilities. These results, and others we have examined, indicate that tastes, skills, and educational experiences are apt to be at least as important as earnings prospects when physicians select their fields of specialization. Hence, on the basis of the empirical evidence now available, the most appropriate theory of physicians' specialty choices should probably contain a combination of psychological, sociological, and economic factors. Accordingly, policies to alter physician specialty distributions should not rely solely on subsidies or other monetary rewards to physicians. If, indeed, physicians are strongly attracted to particular specialties for nonpecuniary reasons, then the levels of compensation that would be necessary to persuade sizable numbers of them to select fields other than those they prefer are likely to be impractically large.

NOTES

1. See Levine (1976) for a review of this literature. The sociological approach underlies much of the research on physicians' specialty choices discussed in preceding chapters.
2. It should be emphasized that even this level of generality greatly simplifies the actual decision. For instance, the model is static (i.e., the decision is assumed to occur once and for all), and it treats the "wage rates" w_i and n_i as if they were known with certainty.
3. In particular, these include the assumptions that the marginal utilities of pecuniary and nonpecuniary income are nonnegative and nonincreasing; and that the physician is willing to sacrifice some, but progressively less, pecuniary income for each increment in nonpecuniary income (and vice versa).
4. This does not preclude the possibility that the actual decision occurs earlier, nor does it preclude the possibility that decisions can be revised during training. It simply states that the specialty choice will be made before the end of the physician's residency training.
5. Inter alia, Fishman and Zimet (1972) examined income expectations among freshman medical students at the University of Colorado. The students were asked to estimate their gross income 10 years after completing training, and their estimates averaged nearly 25 percent lower than the actual median gross income of physicians at the time of the study. Although not necessarily indicative of income perceptions when specialty decisions are made, this re-

sult may be indicative of the degree of medical students' ignorance of market opportunities.

It should also be pointed out that specialty planning takes place when the most immediate influences may not involve future income expectations. That is, individuals may be forced to narrow their range of alternatives in the course of selecting elective courses, a first-year or later graduate program, or a graduate hospital. All such choices may occur under the pressure of time and in response to the attractiveness or availability of specific training opportunities. Hence, specialty planning need not always be "rational" in the strictest possible sense of the term.

6. A number of efforts have been made to measure physicians' lifetime earnings and to compare them with lifetime earnings in nonmedical occupations (Friedman and Kuznets 1945; Sloan 1970b; Fein and Weber 1971; Leffler 1975; Mennemeyer 1978). An important question addressed by these studies is whether medical school barriers to entry have resulted in excess profit for physicians. Sloan (1970b, 1976) suggested an affirmative answer. However, Lindsay (1973, 1976) argued that Sloan had overestimated physicians' earnings vis-à-vis those in other occupations by failing to adjust for differences between physicians and other professionals in hours worked per week. Since physicians work longer hours than other professionals, their higher lifetime incomes are at least partly compensation for longer work weeks. After adjusting Sloan's figures for differences in hours worked, Lindsay reported that lifetime earnings in medicine were about the same as those in comparable occupations. Mennemeyer (1978) constructed another set of (work-hours-adjusted) earnings estimates for medicine and seven other occupations, and found that physicians' lifetime incomes were lower than those of dentists, about equal to those of lawyers, and higher than those of pharmacists, physical/life scientists, social scientists, university teachers, and veterinarians. All of these earnings comparisons were based on pre-1970 income data; and in view of the large increase in medical school capacity that has occurred since 1970, it is conjectural whether the conclusion that there are some monopoly returns to medical training would still be valid.

7. For instance, in the twentieth year of the earnings span, the discount factor $[1/(1 + r)]^t$ is .377 if $r = .05$, .149 if $r = .10$, and .013 if $r = .15$.

8. See Chapter 3. It was also observed in Chapter 3 that physicians with families are disproportionately likely to enter general practice because they have high preferred rates of current (as opposed to future) consumptions. Such preferences are tantamount to placing a high discount rate on future income. It can be shown that increasing the value of r tends to increase the range of earning spans over which career option 1 yields a higher present value of lifetime earnings than option 2. For two otherwise identical physicians, this means that the one with the higher discount rate will find option 1 (curtailing training) a more attractive alternative than will his or her colleague.

9. In general, the expression for w_i will depend on the year t in the physician's productive life. For instance, to make it compatible with the lifetime earnings expression given above, one can write

$$y_{it} = w_{it} x_i s_t h = [\sum_{k=1}^{k} p_{ikt} a_k + B_t] x_i s_t h, \quad i = 1, \ldots, l.$$

The form of this representation is obviously not unique—e.g., the shadow prices of skills may vary with factors affecting B_t, the expression itself may be nonlinear, and so forth. However, the form of the expression does not affect its general implications.

10. As a result, borrowing in order to extend the training period yields a lower lifetime earnings stream (net of interest payments) to physicians who borrow in the marketplace than to self-financing physicians.

11. Also see Kehrer (1976) for evidence on this point. She reported that, unlike men, women physicians have backward-bending labor-supply curves—a further sign of the high value women physicians attach to having time available for activities other than the practice of medicine.

12. Sloan also calculated the present value of lifetime earnings for general practitioners and found them to be mostly higher than those for the specialties. Presumably, this was due to higher incomes in general practice than in the specialties during the assumed four years of residency training. Sloan observed that this finding cast doubt on income motivation as a reason for seeking specialty training. He speculated, however, that in this respect specialists may have had higher anticipated net incomes than those used in his computations. Also, his assumption about the length of residency training may have biased downward his estimates for the lengths of specialists' productive lives and their lifetime earnings. Data presented by Balfe et al. (1971) indicate that the average length of residency training for specialists was closer to two than four years in the late 1960s. The assumption of a two- rather than four-year residency would greatly increase specialty lifetime earnings. (For other efforts to estimate specialty lifetime earnings, see the text below.)

13. This specification has other shortcomings as well. For example, if the residency markets had been in equilibrium, so that $R_t = P_t$, it would have been logically impossible for E_{t-1} to account for any of the interspecialty variation in R_t. Variation in P_t would have completely "explained" variation in R_t. Thus, the associations between R_t and E_{t-1} that Sloan obtained are due to the existence of excess supplies of residency positions. Although it is difficult to determine exactly how interspecialty differences in excess supplies of residency positions affected his estimates of the coefficient on E_{t-1}, the direction of the bias is probably toward zero.

14. Sloan did estimate an additional equation in which R_t was regressed on E_{t-1}, the excess supply of practice openings in the field, and a weighted measure of physicians' dissatisfaction with the field derived from a *Medical Economics* survey of practicing physicians. The last two variables were proxies for psychic income in the field. All three variables entered the regression negatively, but Sloan concluded that the results were questionable because of the small sample size (i.e., nine observations) and ambiguities in the psychic income proxies.

15. Note the contrast between this use of the variable and Sloan's.

16. In statistical terms, this means it is likely that Y_i/Y_j contained a large component of measurement error. The direction of bias due to measurement error is difficult to determine in multiple regressions, but Hadley's equations appear to exhibit bias from this source.

17. The basic theoretical papers on the multinomial logit model are by Mc-Fadden (1973) and Nerlove and Press (1973). Other types of probabilistic choice models have also gained currency, but they have not been as popular as logit models. For a review of the methodological literature in the area, see Hensher and Johnson (1981).

18. It is difficult to say what type of behavior is indicated by the desire to practice in an area of high medical need. Presumably, the desire reflects altruistic feelings, but it may connote pecuniary motives as well.

19. In this chapter and the next, we will occasionally use the terms *exogenous* and *endogenous*. "Exogenous" applies to a variable whose value is determined outside the relationships postulated by a behavioral model; loosely speaking, it means "fixed." "Endogenous" applies to a variable whose value is determined by the relationships the model encompasses.

20. They were, however, generally similar to findings reported by other researchers. For example, the probability of choosing general practice was significantly positively associated with older age at medical school graduation, and signficantly negatively associated with graduation from a private or research-oriented medical school. The probability of choosing internal medicine was significantly negatively associated with older age at graduation, and significantly positively associated with graduation from a private or research-oriented school. Despite their markedly different implications regarding physicians' income motives, each of Hay's two models correctly predicted the specialty choices of 63 percent of his sample physicians. The equal success rates clearly show that the plausibility of alternative models cannot be judged solely on the basis of their forecasting accuracy.

SEVEN

Econometric and Statistical Studies of the Geographic Distribution of Physicians

Most statistical studies of physicians' location patterns have employed some form of regression analysis. The dependent variable has usually been a measure of physician concentration in the geographic area of interest or the number of physicians entering that area. The explanatory variables have been measures or proxies of area-specific conditions which are hypothesized to determine physicians' expectations regarding the pecuniary and psychic income opportunities afforded by going into practice in different geographic areas. In some instances, other explanatory variables have been included to capture the effects on practice location decisions of physicians' tastes for different practice and living conditions. Not surprisingly—in view of the wide range of potential approaches—no two physician location studies have used precisely the same analytical models. Their differences in theoretical specifications, estimation procedures, and data employed all contribute to the diversity of the results obtained. Thus, in order to interpret the available evidence, it is essential to take into account differences in the various study methodologies as well as their empirical findings.

A METHODOLOGICAL OVERVIEW OF PHYSICIAN LOCATION STUDIES

In one sense, studies of practice location choice can be regarded as a segment of the larger (and older) economic literature on population location, which deals primarily with the gross or net migration of persons between geographic areas. This literature holds that the basic determinants of migration are discounted lifetime earnings differentials between points of population origin and potential destination, both implicit and explicit search costs and migration costs, and individuals' tastes. Hence, statistical models of population migration are typically aggregative models which regress the volume of migration into (or between) geographic areas on variables representing these influences.[1]

Physician location studies borrow from the theory of population migration insofar as they employ the same basic determinants of location choices. However, they differ from the population studies in terms of emphasis. Ordinarily, they use one of three fundamental types of models: (1) macro (aggregative) or micro (individual) models of the choice of first practice location; (2) macro models explaining the geographic distribution—i.e., the number or stock—of physicians; and (3) macro models of the change in the distribution of the stock of physicians. Studies using the second type of model are by far the most common. Physician "migration" is explicitly treated only in studies of movement from various training (e.g., medical school or graduate hospital) locations to first or later practice locations. Very little is known of the inter- or intrastate migration of established practitioners.[2]

As is true for specialty choices, few theoretical models have been developed to account for physicians' choices of practice locations. The prototype was set forth by Rimlinger and Steele (1963), who argued that geographic markets for physicians are equilibrated by physician net earnings. They contended that the number of physicians increases in markets where net earnings are high in the short run and decreases in markets where net earnings are low. Since competition tends to reduce incomes as labor supplies increase and to raise them as supplies contract, net earnings approach equality, ceteris paribus, in all areas in the long run. By the same token, the numbers of physicians in different areas reach their equilibrium values when geographic net real earnings differentials vanish.

Clearly, though, the ceteris paribus assumption is not realistic. In particular, different geographic areas do not offer identical levels of psychic benefits to physicians. Those areas that are considered undesirable by large numbers of physicians may fail to attract additional practitioners even if they provide above-average pecuniary income opportunities. Consequently, net earnings differentials between localities may persist indefinitely, and psychic benefits must be introduced as an additional factor equilibrating physician supplies.

Following this general line of reasoning, physician location studies ordinarily hypothesize that the number of physicians in an area increases in response to either the pecuniary or the psychic attractiveness of the area. However, it should be emphasized that this proposition applies to the *flows* of physicians entering an area and not to the *stocks* of physicians already there. Because of the monetary and psychic costs of moving from one place to another, the stocks of physicians are unlikely to adjust very quickly to geographic changes in pecuniary and psychic income opportunities. As a result, practicing physicians are apt to exhibit at least some degree of geographic immobility. For that reason, we cannot necessarily expect to observe any particular *cross-sectional* relationship between geographic stocks of physicians and current measures of area pecuniary or psychic benefits.[3]

The principal elements of the individual physician's location decision can be modeled by slightly modifying the utility-maximizing framework set forth in Chapter 6. Consider the choice of a practice specialty and a first practice location. As before, let there be *l* specialties indexed by $i (= 1, \ldots, l)$. Let g denote either an index of potential geographic locations or a set of variables that characterize the locations (e.g., degree of urbanization, number of hospital beds per capita, etc.). Then let G denote the set of all possible locations.

Physicians can be regarded as selecting the location g, specialty i, and number of work hours, sh, that maximize their utility function

$$U[w_i(g)x_i sh + W - mC, h(1 - s)L(g) + n_i(g)x_i sh - m\overline{C}],$$
$$g \text{ in } G, \quad i = 1, \ldots, l.$$

As before,

$w_i(g)=$ the hourly pecuniary rate of earnings in specialty i at location g,

x_i = 1 if the physician selects specialty i, 0 otherwise,

s = the proportion of time spent working ($0 \leqq s \leqq 1$),

h = the maximum of hours available for work or leisure,

W = nonlabor income,

$L(g)=$ the hourly psychic benefits derived from leisure at location g,

$n_i(g)=$ the hourly psychic benefits derived from practicing in specialty i at location g,

C = the pecuniary cost of moving from the physician's present (e.g., graduate training or military service) location,

$\overline{C}$ = the psychic cost of moving from the physician's present location, and

m = 1 if the physician moves from his or her present location, 0 otherwise.

The first element of the utility function should be viewed as the present value of the physician's pecuniary lifetime earnings. The second should be viewed as the present value of lifetime psychic benefits. The choice of location affects utility through the rate of pecuniary income $w_i(g)$ and the two rates of psychic benefits $L(g)$ and $n_i(g)$. $L(g)$ reflects the influence of the various "personal" location factors described in Chapter 3—e.g., climate or geography, recreational resources, quality of life, and even the attachments formed during prior contact with a geographic area. The $n_i(g)$ denotes the influence of "professional" location factors other than lifetime pecuniary earnings—e.g., work load, professional isolation, etc.

Obviously, any of the pecuniary and psychic benefits can differ sufficiently across location characteristics to make the value of the utility function vary sharply with g, thereby giving the physician strong location preferences. They may also make the choices of practice location and specialty interdependent. For instance, a physician may have a strong preference for rural communities, which means that $L(g)$ is large when g denotes ruralness but small when g denotes urbanness. But if $w_i(g)$ or $n_i(g)$ are low in value for "rural g" when i signifies any specialty other than general practice, it may easily be that the utility function is maximized when g denotes a rural community and i denotes general practice. In this case, the physician would choose a career in general practice at a rural location. Many types of trade-offs among the effects of these three influences can also occur, indicating that—given the physician's tastes (i.e., the shape of his utility function)—specialty and location preferences interact.

Subsequent specialty and location decisions follow the same process as the physician's initial decisions, except that the values of the arguments in his or her utility function change. After entering practice, the physician can be assumed to make new career decisions either continuously or at periodic intervals. For simplicity, suppose that the only type of choice under consideration is locational: that is, (1) whether to stay in the present location (say g^o) or to move, and (2) which new location to select if the decision is to move.

Private practitioners normally begin practice at a below-average annual net income until they acquire a clientele or a system of referrals. Once they are established, their pecuniary income at the present location, $w_i(g^o)$, is larger than it would be if they were just entering practice there. Unless the physician has discovered unusual earnings opportunities at other locations after beginning practice, a move to a new location will consequently tend to depress his or her lifetime net earnings. And the depressing effect will be magnified by the amount of pecuniary moving costs, C. Likewise, the lifetime psychic benefit the physician expects to receive by relocating is diminished by the psychic moving cost $\overline{C}$. Indeed, psychic moving costs—which probably increase with the time spent at the initial location (e.g., as a result of friendship ties, averseness to the risk of entering unfamiliar areas, etc.)—may be the greatest barrier to migration. In any case, the physician will relocate only if the anticipated increment in utility exceeds the loss due to moving costs.[4] Therefore, a comparison of physicians' first and later practice location decisions mainly indicates that new physicians are likely to be more mobile than established practitioners.

One of the more notable features of the 30-odd empirical studies on physicians' location behavior is the great variation in methodology, summarized in Table 7-1. The table shows considerable differences in measures of physician supply, geographic units, data bases, and statistical procedures. The remainder of this section discusses the general aspects of the research methods that have been used in these studies and the implications of the empirical results obtained.

Measures of the Geographic Supply of Physicians

Aggregative studies of physician location have used one or more of four principal measures of physician supply: (1) the number of physicians residing in the area; (2) the area's physician-population ratio; (3) the change in (or growth rate of) measures 1 or 2; and (4) the number of physicians for whom the area is their first practice location.

Several points need to be emphasized in connection with these measures. First, they apply to different dimensions of physician supply and to different location decisions. For example, let P_t stand for the number of physicians located in the area in year t; M_t for the net in-migration of established practitioners; D_t for the number of deaths and retirements; and N_t for the number of physicians for whom the area is their first practice location. Then measure 1 is $P_t = P_{t-1} + M_t + N_t - D_t$, and measure 2 is the same expression divided by population. Measure 3, the change in the physician stock, is $P_t - P_{t-1} = M_t + N_t - D_t$ (or $[M_t + N_t - D_t]/P_{t-1}$ when written as a growth rate), but a somewhat more complicated expression if it is defined on a per capita basis. Notice that the change in the physician stock is not the same as total net in-migration, $M_t + N_t$, because it includes losses due to deaths and retirements. Indeed, if total net in-migration per year is small, a 1 to 3 percent annual attrition rate due to physician deaths and retirements may lead the change-in-stock measure of physician supply to greatly understate the volume of net in-migration. Finally, measure 4 is just N_t.

These various measures of supply represent groups of physicians who make their location decisions at different dates and different career

TABLE 7-1 Characteristics of Physician Location Studies

Study	Geographic Unit	Dependent Variables	Specialty Classifications	Type of Model
Ball and Wilson (1968)	Multicounty "state economic area"	Number of nonfederal office-based MDs per capita in 1962	GPs, specialists	Single-equation regression
Benham et al. (1968)	State	Number of MDs (U.S. census definition); MDs per capita; and decennial changes in both variables, 1930–60	GPs, specialists in some regressions; none in others	Single-equation regression
Blair (1975)	County (northeastern U.S.)	Number and number per capita of nonfederal office- and hospital-based MDs in 1970	GPs, specialists	Single-equation regression
Breisch (1970)	SMSA	Percentage of all graduates of medical school practicing in SMSAs in 1966	None	Single-equation regression
Busch and Dale (1978)	County (in Kentucky)	Numbers of physicians per capita in 1950, 1960, and 1970; changes in the variable, 1950–60 and 1960–70	None	Single-equation regression
Coleman (1976)	County	Number of nonfederal patient care MDs per capita in 1970; ratio of MD in-migrants, 1965–70, to population in 1970; degree of urbanization of 1972 county locations of 1965 USMGs	GPs, other primary care MDs, referral specialists	Single-equation regression

Dougherty (1970)	County (Arkansas)	Percentage of all state MDs practicing in county in 1967	None	Single-equation regression
Elesh and Schollaert (1972)	Census tract (Chicago)	Number of MDs in private practice in 1960	GPs, specialists	Single-equation regression
Evashwick (1976)	Rand-McNally nonmetropolitan trade area	Numbers of nonfederal office-based MDs per capita in 1960 and 1970; change in MD-population ratio, 1960–70	None	Single-equation regression
Fein and Weber (1971)	State	Various measures of 1950–59 USMGs locating in their medical school states in 1967	None	Single-equation regression
Feldman (1979)	State	Number of office-based MDs per capita in 1971	GPs, medical specialists, surgical specialists, and other specialists	Simultaneous-equation regression
Fuchs and Kramer (1972)	State	Number of nonfederal office-based MDs per capita in 1966	GPs, specialists (weighted data)	Simultaneous-equation regression
Gober and Gordon (1980)	City (Phoenix)	Measure of dispersion of office-based practitioners in 1970	GPs, internists, pediatricians, obstretrician-gynecologists, and other referral specialists	Centrography

Continued

TABLE 7-1 Continued

Study	Geographic Unit	Dependent Variables	Specialty Classifications	Type of Model
Guzick and Jahiel (1976)	New York City Health Area	Number of office-based MDs in 1972–73	GPs, several categories of specialists	Single-equation regression
Hadley (1975)	State	Binary variable coded 1 or 0 depending on whether MD located in state of prior educational contact (1972 locations of 1960 USMGs)	GPs, specialists	Single-equation regression
Hambleton (1971)	State, county, ZIP-code area	Number of nonfederal office-based MDs per capita in 1966	GPs, specialists	Single-equation regression
Heald et al. (1974), Cooper et al. (1975)	County	Degree of urbanization of practice counties of 1965 USMGs	GPs, primary care specialists, other specialists	Single-equation regression
Held (1972)	State	Measures of migration of 1955–65 USMGs from state of premedical school residence to state of practice divided by 1955–60 white male migration between same states	GPs, specialists	Single-equation regression
Joroff and Navarro (1971)	SMSA	Number of nonfederal office-based MDs in 1966	GPs, internists, pediatricians, surgeons, other medical specialists	Automatic interaction detector procedure

Study	Unit of analysis	Dependent variable	Physician categories	Method
Kaplan and Leinhardt (1973)	Census tract (Pittsburgh)	Number of noninstitutional MD offices in 1970	None	Single-equation regression
Lave and Lave (1974)	State	Number of MDs per capita, 1950 and 1970 (definition of physicians not stated)	None	Single-equation regression
Lee and Wallace (1970)	State	Number of MDs per capita in 1960	None	Simultaneous-equation regression
Marden (1966)	County/SMSA	Number of nonfederal private MDs in 1960	GPs, specialists	Analysis of residuals from regresson of MDs on population
Marshall et al. (1971)	County (Kansas)	Number of MDs per capita in 1960 (definition of physicians not stated)	None	Single-equation regression
Reskin and Campbell (1974)	SMSA	Number of nonfederal private MDs in 1966	GPs, internists, pediatricians, surgeons, obstetricians, others	Analysis of residuals from regression of MDs on population
Rosett (1974)	SMSA	Number of nonfederal office-based MDs per capita, 1967–70	GPs, surgeons, medical specialists, others	Single-equation regression
Rushing (1975)	County	Number of nonfederal MDs in 1966; measures of movement of 1960 USMGs to counties of practice in 1972	GPs, full specialists, limited specialists	Simple regression

Continued

TABLE 7-1 Continued

Study	Geographic Unit	Dependent Variables	Specialty Classifications	Type of Model
Scheffler (1971a, 1972)	State	Number of nonfederal patient care MDs per capita; annual data 1956–67, average of years 1963–67	GPs, surgeons, medical specialists	Single-equation regression
Sloan (1968)	State	Number of active nonstudent MDs in 1960	None	Single- and simultaneous-equation regression
Sloan and Yett (1970)	State	Number of 1959–63 USMGs located in state in 1967	GPs, internists, pediatricians general surgeons, obstetricians	Single-equation regression
Steele and Rimlinger (1965)	County	Growth rate in the number of MDs, 1950–59	None	Single-equation regression
Wacht (1972)	County (south-eastern U.S.)	Number of nonfederal office-based MDs in 1970	GPs, surgeons, other specialists	Single-equation regression
Watson (1980a, 1980b)	State and SMSA or County (in Utah)	Choice of location in Utah and type of county by Utah graduates, 1964–69	None	Discriminant

Werner et al. (1978)	County (MD-shortage vs. non-MD-shortage)	Probability that a 1965 graduate locates in shortage county	GPs, specialists	Logit
Wilensky (1979)	State and SMSA	Probability that a 1960, 1965, or 1968 Michigan graduate locates in Michigan and Michigan SMSA	None	Single-equation regression
Yett and Sloan (1974)	State	Percentage of USMGs entering practice in 1966 who located in state	GPs, specialists	Single-equation regression

stages. The physician stock in an area is the result of location choices going back perhaps as much as several decades. The change in the physician stock captures the effects of recent location decisions, but reflects both first-time and second or later choices. The number of first-time practitioners entering the area, N_t, reflects only recent, first-time location choices. Hence, if one specifies a particular predictor variable to explain the geographic distribution of physicians, there are no a priori reasons for believing that each of these supply measures will show the same relationship with it.

A second point that should be emphasized is that the physician-population ratio—the most frequently used of the four measures—is different in kind from the others. This ratio is important because it is an indicator of the population's access to physicians' services. However, geographic differences in the physician-population ratio depend on the location behavior of the general population as well as on the location behavior of physicians. Suppose, for example, the determinants of population location and physician location were identical. Then it would be impossible to estimate a statistical model of the physician-population ratio because the ratio would be a constant over all areas. In fact, the physician-population ratio does vary geographically, but, as this example suggests, one must interpret carefully the meaning of differences in the ratio. The physician-population ratio is best regarded as a measure of access to care or as a descriptor of physician location choices *relative* to those of the general population. In either case, it is not a "pure" measure of physician location behavior, as is, say, in-migration by physicians beginning practice.

The third point is that the various physician supply measures are not equally relevant with respect to policy. Most recent policies to influence physicians' location choices have been directed at new physicians.[5] Thus, it is not surprising that many recent studies have focused on the behavior of this particular target group. In this context, the most relevant measures of physician supply are the numbers of new physicians entering an area or the total net numbers of physicians migrating into an area. Evidence derived from the behavior of the geographic stocks of physicians is of limited applicability to most of the recent types of physician location policies.

Stratifying the Supply of Physicians

Considerable evidence—including some reviewed in preceding chapters—shows that there are distinct subpopulations of physicians whose location behavior is not homogeneous. In certain instances the characteristics of important subpopulations are readily identifiable and should be used to stratify physician samples.

For example, descriptive findings show that the location patterns of foreign medical graduates (FMGs) are different from those of U.S. medical graduates (USMGs). FMGs appear somewhat more likely than USMGs to practice in urban areas, to remain in the states of their graduate training, and (possibly) to be constrained by interstate differences in licensure requirements (Butter 1976; Butter and Schaffner 1971; Ernst et al. 1978; Goldblatt et al. 1975; Schaffner and Butter 1972).

Another important characteristic related to location is the type of employment or practice setting. Hospital-based physicians will obviously be more drawn toward areas where attractive hospital facilities are available than will be office-based practitioners. Physicians employed by the federal or state governments will concentrate more in areas providing government employment than will other physicians. Resident physicians will cluster in communities where there are teaching hospitals.

Another characteristic related to location is the physician's specialty. General practitioners are known to be less influenced than other physicians by proximity to hospitals, and to be relatively less likely to choose urban communities. Conversely, pathologists, radiologists, and other referral specialists can be expected to choose urban communities where there are ample hospital facilities and supplies of other physicians to provide referrals. Since, for example, internists are much more dependent on hospital facilities than pediatricians[6]—but less so on the numbers of children in a given area—it is not even clear that primary care practitioners share a common group of significant location influences.

Most location studies define physicians as nonfederal, office-based practitioners, and general practitioners are usually segregated from specialists. However, some of the studies listed in Table 7-1 did not follow these practices. In addition, there have been few efforts to separate USMGs from FMGs except where special data bases were developed. The danger of such unstratified samples is that their results tend to vary with the sample composition, and may not apply particularly well to any of the aggregated subpopulations.

Estimation Procedures

The most common type of statistical location model is the single-equation regression estimated by ordinary least squares (OLS), in which the measure of area physician supply, say Y, is specified as the dependent variable. Area-specific exogenous variables, say $X_1, \ldots, X_k, \ldots, X_n$, are chosen and the linear (or log-linear if Y and the X_k are logarithms) equation

$$Y = a_o + \sum_{k=1}^{n} a_k X_k$$

is estimated. The signs, magnitudes, and statistical significance of estimates of the a_k then tell in what directions, how strongly, and how importantly the exogenous variables X_k affect physician supply.

Although researchers often define the regression simply as a "location model," its conceptual prototype is a market supply function for physicians. Accordingly, one would normally wish to specify one of the X_k as the area-specific price of physicians' labor. In particular, with Y_s (the observed Y) denoting the market supply of physicians, l annual physician net income (the price of physicians' labor), and u a random disturbance term, one might estimate the supply function

$$Y_s = a_o + a_1 l + \sum_{k=2}^{n} a_k X_k + u \tag{1}$$

by OLS.

Ordinarily, one would expect the coefficient a_1 to be positive, indicating that the number of physicians supplied to the area increases as net income increases. But it by no means follows that the OLS *estimate* of a_1 will be positive because of a well-known problem in econometrics called *simultaneous-equations bias*. That is, one can posit an area demand function for physicians in which the number demanded by the area's population also depends on physician net income. One can further specify an equilibrium condition stating that physician net income in the area rises or falls so as to equilibrate the numbers of practitioners demanded and supplied.[7] In short, this new system contains the numbers of physicians demanded and supplied and physician net income as jointly dependent (or endogenous) variables. Therefore, estimating the physician supply function (equation 1) by OLS amounts to fitting a single equation from a simultaneous system and erroneously treating physician net income as exogenous.

Under these circumstances, physician net income is correlated with the disturbance term in equation 1, and it can be shown that this causes the OLS estimator of a_1 to be biased downward (e.g., Malinvaud 1970). Consequently, fitting the supply function by OLS understates the impact of physician net income on area physician supply, and it does so with respect to both large and small samples. One can thus expect single-equation market models estimated by OLS to "demonstrate" that physicians' location patterns are insensitive to geographic differences in physician net income.

The underlying difficulty is that physician net income in an area depends partly on the supply of physicians, and the same may well be true for other variables which have been designated as exogenous in market models of physician location. For instance, some studies using models like equation 1 specify area hospital capacity, the number of group practices, or the number of support personnel as exogenous variables. However, each of these variables should probably be regarded as endogenous because each partly depends on physicians' market behavior. Insofar as the variables are endogenous, OLS estimates of equation 1 will tend to give distorted interpretations of their effects on physicians' location choices.

As a rule, the foregoing observations do not apply to studies where the individual physician is the analytic unit because aggregative or market-level explanatory variables are rarely affected by the behavior of a single individual. Nevertheless, it is fair to say that too little use has been made of simultaneous-equations models in aggregative or market-level studies of physician location. This is not to say that multiequation models are automatically superior to single-equation regressions: they also may be susceptible to specification errors or other conceptual and econometric problems.[8] Even so, the markets for physicians and physicians' services are complex institutions consisting of many interrelated phenomena. Physicians' location behavior is only one of those phenomena, and to attempt to isolate it—as single-equation methodologies do—from the rest of the market's components is neither realistic nor likely to produce totally reliable empirical results.

The Choice of Explanatory Variables

Literally dozens of different explanatory variables have been used as predictors of the geographic supplies of physicians. Their substantive implications for physicians' location behavior are discussed below. Here we draw attention to two problems relating to the *types* of explanatory variables used in the statistical studies of physician location decisions.

The first such problem is measurement bias caused by the use of proxies rather than conceptually correct explanatory variables. Many of the influences operating on physicians' location choices are difficult or impossible to measure empirically. Moreover, it may often be difficult to obtain data on the variables that can, in principle, be quantified. For example, the area-specific lifetime earnings expectations of physicians are not observable. As surrogates for them, researchers have employed either the current average gross or net income of physicians in practice or socioeconomic traits of the area population relating to its demand for physician services (e.g., per capita income, population density, etc.). Each of these surrogates approximates physicians' "true" lifetime earnings expectations with an error which is unobservable, and the sampling distribution of each depends on the proxy itself.

Although it is known that these measurement errors tend to bias the estimators of regression coefficients, neither the amount nor even the direction of the bias can be determined without knowing the sampling distributions of the errors. Ordinarily, some degree of measurement error bias is considered acceptable in econometric studies because proxy variables are all but unavoidable. However, findings based on reasonably accurate proxies can be regarded as more reliable than those based on crude ones. Thus, for instance, the use of different proxies for the same locational influence on physicians can produce different qualitative results. This may account for some of the disparities in the evidence on physicians' location patterns.

The second problem arises from multicollinearity—or high intercorrelations—among the explanatory variables. Multicollinearity inflates estimates of the standard errors of the coefficients on the correlated variables. Consequently, it causes the statistical significance of the variables to be understated. When explanatory variables in a physician location model are highly intercorrelated, one may conclude falsely that one or more of them (and the location influences they represent) do not affect physicians' location choices. In addition, any one or more of the correlated variables may "explain" variation in area physician supplies about equally well. This means that one can select one or more of the correlated variables as predictors in a location regression, eliminate the others, and conclude that the selected location influences are significant while the others are not.

The problem of multicollinearity in physician location studies is not a trivial one. It is well known, for instance, that certain socioeconomic traits of area populations are closely intercorrelated. This is especially true for traits associated with the area's relative affluence—e.g., population income per capita, the degree of urbanization, educational level, and racial composition. The number of medical schools in an area may also be associated with its level of affluence (e.g., Fuchs and Kramer 1972). Rushing (1975) has even argued that the high intercorrelations among area socioeconomic characteristics vitiate the usefulness of regression methodologies for modeling physicians' location choices.

Multicollinearity, measurement error, and the other statistical problems discussed in this section are not unique to studies of physicians' practice location choices. They are common in all kinds of empirical analyses. Some are unavoidable, and all have been recognized by researchers.[9] Nevertheless, the fundamental question is what the studies listed in Table 7-1 tell us about physicians' location behavior. Typically, single-equation models account for 75 percent or more of the geographic variation in physician stocks or physician-population ratios. This suggests that physicians' practice location behavior is reasonably well understood. But the validity of the evidence is weakened when it is derived from biased estimation techniques, unclear conceptual models, or inconsistent groups of findings. Therefore, the methodology of a study can be as important as its numerical or qualitative results. Unfortunately, it is not always easy to see how the methodology of a specific study contributed to its findings. Because of that, one can often say only that a given body of evidence is of doubtful validity, and that the issues it addresses ought to be investigated further.

PHYSICIAN INCOME AND PRACTICE LOCATION

Economic theory holds that the flow of physicians into a geographic area should be largest—other things being equal—where physicians' pecuniary earnings opportunities are highest. On the other hand, the relationships between stocks of physicians (or physician-population ratios) and earnings opportunities are much more difficult to estimate because the stocks may be slow to adjust to changes in an area's income opportunities. Consequently, the stocks of physicians may exhibit only weak cross-sectional correlations with an area's *current* physician income level, or the observed associations may be quite different from those that would prevail after all adjustments had taken place. Several studies have used statewide averages of practicing physicians' gross or net annual incomes as proxies for earnings opportunities, and have attempted to relate flow or stock measures of physician supplies with them. Not surprisingly, the results are mixed.

The earliest work along these lines was done by Sloan (1968), who estimated both single- and simultaneous-equations models of the numbers of active, nonstudent physicians practicing in states. In his single-equation regressions, he found the stock of physicians to be weakly positively associated with estimated physician net income in the state. However, estimates of his simultaneous-equations model indicated that the stock of physicians in the state was negatively correlated with estimated physician net income. Although it is hard to interpret these conflicting results, evidence weakly corroborating the second finding was reported by Yett and Sloan (1974). They found that the proportions of new general practitioners and specialists choosing first practice locations in states were each negatively, but nonsignificantly, related to mean physician net income in those states.

Additional results that contradict the conventional location theory were obtained by Held (1972) and Hadley (1975). Held estimated a model in which the dependent variable was the ratio of the number of 1955–65 medical graduates entering a state to the number of white males entering the same state during 1955–60. His findings showed that the ratio was not significantly correlated with the average net income of solo practitioners in the state in 1966. Although this indicates that physician in-migration into states relative to the in-migration of white males was not affected by practice income opportunities, one can clearly question the use of 1966 incomes as a proxy for the income opportunities perceived by physicians in the previous decade. Moreover, since the physician in-migration rate was defined relative to the rate of white males, the more appropriate earnings proxy is arguably a measure of physician income opportunities relative to those of white males generally.

Using a probability model of individual location choices by 1960 medical graduates, Hadley (1975) reported that there was no significant association between the likelihood of selecting a particular state and the relative net income opportunities in the state. However, he failed to give an explicit definition of relative net income opportunities, and described the variable only as the ratio of mean net physician incomes in the state chosen by the physician and in one "alternative" state. Because of the ambiguities in the variable—and the fact that it restricts income comparisons to two states from a choice set of 50—there is no way to determine whether it actually captured state earnings differentials as perceived by physicians. Indeed, it is difficult to see how such a variable would be related to location choice probabilities if the economic theory of practice location were correct.

In contrast to these findings, studies by Lee and Wallace (1970) and Fuchs and Kramer (1972) both found significantly positive associations between state physician-population ratios and measures of physician income in the state. Each specified its geographic supply function in the context of a simultaneous-equations model, and for that reason one might attach greater credibility to their results than if the evidence had been obtained from single-equation regressions. But Lee and Wallace defined their earnings variable as physicians' gross annual income, and did not adjust for type of specialty. Gross income may or may not accurately reflect net earnings (i.e., after expenses, which may also vary geographically). Also, pooling across specialties may introduce aggregation bias into the results. Fuchs and Kramer adjusted their model for specialty differences, but they defined their earnings variable as gross annual income per patient visit—physicians' average revenue. Again, this is a dubious proxy for physicians' perceptions of the prices they can expect to receive for their time.

Wilensky (1979) estimated a location choice probability model similar to Hadley's, but with the choice probability defined as the likelihood of the physician's selecting Michigan as a state of practice. Also like Hadley, she specified the physician earnings variable as the ratio of net physician incomes in the subjects' state of practice and either (1) their reported second choice of a practice state or (2) their state of most recent prior contact. However, unlike Hadley, she found that the probability of locating in Michigan was significantly positively associated with the income variable. The disparity here may be due to differences in data,[10] but it may also be due to the nature of the earnings proxy.

Only one study has attempted to explore the effects of earnings opportunities on intrastate practice location choices. Werner et al. (1978) estimated a model predicting the probability that a physician chooses a physician-shortage county as opposed to a nonshortage county. However, they used an attitudinal variable—physicians' description of the strength of area income potential as a factor in their location decision—rather than measured physician income to test for income motivation in location choices. The type of county chosen was not found to be significantly associated with this variable, indicating that physicians with strong income motives were about equally likely to select shortage and nonshortage counties.

In quantitative terms, then, about half of the existing evidence shows that physicians' location decisions are insensitive to earnings expectations, while the other half supports conventional location theory. In addition, even some of the supportive evidence indicates that earnings expectations are less important than nonpecuniary factors in shaping physicians' location decisions.

However, a judicious evaluation leads to the conclusion that the insensitivity of physicians' location choices to earnings opportunities has been neither proved nor disproved. All of the studies discussed here relied on proxy measures of earnings opportunities that are vulnerable to criticism. For example, although it is clearly the case that geographic earnings differentials should be measured in terms of real rather than money incomes, none of the studies attempted to deflate physicians' money incomes by area-specific cost-of-living indexes. Consequently, the findings discussed here should be considered tentative. Their implications may well have to be revised as new data and new evidence appear.

POPULATION SOCIOECONOMIC ATTRIBUTES AND PHYSICIAN LOCATION

Regression studies of practice location commonly include one or more socioeconomic traits of area populations among their explanatory variables. Socioeconomic traits are sometimes viewed as proxies for the quality of living conditions in the area. However, more often they are intended to reflect the strength of the demand for medical services and, hence, are interpreted as surrogates for physicians' earnings opportunities.

The traits most frequently used in physician location studies are: (1) the size, density, or degree of urbanness of the population; (2) per capita or mean family income; (3) the percentage of elderly people in the population; (4) the average educational attainment of the population; and (5) the racial composition of the population. Research on the demand for physicians' services has generally found that the quantity of services demanded increases with population size or density, per capita or family income, the percentages of elderly and whites in the population, and the educational level of the population.[11] On the basis of the argument that large demands for services imply above-average physician income opportunities—at least until supply adjusts in the long run—it is usually assumed that large values of these variables represent favorable physician income expectations. And, since it is reasonable to suppose that physicians are attracted into areas by above-average income opportunities, most studies have hypothesized positive partial correlations between measures of physician supply and these socioeconomic variables. Obviously, population socioeconomic traits may be indicative of general living conditions in an area as well as the income opportunities it affords. Thus, one would expect some tendency for physicians to be attracted to affluent, urban communities for nonpecuniary reasons, regardless of the pecuniary incentives.

Empirical evidence on the relationships between physicians' locations and area socioeconomic characteristics varies across studies. However, certain findings have been reported more consistently than others. We now consider separately the findings on each of the five characteristics listed above.

Population Size, Density, and Urbanness

The pattern of physicians' location behavior in relation to population size and density differs depending upon the measure of physician supply, the geographic unit employed, and physicians' specialties. Population size is the strongest single correlate of the *number* of physicians practicing in states, SMSAs, or counties (Marden 1966; Benham et al 1968; Reskin and Campbell 1974). The change in population size may also be the strongest single predictor of a change in the physician stock in states and counties (Steele and Rimlinger 1965; Benham et al. 1968; Fein and Weber 1971). In all such cases the reported relationship between physician supply and population is positive.

By contrast, results are mixed with respect to correlations between the physician-population ratio and population size. County-level studies by Joroff and Navarro (1971) and Blair (1975) indicated that the ratio increases with population size, but a state-level study by Benham et al. (1968) found a significantly negative correlation between the change in the physician-population ratio and the change in population.

Because of the strong association between the stock of physicians and population size, many studies have hypothesized that physicians are more likely to settle in urban or densely populated areas than in other areas. Much of the evidence supports this hypothesis, but some does not —probably because of methodological differences. The findings vary depending on the measures of physician supply, the geographic unit used, and whether or not the physician supply measures are stratified by specialty.

For example, state-level studies by Benham et al. (1968) and Lee and Wallace (1970) found that physician-population ratios were negatively, and not significantly, associated with state population densities and the percentages of state populations living in urban areas. Wilensky (1979) also reported that a Michigan-trained physician's likelihood of practicing in Michigan was unrelated to the degree of urbanization. Studies by Joroff and Navarro (1971) and Evashwick (1976) have indicated that county physician-population ratios are not significantly related to population density. But Lave and Lave (1974) reported a significantly positive partial correlation between a state's physician-population ratio and the percentage of its population living in urban areas.

Because of differences in sample composition and methodology, it is extremely difficult to compare these six studies. Nevertheless, it is noteworthy that five of the six did not stratify physicians by specialty, and the one that did (Evashwick 1976) restricted its sample to rural areas where variations in population density are not large. In Chapter 3 it was shown that general practitioners appear to be less likely than specialists to locate in urban areas. Thus, to the extent that an unstratified physician sample contains a large proportion of general practitioners, it will give misleading estimates of physicians' overall propensities to locate in urban areas.

The available evidence implies that this is indeed the case. County-level regressions where physicians are stratified by specialty report significantly positive correlations between measures of specialist supply (such as specialist-population ratios) and either population density or population urbanness. Conversely, correlations between measures of general practitioner supply and urbanness proxies are either not significant, negative, or both (Ball and Wilson 1968; Dougherty 1970; Blair 1975; Coleman 1976). At the state level, specialist-population ratios and flow measures of specialist supply also tend to be more highly positively correlated with urbanness than general practitioner-population ratios and flow measures of general practitioner supply (Scheffler 1971a, 1972; Yett and Sloan 1974).

Whether the area under consideration is large or small, and whether it is predominantly urban or rural, also affects the empirical results. For instance, one would expect the degree of urbanness of an area to be a more important factor in intrastate practice location decisions than in interstate decisions. A physician may prefer a predominantly rural to a predominantly urban state, but he may still choose to practice in an urban center of the rural state. In either case, a physician who prefers to practice in a city may choose to locate in a more densely rather than less densely populated section of the city.

The statistical findings on these points are inconclusive. Wilensky (1979) found that the degree of the state's urbanness had no effect on Michigan-trained physicians' choices of state locations, but they were significantly more likely to practice in their residency or medical school SMSAs if those SMSAs were highly urbanized. Wacht's (1972) results implied that physicians who selected rural and suburban counties preferred those with the largest populations, but those who were attracted to SMSAs showed no preference in terms of population size. This may mean that, having decided to practice in a non-SMSA county, a physician is more likely to choose one where the population is clustered than where it is thinly scattered. However, Marden (1966) obtained the opposite result, that differences in population explain the distribution of physicians across SMSAs better than they do the distribution of physicians across rural counties.

Three studies of the distribution of physicians within cities produced still another set of results. Elesh and Schollaert (1972), Guzick and Jahiel (1976), and Gober and Gordon (1980) all found that specialists were less likely than general practitioners to have offices in those intracity areas with the largest populations. But they also found that neither population size nor density appeared to be a major determinant of office locations. Indeed, Gober and Gordon showed that, in Phoenix, offices were clustered around hospitals regardless of physicians' specialties— and not particularly in areas having high population concentrations. What these patterns reflect is that population size is not the only factor that will determine whether a practice location is a viable one. Hence, specialists who draw on large populations and depend on hospital facilities tend to situate in central areas close to hospitals. General practitioners and other primary care physicians who are less dependent on hospital practice display weaker tendencies to cluster in central locations.

It is notable that much of the evidence concerning physician location in relation to population size or urbanness is conflicting. However, it is fair to conclude that the *number* of physicians in a state or county is positively correlated with the area's population. Whether there is a similar association with the degree of urbanness of the area is an open issue. For the most part, the findings showing that population density does not affect physicians' location decisions are from data pooled across specialties. And, since location patterns vary by specialty, these results cannot be regarded as reliable. Population density within cities does not seem to be a significant influence on intrametropolitan practice location decisions, although it does seem to be more important for general practitioners than for specialists.

Per Capita and Family Income

The two measures of consumer affluence most commonly employed by researchers in this field are (undeflated) per capita income and median family income. Nearly all of the studies using stock measures of physician supply (summarized in Table 7-1) have obtained significantly positive associations between these income measures and the physician stock or the physician-population ratio.[12] Some of the correlations are not very significant, but this may be due to the effects of multicollinearity between the income measures and other socioeconomic traits of the area.[13]

On the other hand, studies using flow measures of physician supply have obtained mixed results with respect to the effects of population income. Several found that physicians having prior contact with a state are more likely to locate in that state when its per capita income is high relative to other states' (Fein and Weber 1971; Yett and Sloan 1974; Wilensky 1979). One study reported a positive correlation between the growth rates of county physician stocks and county per capita incomes (Steele and Rimlinger 1965). By contrast, Wilensky (1979) found that the probability that a Michigan-trained physician will locate in an SMSA of prior educational contact falls significantly as SMSA per capita income increases. Two other studies have indicated that changes in state or county physician-population ratios are either negatively or not significantly related to per capita income (Benham et al. 1968; Evashwick 1976). And Coleman (1976) found that the rate of net physician in-migration into counties was negatively associated with county per capita income.

Thus, although the hypothesis that physicians choose to practice in affluent states and counties is a plausible one, it is consistently supported only by location studies using stock rather than flow measures of physician supply. Indeed, two of the studies produced positive partial correlations between stock measures of supply and per capita income, but negative partial correlations when flow measures were used instead (Coleman 1976; Evashwick 1976). Although we have argued that flow measures of physician supply are conceptually preferable to stock measures, there are no obvious explanations for why they give inconsistent results. One possibility is that the affluence of an area leads to high densities of physicians which, in turn, discourage new practitioners from entering the area. At any rate, until these inconsistent results can be satisfactorily explained, there are grounds for reservations concerning the validity of the evidence on this point.

The possibility that general practitioners and specialists respond differently to population income levels has been explored by a number of researchers. The majority of studies indicate either that the stocks of both types of physicians are positively correlated with area per capita income, or that specialists are somewhat more attracted than general practitioners to high-income areas (Ball and Wilson 1968; Benham et al. 1968; Hambleton 1971; Yett and Sloan 1974; Blair 1975; Coleman 1976).

The evidence with respect to the influence of consumer income on physician location within metropolitan areas is also inconclusive. Kaplan and Leinhardt (1973) found that the distribution of physicians' offices among census tracts in Pittsburgh was unrelated to median family incomes. Likewise, using a sample of ZIP-code areas in 15 large cities, Hambleton (1971) found that the numbers of general practitioners and specialists per capita were not significantly associated with family income levels.

However, other studies of metropolitan areas by Elesh and Schollaert (1972) and Guzick and Jahiel (1976) reported that the reverse is true. Elesh and Schollaert found that the stocks of general practitioners and specialists in Chicago were both significantly positively correlated with the percentage of families earning more than $10,000 per year. And Guzick and Jahiel showed that the stocks of all physicians and of general practitioners in New York City were both highly positively correlated with median family income.

Since they apply to physician stocks rather than physician offices (which may be group practices) or the physician-population ratio, the Elesh-Schollaert and Guzick-Jahiel findings give the most reliable picture. They indicate that, other things being equal, physicians do gravitate into high-income metropolitan neighborhoods, but it is not clear whether there is a significant difference between specialists and general practitioners in this regard.

Age Distribution of the Population

About a third of the studies shown in Table 7-1 employed explanatory variables describing the age distribution of the area population. All but one used geographic units smaller than the state, and nearly all defined age distribution as the percentage of the population aged 65 (or 66) and older. The results consistently indicate that the stock of *general practitioners* is significantly positively correlated with the percentage of elderly in the population (Marden 1966; Hambleton 1971; Joroff and Navarro 1971; Elesh and Schollaert 1972; Reskin and Campbell 1974; Blair 1975; Coleman 1976; Guzick and Jahiel 1976).

Stock measures of the total supply of physicians also appear to be positively correlated with the percentage of elderly, but the results concerning specialists vary. Some studies have shown that the stock of specialists increases with the percentage of elderly persons (Blair 1975; Coleman 1976), but most report no significant correlation between the two variables. These findings imply that concentrations of physicians in counties or city neighborhoods with large proportions of the aged are due to the location behavior of general practitioners more than that of specialists.[14]

Two studies sought to identify an association between changes in the physician-population ratio and the percentage of elderly in the population. Coleman (1976) and Evashwick (1976) both found the relationship to be either negative or nonsignificant. These findings conflict with those indicating that physicians locate in areas having disproportionately large percentages of elderly persons.

Educational Attainment of the Population

Several studies have explored the relationship between the distribution of physicians and the median number of years of schooling completed by an area's population. On balance, the results indicate a weak tendency for physicians to prefer situating in areas where the population is well educated. However, no consensus exists concerning whether the general level of education has the same or different effects on the distributions of general practitioners and specialists.

County-and SMSA-level studies by Marden (1966), Joroff and Navarro (1971), and Blair (1975) reported that specialists are relatively more concentrated in areas of high educational attainment than are general practitioners. Reskin and Campbell (1974) reached the opposite conclusion, while Coleman (1976) found that general practitioners, other primary care practitioners, and referral specialists are all attracted by well-educated populations. Elesh and Schollaert (1972) found that both general practitioners and specialists were most concentrated in those sections of one metropolitan area where the population's educational level was highest.

Racial Composition of the Population

Comparatively little is known about the influence of the racial composition of the populations of different areas on physician location; and
the evidence that does exist is mixed. Hambleton (1971) found that state
and county general practitioner-population ratios are negatively correlated with the percentage of nonwhites in the populations. Marden
(1966) reported a similar result for SMSAs, but Joroff and Navarro
(1971) and Blair (1975) found no significant relationships between general practitioner concentration and the racial compositions of county
populations. Only one of the four studies found a significant (positive)
association between the concentration of specialists and the nonwhite
proportion of the population.

Three metropolitan area studies also produced conflicting results.
Kaplan and Leinhardt (1973) failed to find a significant relationship between the distribution of physician offices and the racial composition of
census tracts in Pittsburgh. However, Guzick and Jahiel (1976) obtained
positive, and generally significant, correlations between the number of
physicians and the percentage of blacks in New York City Health
Areas.[15] The same type of finding was reported by Hambleton (1971) in a
study of metropolitan ZIP-code areas.

The central issue connected with the racial composition of metropolitan areas is its role, if any, in producing inner-city physician scarcity.
Although the evidence is not abundant, what there is does not support
the view that race of the patient population is a significant factor. The
findings to date imply that economic causes—principally consumer pov-
erty—are much more important. Physicians' residential living tastes,
which appear to lead them (like other high-income professional groups)
to prefer suburban home locations, may be important as well. One cannot ignore the possibility that home location preferences are related to
community racial composition. However, it is most unlikely that this
factor alone could account for the historical movement of physician supply from the inner city to the suburbs, and the possible roles of other factors are not yet clear.

Other Socioeconomic Characteristics

Many other population and area characteristics have also been used
as predictor variables in physician location regressions. Basically, they
were selected to represent: (1) measures of the physical causes of medical
service demands (per capita numbers of bed disability days, workdays
lost, and acute illness conditions); (2) the stability of medical service demands and, hence, physicians' expected net incomes (the unemployment

rate, the composition of employment in the area); and (3) additional demand proxies such as the percentage of women in the population, Medicare payments per capita, and the percentage of the (city) area that is commercially zoned.

With the exception of findings on the percentage of commercially zoned land, the results have not been replicated or are not statistically significant. Elesh and Schollaert (1972), Kaplan and Leinhardt (1973), and Guzick and Jahiel (1976) all found that metropolitan physicians were concentrated in census tracts or similar areas with large percentages of commercially zoned land.

HOSPITAL FACILITIES AND PHYSICIAN LOCATION

More than half of the studies shown in Table 7-1 examined the impact of the availability of hospital facilities on physicians' location patterns. The customary measures of local supplies of hospital resources are the number of hospital beds and the number of beds per capita.[16] Although the findings are not fully consistent, they suggest several tentative conclusions.

First, the stock of specialists and the specialist-population ratio are positively correlated with the volume or per capita volume of hospital capacity, but the stock of general practitioners and the general practitioner-population ratio are not—except, perhaps, in urban areas. Second, the overall stock of physicians and the total physician-population ratio are weakly positively correlated with measures of hospital capacity. This result simply reflects the predominance of specialists in the physician population. Third, *urban* general practitioners are as likely as urban specialists to be located near concentrations of hospital capacity. This finding conflicts with the results for rural general practitioners, but no attempt has yet been made to explain it.[17]

The evidence indicates that most physicians are attracted to specific areas by the presence of hospitals. However, it does not establish a clear cause-effect relationship between physician supply and hospital capacity, since physicians may be instrumental in expanding an area's hospital capacity after they have settled there. Hence, partial correlations between area hospital capacity and measures of the physician stock do not necessarily show that physicians locate near hospitals.

Support for this view has been provided in several studies using flow measures of physician supply rather than stocks. Yett and Sloan (1974) and Evashwick (1976) each reported that flows of physicians were not significantly correlated with the volume of hospital capacity (or the change in hospital capacity) in states or counties. Busch and Dale (1978) found that the change in the physician-population ratio in Kentucky counties between 1950 and 1960 was only weakly positively related with the number of hospital beds per capita. And Wilensky (1979) showed that the likelihood of a Michigan-trained physician's locating in an SMSA of prior educational contact was significantly negatively associated with the number of interns and residents in the SMSA (a proxy for teaching hospital capacity).[18]

The simplest theory postulating a relationship between the numbers of specialists and hospital beds is based on economies of scale in producing medical services. In particular, physicians should produce in hospitals the types of services they cannot produce efficiently or profitably in their offices. Surgical services, as well as many types of diagnostic and therapeutic services, normally involve the use of expensive capital equipment, beds, and personnel, while generalized ambulatory care does not. Thus, one would expect referral specialists to locate near the hospitals whose resources they use. Conversely, the incentives for general practitioners to do so should be much weaker.

Rosett (1974) advanced a different argument based on the proposition that a hospital may be either a source of benefits or a source of competition to an office-based physician.[19] He observed that hospital services are a collective good to physicians (i.e., that they are shared by all office-based physicians in the market area who are entitled to admit patients). Consequently, an increase in hospital capacity in a given market may yield only a small or negligible increase in benefits to individual practitioners. Rosett went on to assert that whether or not office-based physicians are induced to locate near hospitals may depend on the total amount of hospital benefits, the number of physicians sharing them, and the extent to which office-based physicians regard hospitals as competitors in the sale of outpatient services.

Rosett tested his hypotheses by estimating four specialty-specific regression equations. As dependent variables, he chose the per capita numbers of general practitioners, medical specialists, surgeons, and other specialists in 27 SMSAs. His principal explanatory variables were the per capita numbers of hospital beds and hospital-based physicians in the SMSA.[20] Both variables, he claimed, are measures of the benefits available to private practitioners, while the second is also a measure of the strength of competition between hospitals and private practitioners.

The coefficients on the hospital beds variable were negative for all four specialties, a finding at variance with the results of most other studies using stock measures of physician supply. But, except in the general practitioner regression, the coefficients on the hospital physicians variable were positive. Rosett interpreted the first set of findings as showing that increasing the number of hospital beds without increasing the number of hospital physicians per bed *lowers* the benefits of hospitals to office practitioners because it reduces the availability of hospital personnel to care for their patients. That is, office-based physicians in areas having large numbers of beds and relatively few hospital physicians must either spend more of their own time with hospitalized patients or accept a lower quality of care for those patients. From this, Rosett concluded that hospitals attract office-based practitioners to an area only if they provide adequate staff to care for patients.

The second set of findings, he contended, reveal office-based physicians' perceptions of hospital physicians as either competitors or joint providers of patient care. If they view hospital physicians as competitors, they are not likely to locate near hospitals. If they view hospital physicians as supporting personnel, they are likely to choose practice locations near hospitals. On this basis, Rosett interpreted the positive partial correlations between his specialist-population ratios and hospital physicians per capita as showing that specialists perceive hospital physicians as contributing to their profits. The negative partial correlation between the general practitioner-population ratio and hospital physicians per capita, he argued, implies that general practitioners regard hospital physicians as competitors.

In another study, Feldman (1979) obtained results which partly contradict Rosett's findings. Feldman used the same four specialty groupings and a similar supply equation for office-based practitioners as did Rosett (although it was specified and estimated within a simultaneous-equations model). However, he found that the supply of office-based practitioners in each specialty grouping was negatively related to a proxy for the number of hospital physicians per capita. He also found that the supplies of office-based physicians were not significantly related to the number of hospital beds per capita, except for general practitioners where the relationship was positive and significant. In terms of Rosett's approach, Feldman's findings indicate that all office practitioners at least weakly perceive hospital physicians as competitors, and only general practitioners are attracted to states by the presence of abundant hospital facilities.

Despite these conflicting results, the hypothesis that hospitals compete with general practitioners and complement specialists has been incorporated into other studies as well. Sloan and Yett (1970) and Hambleton (1971) both reported that specialists tend to be concentrated in areas having large numbers of interns and residents (who represent roughly 60 percent of all hospital-based physicians). Although Sloan and Yett also found a positive correlation between (state-level) concentrations of general practitioners and interns, Hambleton (1971) found that the (county-level) general practitioner-population ratio was negatively correlated with the ratio of interns and residents to population.[21]

Still another economic explanation of the link between office-based specialists and hospitals was advanced by Rushing (1975). He contended that: (1) specialists were historically dependent on general practitioners for referrals; (2) hospital capacity expanded in wealthy, urban communities as part of the overall process of economic and social progress; (3) hospitals have gradually replaced general practitioners as the source of specialists' referrals; and (4) specialists therefore tend to cluster around hospitals while general practitioners do not.

This hypothesis implies that specialists tend to locate in areas having large volumes of hospital capacity *if* the number of general practitioners is small. To test it, Rushing first cross-classified all U.S. counties by the size of their general practitioner-population ratios and degree of urbanization. For each resulting cell or subsample of counties, he then regressed the specialist-population ratio on the number of hospital beds per capita. If his hypothesis is correct, he argued, the coefficients on beds per capita should be larger in counties where the general practitioner-population ratio is small than where it is large.

The results of Rushing's test strikingly confirmed his prediction, indicating that specialists are much more likely to be located near hospitals when general practitioner concentration is low rather than high. Moreover, the relationship held regardless of the degree of urbanization of the county. On this basis, Rushing concluded that hospitals attract specialists because they substitute for general practitioners as sources of referrals.

One can, of course, question this conclusion. In particular, Rushing offered no direct evidence that hospitals actually refer patients to specialists, although it is possible that some unknown numbers of emergency-room or walk-in patients are treated by and/or later referred to private practitioners on hospitals' staffs. Nor is it evident that specialists rely heavily on general practitioners and hospitals as sources of their patients. Primary care specialists obtain new patients in much the same ways as general practitioners do, and may themselves refer patients to other specialists. Even so, the pattern of Rushing's empirical results is striking.

The emerging market theories of physician-hospital relationships suggest that the role of the hospital in physicians' location decisions is more complicated than the one assigned to it in many location studies.[22] The complexity of the role may account for some of the disparities in the empirical findings. Indeed, the fact that there are so many competing views of the matter is itself evidence that the physician-hospital relationship is not yet well understood.

MEDICAL SCHOOLS AND
PHYSICIAN LOCATION

According to the findings described in Chapter 3, the presence of medical schools can affect physicians' location choices in two ways. First, they are a source of medical knowledge and progress for the practitioner, and they may also be an indicator of high professional standards in the locality generally. Thus, the presence of medical schools is likely to attract to the area physicians who are economically or professionally dependent on medical progress, or who wish to practice in a medically sophisticated community.

Second, the medical school is a source of prior contact with the area. Owing to admissions policies favoring state residents, physicians often attend medical schools in or near the area where they were raised, or take graduate training near a medical school even if it is not their own. Thus, the presence of a medical school partially serves as a proxy for upbringing and graduate training attachments in addition to attachments attributable to the medical school itself.[23]

The "medical-knowledge" and prior-contact effects of medical schools both presumably diminish as the distance from the institution increases. The medical-knowledge effect is probably confined to the immediate vicinity (e.g., county) of the school. But the prior-contact effect is apt to remain strong at the state level, especially insofar as it captures the influence of upbringing attachments. Rosett (1974) suggested a third type of medical school effect on location—namely, that schools providing patient care compete with private practitioners. Obviously, the competitive impact of medical schools will tend to be local, possibly not even extending to the county level.

State-level studies report strong positive partial correlations between the aggregate physician-population ratio and the numbers of medical schools, medical school places, first-year places, graduates, and faculty (Benham et al. 1968; Lee and Wallace 1970; Scheffler 1971a; Fuchs and Kramer 1972; Lave and Lave 1974; Busch and Dale 1978; Feldman 1979). In some instances, measures of medical school capacity were the most significant of all predictors of the physician-population ratio. Sloan and Yett (1971) and Held (1972) also found one or more of the capacity measures to be positively correlated with the flows of new physicians into states. However, results are inconclusive as to whether general practitioners or specialists are the more likely to be located in states having medical schools.

The evidence at the county and SMSA levels shows the same overall tendencies, except that specialists appear significantly more likely than general practitioners to cluster near medical schools (Ball and Wilson 1968; Joroff and Navarro 1971; Blair 1975). Studies of 1965 medical graduates by Rand researchers have shown that, regardless of field, the degree of urbanization of the physician's county of practice is significantly positively associated with the presence of medical schools (Heald et al. 1974; Cooper et al. 1975; Coleman 1976). This may indicate that recent general practitioners gravitate more toward locations with medical schools than do older generations of their colleagues. Or it may reflect a greater tendency on the part of urban general practitioners than their rural counterparts to prefer locations nearer medical schools.[24]

These findings are broadly consistent with the medical-knowledge and prior-contact hypotheses of medical school attractiveness. However, they are not sufficient to establish the extent to which each accounts for the observed medical school influence on physicians' location patterns. The apparently weak tendency of general practitioners to settle near medical schools may signify the influence of competition from their clinics. On the other hand, it may simply indicate that general practitioners are less professionally dependent than specialists on access to new medical technology.

LICENSURE BARRIERS AND PHYSICIAN LOCATION

Variations in the requirements of state licensure boards may affect the interstate mobility of physicians. Other things being equal, the highest concentrations of physicians or the largest inflows of new practitioners should occur in states where the licensure requirements are the least demanding. Indeed, some studies have concluded that licensure requirements restrict mobility in such professions as dentistry and the law (Holen 1965; Maurizi 1969).

The most common measure of difficulty of licensure is the failure rate on the state board examination. However, Benham et al. (1968), Sloan (1968), and Scheffler (1971a) all reported that the failure rate is not significantly correlated with state-level physician stocks or changes in stocks. On the other hand, Yett and Sloan (1974) found negative partial correlations between flow measures of *new* USMGs into states and the failure rate. While this suggests that new physicians are less likely to migrate to states where licensure barriers are high, the correlations were generally not statistically significant.

The fact that the majority of USMGs now become licensed by passing the National Board rather than state board examinations[25] also indicates that state licensure requirements probably do not seriously inhibit interstate movement by new USMGs. National Board certification is accepted as a demonstration of competence by nearly all state boards and thus enables physicians to begin practice in virtually any state they choose. Similarly, most state boards participate in multilateral reciprocal licensing arrangements whereby a physician licensed in one state can easily obtain a license to practice in another.

As discussed earlier, the licensure requirements for FMGs do vary from state to state. At present, all states give licensure candidates the same examination (FLEX). Thus, the differences in state licensure requirements for FMGs are probably not related to the type of examination given or to scoring.[26] However, Butter (1976) reviewed state boards' policies toward FMGs and found that some states required a much longer period of graduate training or waiting time for licensure than others. She also indicated that FMGs face greater obstacles than USMGs in obtaining licenses to practice in states other than those of their first licensure.[27] There are no regression studies of the interstate mobility of FMGs vis-à-vis licensure barriers, but a large-sample descriptive study indicated that differential licensure requirements had no effect on the choice of a first state of practice (Ernst et al. 1978). Thus, at this point, it seems reasonable to conclude that licensure barriers do not greatly affect FMGs' state locations at entry into practice, although they may limit the alternatives open to FMGs wishing to move from their first state to others.

QUALITY OF LIVING CONDITIONS AND PHYSICIAN LOCATION

The attitudinal studies discussed in Chapter 3 show that physicians' tastes have an important—perhaps even dominant—role in the choice of practice location. Several econometric studies have also sought to estimate the impact of tastes by including quality-of-life attributes of areas in their location regressions. Broadly speaking, these variables consist of: (1) proxies for the climate of the area; (2) measures of recreational features; and (3) general proxies for the attractiveness of the area, such as per capita income, the rate of population in-migration, the number of dentists per capita, and the average FHA price of land.

The influence of climate was explored by Yett and Sloan (1974), Coleman (1976), and Wilensky (1979). Yett and Sloan regressed flow measures of new physicians entering states on the mean annual number of degree-days (each degree below 65°F). They reported significantly negative correlations between flow physician supply and this proxy for cold climates. Coleman also found negative partial correlations between county physician-population ratios and both the annual number of de-gree-days and the average summer high temperature. However, he indi-cated that county in-migration of physicians per capita was not systemat-ically related to either of the climate measures. Wilensky found that physicians for whom climate was an important locational decision factor were significantly less likely to remain in Michigan than other physi-cians. These results imply that physicians prefer warm winter climates, but that climate is probably not a dominant consideration.

The effects of recreational tastes were analyzed by Hambleton (1971) at the state, county, and ZIP-code levels. As indicators of a locali-ty's recreational assets, he included recreational expenditures per capita, the number of campsites, beach area per square mile of territory, the number of tennis courts, and other similar variables. According to his re-sults, specialists are attracted to geographic areas by recreational re-sources, but general practitioners are not. These findings have not been replicated by other researchers.

The general proxies for quality of life referred to above have been found to be positively related to the stocks and flows of physicians per capita (Fuchs and Kramer 1972; Held 1972; Rosett 1974; Hadley 1975; Wilensky 1979). The main question is whether they capture only the in-fluence of physicians' psychic motives in choosing locations or other forces as well. For example, the concentration of dentists is probably de-termined in much the same way as the concentration of physicians—that is, by market forces in addition to individuals' tastes. Indeed, the num-ber of dentists per capita, consumer income levels, population in-migration, and the price of land may all reflect area market conditions as much as the quality of life in the locality.

The Rand studies (Heald et al. 1974; Coleman 1976) showed that physicians expressing interests in "social life" and "cultural advantages" were significantly more likely to select urban than rural counties. Those with stated interests in "sports and recreation" tended to choose nonur-ban counties. On the other hand, Wilensky (1979) reported that individ-uals' desires for cultural and social opportunities had no effect on Michi-gan physicians' choices of SMSAs where they had prior educational contact. None of these studies found that other types of tastes affected physicians' location choices, although in Wilensky's regressions the de-sire to locate near friends and relatives was a significant predictor of the individual's SMSA of practice.

By and large, these various results do not confirm the attitudinal findings which depict personal tastes as crucial determinants of physi-cians' location choices. However, a serious problem in producing con-vincing evidence on this score is the difficulty of devising proxies for the quality of life in an area. Another problem is that physicians' tastes are not likely to be homogeneous. To the extent they are not, aggregative studies are unlikely to find straightforward, one-directional associations between area attributes and measures of physician supply.

The Rand studies followed an approach different from that of the others—using physicians' questionnaire responses as measures of their location preferences. The results imply that tastes are important predictors of urban or rural practice locations. But it is not readily apparent what physicians mean when they label "social life" or "cultural advantages of the area" as influential location desiderata, or even that all physicians define these terms in the same way.

Thus, done in this manner, the questionnaire approach does not really avoid the problems of aggregative studies. In order to explain or predict actual location choices, stated location preferences must denote well-defined dimensions of physicians' tastes, and the tastes themselves must be related in a comprehensible way to the type of area chosen.[28] In both micro and macro studies of physicians' behavior, the difficulty of unambiguously measuring location preferences limits the strength of inferences that can be drawn from such variables.

SOME UNRESOLVED QUESTIONS

Implicitly or explicitly, many researchers have raised issues regarding physicians' location behavior that cannot now be resolved. In some instances the evidence or interpretations of it are contradictory, while in others the research is fragmentary and its implications are merely suggestive. Some of the more important such issues are the following.

Prior-Contact vs. Market Hypotheses of Location Behavior

Most of the studies listed in Table 7-1 employ proxies for market conditions as explanatory variables in their location regressions. Their central hypothesis is that, given tastes, physicians are either attracted to or avoid localities on the basis of those localities' observable characteristics. By contrast, the prior-contact hypothesis holds that practice location choices are the products of physicians' past experiences with the localities. Out of these experiences physicians form attachments to areas, and the attachments induce them to practice there.

These hypotheses are not, of course, mutually exclusive. However, they emphasize different aspects of location behavior, and they have different policy implications. For example, the market hypothesis argues that we do not need to know physicians' histories of prior area contact in order to predict or influence their location choices. Although it does not rule out the possibility that location tastes can be altered by changing physicians' prior contact, neither does it expressly recognize the possibility. Hence, the market hypothesis leads away from policy options for changing the geographic distribution of physicians by revising the structure of their area contact.

By contrast, the prior-contact hypothesis suggests that we cannot accurately predict location choices on the basis of market or area-specific variables alone, and leads to the conclusion that the distribution of physician manpower can be materially affected by policies that determine the structure of practitioners' prior geographic contact.

Most of the descriptive evidence reviewed in Chapter 3 indicates that prior contact can influence physicians' choice of a place of practice or the urbanness of the community they select. Statistical studies also show a strong propensity for new practitioners to remain in states where they have lived before or during medical school, and where they have taken graduate training (Fein and Weber 1971; Scheffler 1971b; Yett and Sloan 1974; Watson 1980b).[29] Moreover, there are indications that the degree of urbanization of the physician's place of practice is significantly positively correlated with that of his or her place of upbringing and medical school county (Breisch 1970; Heald et al 1974; Watson 1980a).

What is not well understood is the comparative strengths of the market and prior-contact influences in accounting for physicians' location choices. To date, this question has been addressed in only two studies. Yett and Sloan (1974) estimated the probability that a new physician would enter practice in a given state as a function of three sets of explanatory variables: one representing market influences, a second denoting types of prior contact with the state, and a third consisting of both market and prior area contact measures. In terms of R^2, prior area contacts predicted state choices 50 to 60 percent more successfully than the market variables. And the combined set of market and prior area contact explanatory variables predicted state choices only 10 to 20 percent better than the prior-contact proxies alone.

Wilensky (1979) carried out a generally similar analysis on a sample of physicians trained in Michigan. Like Yett and Sloan, she reported that physicians' choices of states of practice were significantly associated with both prior-contact and market variables. But in her equation, the combined set of prior-contact and market variables predicted state location choice probabilities about twice as well as the prior-contact variables alone. Moreover, two attitudinal variables—the importance of nearness to friends and relatives (which may be related to prior contact) and the attractiveness of the climate—were more significant predictors of the location choice probabilities than either the prior-contact or market proxies.

Obviously, two sets of results—one of them based on a restricted geographic sample—are not a sufficient basis on which to judge the relative importance of prior area contact and market factors in explaining physicians' location behavior. Furthermore, as we have emphasized, the apparent effects of prior contact may actually reflect other aspects of location decisions besides inertia and area attachments. A physician may decide to locate in a state because it offers exceptional economic opportunities, a desirable professional environment, a pleasant climate, and so forth. If he does so before medical school or graduate training, he may also elect to take part or all of his medical education in the state. In such cases area attachments are themselves responses to market stimuli. Analyzing physicians' location choices at different career stages is a promising approach to reconciling the market and prior-contact hypotheses.

Urbanization

The economic rationale for using urbanization as a physician location predictor is that high population densities mean larger market demands for medical services and, other things being equal, larger net income opportunities for physicians. Hence, greater net income opportunities attract physicians to high-density urban areas.

Most of the findings reviewed above show that stocks of specialists (who compose the great majority of all physicians) and specialist-population ratios are larger in urban than in rural areas. This would seem to confirm the urban concentration hypothesis. However, other results also discussed above—particularly those using flow measures of physician supply—indicate that urbanness is not a strong factor influencing physician location at the state level.

In addition, there are conflicting interpretations of the impact of urbanization on physician supply. For example, in an analysis of counties in Kansas, Marshall et al. (1971) found that physicians avoided locating in rural areas regardless of whether they had high or low levels of service demands (as measured by socioeconomic variables). Their conclusion was that urbanization by itself is the single most powerful predictor of county location choices. The implication is that location tastes, rather than market opportunities, lead practitioners to select urban communities.

On the other hand, case studies and descriptive summaries of trends in metropolitan physician supplies favor a combination of the taste and market opportunity hypotheses of location (Dorsey 1969; Dewey 1973; Rushing and Wade 1973; Rushing 1975; Miller et al. 1978). They note, in particular, that the dominant metropolitan migration pattern from 1940 to 1970 was a movement of physicians from central cities to the less densely populated suburbs. Dorsey and Dewey attributed this shift to the declining socioeconomic status (SES) of the central city, stressing that physicians tend to locate their offices in upper-SES neighborhoods.[30] Dewey contended further that the migration was also prompted by physicians' desires to live in upper-SES suburban communities and their unwillingness to travel long distances between home and office.

What complicates the matter is that central cities have experienced substantial changes in physician specialty composition and setting as well as losses of practitioners. All studies show sizable losses of office-based general and primary care practitioners, but gains in hospital-based physicians (chiefly interns and residents), specialists, or both.[31]

Rushing (1975) and Miller et al. (1978) argued that these shifts had three major causes: (1) the overall decline of general and primary care practice up to the early 1970s; (2) a net outflow of office-based physicians from the central city to the suburbs; and (3) a rapid growth of urban hospital capacity. They differed, though, on the relative importance and interpretations of these factors. Rushing held that central cities had attracted new specialists by virtue of the growth of hospital capacity and the complementary relationship between hospitals and specialists. On the other hand, Miller et al. showed that only cities in the South and West had successfully attracted new specialists, and that cities in the Northeast had experienced large outflows of specialists from core areas.[32] They contended further that the replacement of office-based practitioners by hospital physicians was a coincidence due to the growth of teaching hospitals in central cities. Whatever the correct explanation is, there are considerable differences between the central areas of cities and suburbs in access to office-based and primary care practitioners.

These various findings raise numerous questions concerning the relationship between physician location and population density. For example, does population density have the same role in the physician's location decision as to a state, county, and metropolitan area of practice? The evidence to date indicates it does not, but the results are not sufficiently consistent to view this as an unequivocal answer. Further, is there some threshold range of population densities above which concentrated populations are no longer attractive to physicians, and below which an office practice is not economically viable? If so, physician density is likely to be nonlinearly related to population density. Finally, how is the physician-to-population relationship affected (if at all) by the presence of hospitals? Do hospitals compete with office-based practitioners in central cities, complement them, or neither? Some state- and city-level studies indicate that physicians are attracted into areas by the presence of hospitals. Are teaching hospitals an exception? The migration of physicians to suburbs has been accompanied by the growth of teaching hospitals in central cities. Would the migration have been as large if there were fewer teaching hospitals in central cities posing less of a threat of competition to office-based practitioners? Clearly, population density alone cannot account for the intracity distributions of office-based physicians.

Other Issues

The possibility of regional variation in physicians' location behavior was raised by Lave and Lave (1974) and Evashwick (1976). Both found regional differences in the physician-population ratio after standardizing for the influences of socioeconomic and medical status characteristics among geographic areas. But neither study standardized for specialty. The observed differences may have been the result of regional variation in specialty composition.[33]

Although the size of the physician's anticipated work load has often been described as an important location factor, its effects have not been extensively investigated. At the state level, Fuchs and Kramer (1972) reported that the number of physicians supplied per capita was negatively but not significantly associated with the mean number of patient visits per physician. Likewise, Yett and Sloan (1974) found that mean hours worked by physicians in private practice in a state had no statistically significant influence on the number of new practitioners who located in the state.

Several studies using flow measures of physician supply sought to estimate the effects of potential competition by including the number of established physicians per capita among their explanatory variables. If potential competition is an influential determinant of practice location, the change in the physician stock and the flow of new practitioners should both be negatively correlated with the stock per capita. In state-level studies, Benham et al. (1968), Sloan and Yett (1970), and Held (1972) found regression coefficients on the stock per capita to be nonsignificant or positive. Wilensky (1979) also reported that physician concentration did not significantly affect the retention probabilities of Michigan-trained physicians. Conversely, at the (rural) county level, Evashwick (1976) found the coefficient on the per capita stock to be significantly negative. These conflicting results deserve further research attention, particularly in view of their policy implications and the fact that competition with hospital-based physicians has been hypothesized to influence practitioner location decisions.

Despite physicians' purported desires to locate near or join group practices, results bearing on the locational influences of group practice opportunities are also mixed. In five of eight geographic regions of the country, Evashwick (1976) found that the 1960–70 change in the rural physician-population ratio was significantly positively related to the 1960 percentage of physicians in group practices. This implies that to some extent rural physicians prefer to locate near established groups. Heald et al. (1974) also reported that 1965 medical graduates who preferred to practice in groups were more likely to choose rural than urban communities. But using other subsets of the same data, Coleman (1976) obtained nonsignificant correlations between group practice preferences and a rural practice location.

Busch and Dale (1978) produced even more perplexing results in a study of county physician-population ratios in Kentucky. According to their estimates, the physician-population ratio was positively and non-significantly related to the percentage of physicians practicing in groups, but changes in the physician-population ratio from 1960 to 1970 were significantly negatively associated with the percentage of physicians in groups. Moreover, the negative partial correlation between the change in the physician stock and the group practice variable applied to both rural and urban counties. These results indicate that migrating physicians avoid counties where large fractions of physicians are already in group practices.

Other important location patterns have either not yet been explored in regression studies, or else the evidence on them is too thin to be considered reliable. These include the location behavior of recent medical graduates and that of family practitioners, women, and minority physicians.

SUMMARY

Statistical analyses of geographic physician supply are notable for the diversity in their measures of labor supply, geographic units, stratification procedures, estimation methods, and selection of explanatory variables.

The bulk of the evidence indicates that the determinants of the *distribution* of physicians are not the same at the state, county, and intracity levels. Moreover, in states and counties the correlates of general practitioners' and specialists' locations appear to differ systematically. As yet this fact has received little attention, but there are no important indications that the location patterns of primary care practitioners other than general practitioners differ from those of non–primary care specialists.

At the state and county levels, specialists—the great majority of practicing physicians—are attracted to areas with large, urban, and relatively affluent populations. They also tend to cluster in areas having medical schools and abundant hospital facilities. By contrast, general practitioners are much more likely to locate in rural areas where populations are elderly and there are fewer hospitals or medical schools.

Within metropolitan areas, the distributions of general practitioners and specialists are similar. Most findings show that both groups prefer to locate in high-income, affluent areas of a city, and both groups tend to cluster near hospitals as well. However, the evidence is mixed as to the effects of intracity population density on physician location. Several studies indicate that practitioners concentrate near high-density population centers. On the other hand, descriptive analyses documenting the migration of physicians from central cities to the suburbs suggest that population density is not a major factor in office location choices. The relationship between office locations and population density may also vary regionally. This would mean that case studies of single cities do not accurately depict overall urban location patterns. Even so, there is no systematic evidence that physicians avoid black or other minority neighborhoods as such. The causes of relative physician scarcity in central cities—or the tendencies for hospitals to be the major providers of physicians' care in such areas—seem to be partly economic, and partly the result of institutional and other factors not specifically related to the racial makeup of central city populations.

In view of the large volume of research on physicians' location choices, one might well imagine that most of the issues would have been thoroughly explored. But such is not the case. At least some contradictory empirical evidence exists with respect to practically every general statement that can be made about physicians' location choices. Undoubtedly, the contradictions are in some measure due to differences in research methodology. Much of the literature is characterized by intuition rather than rigorous theory, and by statistical models selected to accommodate the data that were available.

The list of important policy-relevant issues that cannot be regarded as satisfactorily resolved includes:

1. *The type of optimizing behavior physicians most often pursue.* Although one can assume that physicians select practice locations in order to maximize utility, little is known about the probable shapes of their utility functions. For instance, if physicians tend to be satisficers with respect to certain area characteristics, their utility functions should be sensitive to changes in these characteristics up to threshold values, but insensitive to them once the thresholds have been passed. Empirically, this means that the relationships observed between location choices and utility-generating area attributes should be nonlinear. That is, one would expect to observe physicians tending to avoid areas where the utility-gen-

erating attribute levels are below the thresholds, but not necessarily being attracted into areas where these attribute levels are high. If—to give an illustration—an area's hospital capacity was already well above the threshold level, then a program to build new hospitals would not be likely to induce large numbers of new physicians to settle in the area.

2. *How to choose a measure of physician supply that accurately reflects location behavior.* Not only are there conceptual differences between the stock and flow measures of physician supply used in location studies, but in some cases the different measures yield qualitatively different implications with respect to physicians' location behavior. Hence, policymakers desiring to influence such choices may well feel compelled to rely on conventional wisdom as to which results are the most reliable.

We have argued that since stock measures of physician supply describe the distribution of established practitioners, they are not appropriate for analyzing the behavior of new physicians—who are, after all, the principal targets of location policy. In addition, the majority of studies using stock (or change-in-stock) measures of supply also employed single-equation regression models. Such models are subject to two kinds of bias. First, they are likely to give distorted estimates when endogenous influences such as physician net income, hospital capacity, and measures of group practice opportunities are treated as if they were exogenous variables. Second, even when these endogenous variables are not used as predictors, single-equation regressions can still yield distorted estimates if the exogenous variables they do contain are correlated with the omitted endogenous variables. Therefore, future research should focus on improving the statistical specifications of models of physician migration, changes in the physician stock, or the locational behavior of individual physicians.

3. *The sensitivity of physicians' location choices to pecuniary income opportunities.* Much of the evidence on the issue shows that physicians' location patterns are not sensitive to prevailing net practice incomes. However, their location choices do appear to be positively related to net income proxies such as the area's population size, its per capita income, and the size of high-utilization subpopulations such as the elderly. Unless these characteristics are viewed as being strictly indicators of the quality of living conditions in different areas, the two sets of findings give contradictory implications regarding the relationship between pecuniary motivation and practice location choices. The first set of results has been cited as evidence that locational policies based on raising physicians' earnings in medical shortage areas are apt to be ineffective. The second set of results has been used to argue that policies to hold down health insurance reimbursement for low-income families further discourage physicians from settling in medical shortage areas. Clearly, this issue needs to be reconsidered in future research.

4. *The role of hospital capacity in physicians' location choices.* The traditional theory holds that most medical practices are to some extent dependent on the availability of hospital resources, and that, consequently, physicians prefer to locate near hospitals. This view is strongly supported by attitudinal studies of physicians. However, statistical analyses indicate that the physician-hospital relationship is more complex than this argument implies. In addition to providing benefits to office practitioners, hospitals—especially teaching hospitals—may compete with them for outpatient clientele. The net effect is not predictable on a priori grounds alone. Still other researchers have emphasized that physicians who are new to an area may be blocked from obtaining admitting privileges in the hospitals they would prefer by those already on the staffs. Thus, a positive correlation between areas' physician-population ratios and hospital capacities need not imply the same association with the flow of new physicians into the same areas. Most physician location studies have not attempted to integrate market theories of physician-hospital relationships into their models. The few that have done so have, unfortunately, estimated their models with state-level data, which is not likely to be the appropriate designation of a single medical services market. For all of these reasons, the extent and nature of hospitals' causal influences on physicians' location choices is still not well understood.

5. *Market forces versus prior-contact influences on physician location.* Since aggregative data do not contain detailed background information on physicians, studies based on such data have excluded prior-contact influences as predictors of location choices. On the other hand, most recent studies using micro data on individual physicians have included measures of prior area contact as predictors of location choices. Consequently, the two types of studies give different pictures of the choice behavior. The former indicate that market factors and tastes (aside from prior contact) are the determinants of location choices, while the latter report that prior contact is a highly significant influence as well. If a physician's educational contact with an area is itself causally affected by his or her plans to practice there, then the aggregative studies portray location behavior more accurately than the micro studies. That is, if anticipated practice location choices themselves cause prior contacts to occur, then measures of prior contact are either redundant or irrelevant in specifying physician location equations. But to the extent that physicians' prior contacts cause subsequent practice location choices, then the aggregative studies give an incomplete and misleading impression of physicians' location decisions. In order to clear up this issue, future research should employ methodologies where prior-contact influences are not automatically excluded, and where the direction of causation between prior contact and practice location choices can be tested.

NOTES

1. See Greenwood (1975) for a review of this literature.
2. Small-sample studies of rural or mostly rural practitioners by Fein (1956), Hassinger (1963), and Cordes (1978) indicate that 40 to 50 percent of these physicians leave their first practice locations. Heald et al. (1974) reported a figure of only 5 percent using a large national sample of urban and rural practitioners, but none of their subjects had been in practice longer than several years.
3. As an example, consider two localities, A and B. Suppose A has been popular with physicians and has attracted a large stock, while B has been unpopular and has attracted only a small stock. But suppose that A begins to experience a loss of population while B experiences a rapid rise. Inasmuch as the population changes should alter physicians' net incomes (through their effects on medical care demands), net incomes should increase in B relative to A— perhaps even surpassing the net income level in A. If the Rimlinger-Steele hypothesis is correct, physicians would then tend to move into locality B and out of locality A. However, if one were to compare the stocks of physicians in A and B with physician net incomes in the two localities, one might easily find the larger "supply" of physicians situated in the locality with the lower net earnings.
4. There are also obvious barriers to specialty switching, since changing specialties normally requires resumption of training and the consequent loss of practice income.

   The observations in the text above suggest that changes of location or specialty are more likely to be induced by psychic than pecuniary motives. Interestingly, this seems to be true in the only midcareer specialty changes that have been studied—the switch out of the primary care fields, usually in rural locations. The reasons for switching are described as desire to avoid excessive work loads, irregular work hours, professional isolation, etc., but never as unsatisfactory earnings. See, e.g., Crawford and McCormack (1971).
5. See Chapter 8.
6. See, e.g., the breakdowns of office and hospital visits by specialty reported in Cantwell (1976) and Glandon and Shapiro (1980).
7. More specifically, let the two additional equations be

$$Y_d = b_o + b_1 I + \sum_{m=1}^{M} b_m V_m + v \qquad \text{(demand function)},$$

$$Y_s = Y_d \qquad \text{(equilibrium condition)},$$

where Y_d is the number of physicians demanded by the area population, the V_m are exogenous variables affecting the demand, and v is a random disturbance term. The reader familiar with economic modeling will recognize that the demand function here is an oversimplification. Presumably, the demand function for physicians depends on the prices of physicians' services rather than on physician net income. However, making the model more realistic would necessitate at least one other equation linking physician net income with fees or the net (of insurance reimbursement) prices of physicians' services. The simple illustrative model given here is adequate for the purpose at hand, since fee levels and the net prices of services typically move in the same direction, ceteris paribus, as physician net incomes.

8. For example, one of the most sophisticated physician location (and pricing) models was estimated by Fuchs and Kramer (1972). Their model contains four behavioral equations defining (1) the demands per capita for physicians' services, (2) a supply function for physicians per capita, (3) output per physician, and (4) the rate of health insurance reimbursement. The model was fitted by two-stage least squares (a simultaneous-equations estimation method) to cross-sectional data on states.

   Ramsey (1980) has described the Fuchs and Kramer model as ambiguous because it failed to include an explicit supply function for physicians' services (paralleling the demand-for-services function) and an explicit demand function for physicians (paralleling the supply function). It is difficult to tell how these omissions may have affected estimates of the model. Because of the lack of essential data—a problem in many physician location studies discussed below—Fuchs and Kramer were also forced to construct the values of some of their variables. Newhouse et al. (1979) have argued that these constructions produced biased estimators of the demand-for-service function, but they did not discuss the effects of measurement errors on the rest of the model.

9. Methods for dealing with multicollinearity and data measurement errors can be found in standard econometrics texts such as Malinvaud (1970) and Johnston (1972).

10. For example, Wilensky's (1979) data base included an unspecified number of FMGs, while Hadley's (1975) was restricted to USMGs.

11. For a review of the empirical evidence, see, e.g., Kimbell and Yett (1974).

12. Contrary results have been obtained in state-level studies by Benham et al. (1968) and Lee and Wallace (1970). In each case per capita income was found to be negatively, but not significantly, related to the physician-population ratio.

13. Some studies have also investigated the relations between physician supply and variables characterizing the *distribution* of consumer income. Hambleton (1971), Wacht (1972), and Blair (1975) employed such distributional variables as welfare payments per capita and the percentage of the population with less than poverty-level family incomes, but no clear-cut implications emerged.

14. Other measures of the population age distribution besides the percentage of the aged have been tested as well. These include the number of women of childbearing age, the percentage of the population under age 5, and the percentage of the population under age 18 (Sloan and Yett 1970; Reskin and Campbell 1974; Guzick and Jahiel 1976). Guzick and Jahiel reported that the percentage of the population under age 5 is significantly positively associated with the stock distribution of pediatricians and surgeons in New York

City. But the other measures of age distribution do not seem to distinguish the location patterns of specialists and general practitioners from one another.

15. As was remarked in Chapter 2, Guzick and Jahiel reported that Howard and Meharry graduates were much more likely to be located in predominantly black Health Areas than graduates of other medical schools. They showed further that FMGs were somewhat more likely than USMGs to practice in Health Areas with large percentages of nonblack minorities.

16. Ordinarily, these measures refer only to short-term general hospitals. Other measures of hospital supply that have been used include the number of hospitals in the area, the number of hospitals per square mile, the number of special hospital units (e.g., cardiac care), and the percentage of physicians without hospital admission privileges.

17. Evidence on this point is also somewhat mixed. The general pattern was reported in studies of SMSAs and urban areas by Hambleton (1971), Elesh and Schollaert (1972), Wacht (1972), and Reskin and Campbell (1974). However, Marden (1966), Joroff and Navarro (1971), and Guzick and Jahiel (1976) all found either the number of general practitioners or the general practitioner–population ratio to be unrelated to hospital capacity in metropolitan areas. In fact, unlike other researchers, Guzick and Jahiel found that, regardless of specialty, the distribution of metropolitan physicians is unrelated to the distribution of hospital capacity.

18. These results suggest that the stock of physicians and the stock of hospital capacity should be regarded as jointly endogenous, with each variable specified as being dependent on the other. Unfortunately, to date there have been no simultaneous-equations models of physician location employing such a specification. In the model estimated by Fuchs and Kramer (1972), the number of hospital beds was treated as exogenous. And in the state-level model fitted by Feldman (1979), the number of beds per capita was assumed to be independent of the number of physicians per capita. For additional empirical evidence on this point, see the discussion of the Hill-Burton hospital construction program in Chapter 8.

19. The benefits might be either pecuniary or psychic. In this regard, Rosett suggested that private physicians can obtain longer or more regular leisure hours by relinquishing part of their patient management to hospitals.

20. Also included were per capita income in the SMSA and the number of dentists per capita. Respectively, they were defined as proxies for the demands for physicians' services and the quality of life in the SMSA.

21. Neither study specified the number of hospital beds among its explanatory variables, so that neither provides a further test of Rosett's complete hypotheses. In still another study, Evashwick (1976) used the per capita numbers of hospital beds and hospital-based physicians as explanatory variables. Neither variable was systematically related to the physician-population ratios in 1960 and 1970, or to the change in the ratio between 1960 and 1970. Unfortunately, since the latter study did not stratify by specialty, and confined its sample to rural areas, its results do not apply directly to Rosett's hypotheses.

The tendency for established physicians to settle near concentrations of interns and residents may signify another location influence independent of hospital-physician relationships. That is, it may capture the effects of prior area contact during graduate training. In Chapter 2 it was shown that physicians have a high propensity to practice in areas where they took graduate training. Thus, one would expect to observe above-average concentrations of physicians entering, or located in, states with large volumes of graduate training capacity.

22. Other theories have been presented besides those described here. Pauly and Redisch (1973) argued that physicians organize voluntary hospitals as producers' cooperatives. The cooperative then chooses the number of staff physicians—i.e., those allowed to practice in the hospital—so as to maximize the joint net income of the controlling group of practitioners. One implication of their hypothesis is that the hospital has a demand function for new practitioners in its market area. This contrasts with the usual approach in location studies, where the attitudes of established physicians toward new practitioners are ignored. Shalit (1977) proposed another theory according to which established physicians collusively select the volume of local hospital capacity which maximizes their joint net income. Although his tests failed to confirm the hypothesis, it does emphasize that hospital capacity is not necessarily exogenous to the local stock of physicians.

23. For instance, Scheffler (1971b) argued that attachments formed during graduate training are stronger than those formed during medical school. But since graduate hospitals cluster around medical schools, graduate training attachments would tend to be captured by the number of medical schools in the area.

24. In this regard Coleman (1976) found that rural general practitioners are not attracted into counties by the presence of medical schools.

25. For example, 72 percent of the first licenses issued to USMGs in 1978 were by endorsement of National Board certification (Wunderman 1979).

26. Goldblatt et al. (1975) noted that graduates of the same foreign medical school perform somewhat differently on the state board examination in different states. They indicated that this may be due to different scoring procedures.

27. Most states have reciprocal arrangements whereby a physician granted licensure in one state can easily obtain a license to practice in another. The difficulty FMGs have in obtaining new licenses by reciprocity may be evidenced by the fact that, of the 23,000 physicians in 1973 who were licensed in states other than those where they received professional training or their first licenses, only 226 were FMGs (AMA 1974).

28. Two of the Rand studies point up another methodological pitfall. Heald et al. (1974) and Cooper et al. (1975) used the physicians' stated preference for rural living as a predictor of the urbanness of their county locations. Not surprisingly, the variable was significantly negatively correlated with selection of an urban county. But the result is descriptive rather than substantive. A positive or nonsignificant correlation would occur only if other tastes domi-

nated rural preferences or if the responses were dishonest. The regression estimates are more a test of the validity of the responses than an explanation of the respondents' location behavior.

29. It has also been contended that the influence of market-variable predictors of state location varies with the type of the physician's previous contact with the state (Held 1972; Hadley 1975).

30. For instance, Dewey concluded that Chicago physicians followed the migration of the relatively affluent white population from the Loop to the suburbs. This interpretation is consistent with the results of cross-sectional studies showing that physicians select relatively affluent areas within cities (Elesh and Schollaert 1972; Kaplan and Leinhardt 1973; Guzick and Jahiel 1976).

31. Most studies also indicate that this phenomenon has greatly increased the maldistribution of physicians between central cities and suburbs. Scheffler (1972) offered a contrary interpretation, claiming that there were no significant differences between physician-population ratios in urban and suburban areas. However, his analysis was confined to SMSAs as units and is not relevant to physician distributions within cities.

32. Miller et al. attributed these differences to different degrees of "suburbanization." Northeastern cities, they argued, are in a more advanced stage of "suburbanization" than southern and western cities, and the patterns of physician location within them reflect this type of development. However, they conceded that differences in physicians' market opportunities across cities might also account for the variations.

33. Large regional differences exist in the ratio of general practitioners to all physicians, even in rural counties. See, e.g., Wunderman (1979).

EIGHT

Policies to Influence Physicians' Specialty and Practice Location Choices

An important measure of the success of any policy is the amount by which its benefits exceed its costs. In this respect, the evaluation of policies designed to alter the specialty and locational distribution of physicians requires estimating the quantity of benefits each such program produces, the explicit and implicit values of those benefits, and the program's direct and indirect costs. However, there have been few efforts to define and estimate the benefits and costs of physician manpower policies. For the most part, researchers have sought only to determine whether specific policies actually alter physicians' career choices in the directions intended by policymakers. Even this more narrow objective has been difficult to achieve because of the problems inherent in isolating the effects of a given policy from all of the other factors acting on specialty and practice location decisions. The preceding chapters have shown that, in many instances, the quantitative impacts of these "other factors" have not been clearly established. As a result, there have been relatively few convincing assessments of the impact of a given program on physicians' career choices.

The first state- and privately sponsored programs to influence physicians' specialty and practice location choices were established in the 1940s. Although some federal programs date from the same period, large-scale federal support began with the Health Professions Educational Assistance Act (HPEAA) of 1963. In this and subsequent legislation, federal policy had three principal objectives: (1) to enlarge the total supply of physicians; (2) to induce medical school graduates to practice in physician-scarcity areas; and (3) to increase the number of primary care practitioners.

The first of these goals—motivated by the conviction that a shortage of physicians existed—was the dominant theme of federal legislation in the early 1970s. The Comprehensive Health Manpower Training Act (CHMTA) of 1971 introduced a system of capitation grants for medical schools, which were chiefly intended to increase the numbers of medical school graduates. Also, beginning in the 1960s and carrying over into the early 1970s, many states initiated programs to build new medical schools, at least in some cases for the explicit purpose of training more primary care practitioners. Although the supply of new physicians grew rapidly following this legislation, part of the increase was due to an unexpectedly high rate of foreign physician immigration.

Governmental efforts to expand the supply of physicians can best be characterized as a trial-and-error process, rather than a systematic program based on carefully considered targets and estimates of the responsiveness of medical schools to the funding incentives provided. According to Hadley and Levenson (1980), the Institute of Medicine estimated that CHMTA capitation grants amounted to at most 5 percent of medical schools' total incomes in 1974. The American Medical Association (AMA) reported that federal teaching subsidies (including those paid for graduate training) remained constant at 11 to 12 percent from 1969 to 1974, and then declined to less than 5 percent in 1978 (AMA 1980). Yet, despite the relatively small contribution of capitation grants to their revenues, the medical schools in existence in 1971 increased their numbers of graduates by 48 percent from 1971 to 1978 (AMA 1971, 1980). When the outputs of new schools that became operational after 1971 are added into the total, the overall number of new U.S. medical graduates rose by 65 percent from 1971 to 1978.

Those observers who dissented from the view that government intervention was necessary to correct the "physician shortage" based their arguments largely on the poor quality of projections of "needs" for physicians and lack of knowledge regarding the capabilities of medical schools for supplying new graduates.[1] Second thoughts about the consequences of the CHMTA of 1971 began to proliferate almost as soon as the bill was passed.

In 1976 Congress declared that the overall "physician shortage" had ended. Accordingly, the Health Professions Educational Assistance Act of 1976 had as its stated goals alleviating geographic imbalances of access to physicians and promoting entry by new physicians into the primary care fields. The 1976 act continued most of the features of the CHMTA of 1971 (including start-up and construction assistance for medical schools, support for family medicine departments, and student loans and scholarships), but at stable or reduced rates of funding. Among other things, it made eligibility for capitation grants contingent on schools' setting up or enlarging their primary care residency programs. Specifically, it set national goals requiring that 35 percent of all residencies be offered in the primary care fields in fiscal 1978, 40 percent in fiscal 1979, and 50 percent in fiscal 1980.

Federal policies to increase the supplies of primary care practitioners, as reflected in this legislation, have been directed at institutions rather than at medical students or physicians. Little is known about the states' policies to promote primary care, although they too appear to focus on institutions. According to descriptive and anecdotal evidence, state legislatures have most often addressed the issue by defining as a goal of public medical schools the production of more primary care practitioners, requiring certain curricular features such as preceptorships or clinical courses in family medicine, and setting guidelines for admissions policies. It does not appear that any major state-sponsored programs exist to support primary care training in private medical schools. However, in 1978–79, 16 states offered capitation grants to private schools to encourage them to accept in-state students (Rosenthal 1980).

By contrast, governmental policies relating to practice location choices have been aimed chiefly at individual physicians. Traditionally, loan-forgiveness programs have been the mainstays of both federal and state efforts to recruit physicians for physician-scarcity areas. Under these programs, a medical student or resident is offered an educational loan, and the interest on the loan, the principal, or both are reduced or cancelled if, after completion of training, the physician practices for a specified length of time in an area designated as medically underserved. If the physician accepts the loan but decides not to practice in an underserved area, he or she can "buy out" of the contract by repaying the full amounts of the principal and interest—in some instances with a sizable penalty.

The original federal loan-forgiveness program, created by the HPEAA of 1963, provided for loan cancellation if the borrower practiced for at least two years in a physician-scarcity area so designated by the U.S. Department of Health, Education, and Welfare. Although unsuccessful at their outset,[2] loan-forgiveness provisions have been retained and even expanded in subsequent federal physician manpower legislation. In addition, 25 states have operating loan-forgiveness programs (Hadley 1980), some of which, as described below, seem to have been more effective than their federal counterparts.

While their principles and prototypes are not new, many of the specific programs to influence physicians' specialty and location choices are of relatively recent origin. Because of this, and the length of time it takes to observe the outcomes of such programs, evaluative research on physician manpower policies is still fragmentary and uneven. This is particularly true for federal legislation of the past decade, but it applies in varying degrees to nonfederal programs as well. The existing findings are discussed in the next two sections.

EMPIRICAL STUDIES OF POLICIES CONCERNING SPECIALTY CHOICES

Warner (1975) listed five approaches that have been used to stimulate medical students' or residents' preferences for the primary care specialties. They are (1) curricular innovations, especially the introduction of courses in family medicine; (2) preclinical exposure to primary care; (3) preceptorships and clerkships in primary care; (4) interdisciplinary courses to promote new modes of medical practice; and (5) the establishment of residency positions in family practice and other primary care fields.

In varying degrees, all of these types of programs were started or expanded in most medical schools during the 1970s. The main impetus appears to have come from federal funding, although some efforts predated the federal legislation and were established either by the schools themselves or under mandates from state legislatures. In general, the programs have had two objectives: (1) to encourage students' interests in primary care through increased exposure to it, and (2) to raise the academic status of primary care. In the latter case, it was believed that a greater proportion of medical students would adopt primary care role models for their professional careers once the prestige of primary care faculty and teaching programs was increased.

It is difficult to judge whether these objectives have been—or will be—successfully achieved. Few studies of undergraduate medical curricula have made an effort to assess the impact of teaching programs on physicians' specialty choices. Fewer still have found that specific curricular innovations have been responsible for altering physicians' career patterns. Moreover, all such studies have been beset by the same major methodological problem discussed earlier—namely, that in order to evaluate a program's effectiveness, extraneous factors must be eliminated as potential causes of the program's outcome. As a rule, this can be done only with the use of a suitable control group, experimental design, or statistical methodology that removes the effects of non–policy factors. Otherwise, what may appear to be "policy effects" may not be due entirely, or at all, to the policy under consideration.

Two studies illustrate the foregoing point. In one, Phillips et al. (1978) reviewed the residency specialty choices of graduates of the University of Washington's "family physician pathway" from 1972 to 1977. The pathway is a special two-year clinical curriculum allowing medical students to select courses and clerkships that train them for family practice. During the five-year study period, Phillips et al. reported that 61 percent of the pathway graduates and 33 percent of the Washington graduates overall (including those who had not taken the pathway program) chose first-year residencies in family practice, or else rotating, mixed, or flexible first-year residencies presumably leading into family practice.

Lacking a natural control group, Phillips et al. compared these percentages with data on students' specialty preferences at other medical schools during the early and mid-1970s. They cited three studies (Oates and Feldman 1974; Held and Zimet 1975; and Herman and Veloski 1977) showing that overall an average of 17 to 22 percent of new medical school graduates were choosing family practice. In contrast to these studies, Phillips et al. concluded that the family practice pathway had produced a significantly higher percentage of new family practitioners at the University of Washington.

Phillips et al. themselves stressed the dificulties inherent in appraising the effects of the family practice program. First, initial residency choices are not necessarily indicative of physicians' practice specialties. Second, self-selection of the program by medical students already interested in family practice cannot be ruled out as the "cause" of the success of the pathway. More than one-third of the total number of graduates chose the pathway of their own volition, and 12 percent of the graduates who chose other pathways also selected family practice or similar residencies. Taken together, these figures imply that the study group contained a large proportion of students who were predisposed toward family practice and might well have entered the field even without the special curriculum. Hence, the apparent effectiveness of the curriculum may have been due more to characteristics of the school's applicant pool or admissions policies than to training in family practice.

The second study that illustrates the difficulties confronted in assessing the impact of training programs on specialty preferences is by Simon and Shriver (1964). They explored the effects of training grants on preferences for psychiatry. The grants were given by the National Institute of Mental Health for extracurricular clinical training in psychiatry. The purpose of the grants was to promote a general interest in government service in psychiatry and, secondarily, to encourage teaching and research in the field.

Simon and Shriver selected 558 grant recipients in 1957—the first year of the awards—and observed their specialty preferences at the start of the program, again one year later, and a final time in 1963. They found that 28 percent initially preferred psychiatry, and that 32 percent preferred (or planned to enter) the field at each of the two later observation dates. However, they argued that the truest test of the program was not the percentage increase in the number of students preferring psychiatry but, rather, its effect on the 230 grant recipients who were originally undecided about a specialty. While only 10 percent of recent medical school graduates had entered psychiatry, 23 percent of the previously undecided students in their study chose the field. On the basis of their results, Simon and Shriver concluded that the training grant program more than doubled the number of graduates who elected to specialize in psychiatry.

The problem is that the undecided students were obviously not a random sample of all medical graduates. Since they all applied for the grants many were almost certainly favorably predisposed toward psychiatry. Hence, the 10 percent benchmark figure for the normal rate of entry into psychiatry is inappropriately low for persons already inclined toward the field. This means that the magnitude of their estimate of the grant program's effect on specialty choices is probably overstated. Indeed, if it is assumed that the undecided students were drawn from the same population as the grant recipients who had already decided on specialties, one might conclude that the program discouraged interest in psychiatry. Among the "decideds," 48 percent initially preferred psychiatry. If this percentage is used as the benchmark standard, the rate of entry into the field by the "undecideds" is only half the normal rate.[3]

Many medical schools provide programs for students in family or comprehensive care. Some are short courses in which the student—supervised by a physician and possibly one or more residents—has the responsibility of caring for a family. In others, they are essentially preceptorships or clerkships conducted either in physicians' offices or clinics.[4] The basic goals of these programs are (1) to acquaint students with patient management outside the hospital setting, (2) to familiarize them with comprehensive patient care and community health problems, and (3) to encourage their interest in the primary care fields.

Unfortunately, most studies of these programs simply describe their features or report on students' experiences with them. Attitudinal reports generally show that students regard the programs as worthwhile, come to view primary or comprehensive care more favorably, and use the courses to improve their ability to relate to patients (Beloff et al. 1970; Kaplan and Plotz 1974; Silberstein and Scott 1978). One study, which covered the early record of a program at the University of Rochester, indicated a good deal of student dissatisfaction, principally because the course involved a large caseload and complex or insoluble patient problems (Reed 1970). Another study, which reviewed a community-based clerkship at the University of Kentucky, found that the clerkship had significantly influenced the specialty choices of 30 percent of the school's graduates. However, it did not state how their choices were affected (Burke et al. 1979). Among seniors at Wayne State University who selected family practice residencies, Eagleson and Tobolic (1978) found that preceptorship training was given as the single most important influence on specialty choices. However, they also reported that three-quarters of the students had "considered" family practice before entering medical school. Thus, the preceptorships may have functioned more to consolidate than to influence the students' specialty decisions.

Likewise, studies of the relationship between undergraduate curricula and specialty choices have not been able to establish a definite pattern. Chyatte and Slater (1971) reviewed three years of experience with a course in physical medicine at the Emory University School of Medicine. They found that one-third to one-half of the students who took the course expressed an increased interest in physical medicine after taking the course, but a follow-up survey of the students during their residencies yielded too small a sample to provide clear results regarding their specialty choices.

Herrmann (1972) conducted an attitudinal study of students at the University of Michigan Medical School after the introduction of an all-elective fourth year in 1970–71. The curriculum change was designed to aid students in settling on their specialty choices. And, in fact, the students apparently used it for that purpose. The study did not indicate whether shifts in specialty preferences occurred as a result of the elective year. However, it did emphasize that students enrolled in the elective courses chiefly to gain experience with career alternatives they were already considering. This, of course, suggests that self-selection plays an important part in students' participation in special programs of this sort. It also indicates that the influence of such programs on specialty choices occurs primarily after medical students have already identified their preferred alternatives.

Canning et al. (1974) surveyed students who had participated in a faculty-student discussion group involving community medicine at the University of Utah College of Medicine. They reported that, unlike other students, those who participated in the discussion group did not display an increase in cynicism (as measured by personality tests) during the school year. However, there was no attempt to determine how the experiment affected the students' specialty preferences.

As yet, little has been done to evaluate the subsidies for primary care residency training provided by the HPEAA of 1976. In 1978, the U.S. Department of Health, Education, and Welfare (DHEW) reported that 53 percent of the first-year residency positions offered in July 1977 were for primary care programs as defined by the act (family practice, general internal medicine, and general pediatrics). This percentage exceeded by one-half the 35 percent target set by the act for 1977, and it even exceeded the 50 percent target established for 1980. The fact that the number of first-year primary care positions grew so quickly—and so greatly surpassed the act's targets—led some observers to question the law's importance as a factor promoting the supply of new primary care practitioners.

On the basis of a 1977 survey, Jacoby (1979) found considerable variation in medical school's willingness to offer primary care residencies. Specifically, 9 of the 116 schools surveyed provided 70 percent or more of their first-year positions in the primary care fields, while 15 provided 40 percent or fewer. Some of the variation seemed to be due to characteristics of the medical schools themselves. Using a typology developed by the Association of American Medical Colleges (AAMC), Jacoby reported that prestigious, privately owned institutions tended to offer the smallest percentages of first-year residency positions in primary care. The same kind of schools also tended to offer the smallest percentages of family practice positions. Perhaps significantly, similar relationships have been observed historically between medical schools' eminence and ownership characteristics and their outputs of general practitioners.[5]

The degree to which the federal subsidies have attracted medical graduates into the primary care fields has not yet been determined. However, no school is likely to continue providing residency positions in a specialty that very few graduates elect. Hence, a perceived demand for primary care positions is virtually a sine qua non for a supply of positions to be made available. The increase in students' preferences for the primary care fields that occurred around 1970 could not have been ignored by medical schools. Accordingly, the large increase in the number of first-year residency positions in primary care during 1977 may have been partly due to schools' anticipation of increased demands.[6] It may also have been partly due to pressures within schools to provide new training for primary care and to the anticipation of federal funding. In any event, it is clear that the HPEAA of 1976 assisted medical schools in meeting the new demand for primary care training, whether or not it significantly stimulated the demand.

To date, there is little direct evidence on the effectiveness of new residency training programs in encouraging physicians' interest in primary care. Pozen et al. (1979) studied the introduction of primary care pathways into traditional residency programs in internal medicine and pediatrics at Boston City Hospital in 1974. On the basis of four years' experience with these programs, they reported that the primary care pathways had generally stabilizing effects on residents' plans not to subspecialize. However, they also found that substantial percentages of residents in the pathways did not intend to practice full-time in patient care, and that one-third of those in internal medicine planned to follow academic careers.

Whether federal funding has succeeded in elevating the academic status of family practice in the past decade is another open question. In Chapter 4 it was observed that some authorities have expressed doubts about the matter. On this score, a study conducted by Kimberly and Counte (1978) at an unnamed medical school found that recent medical students still do not regard family practice as a prestigious field. They concluded that the educational system's support of family practice may be both superficial and short-lived.

Thus, at least until new findings come to light, there are reasons for skepticism about policies to promote primary care practice through the support of institutional training in primary care. The fundamental logic of the policies—i.e., that training in a specialty motivates a physician to take up the specialty as his or her career field—has not been proved. For one thing, there are no guarantees that exposure to a primary care program is always (or even typically) a positive experience for the medical student or resident. Moreover, most undergraduate programs in primary care are of short duration. Considerable research has shown that short programs need not have significant or lasting effects on students' specialty preferences, particularly where a predominantly specialty-oriented teaching environment influences specialty choices. Beyond that, most results indicate that the programs attract participants with preestablished interests in primary care. Consequently, their impact may be greatest in terms of persuading marginally undecided students to select a primary care field and discouraging defections to the referral specialties. These would not be negligible accomplishments. However, there are as yet no solid grounds for knowing whether, in fact, they are the principal achievements of the new primary care teaching programs.

EMPIRICAL STUDIES OF POLICIES TO INFLUENCE PRACTICE LOCATION CHOICES

Many longstanding government- and privately sponsored programs exist for influencing the practice location choices of physicians. They have usually sought to recruit physicians into rural communities, central cities (especially black and other minority neighborhoods), or both. The major types of these programs consist of preferential medical school admissions policies, rural preceptorships, student loan forgiveness, and, indirectly, the Hill-Burton Act hospital construction subsidies. A host of newer and generally less well studied programs also exist. These include community-based physician recruitment projects, decentralized graduate training, the National Health Service Corps (NHSC), and others. Dozens of policy recommendations have been made over the past two decades, and many states, private foundations, communities, and other agencies have recently initiated programs to affect the geographic distribution of physicians. Unfortunately, little is known about the effectiveness of these newer efforts, and reports on them are chiefly descriptive. This section focuses on the evaluative evidence relating to 10 of the most common types of physician location policies.

Preferential Medical School Admissions Policies

Publicly owned medical schools have long given preferential treatment to in-state applicants, but in most instances not for the explicit purpose of managing the geographic distribution of graduates.[7] Only two admissions programs for influencing physician location have been systematically evaluated to date. While different in terms of their structure and objectives, both are operated by the state of Illinois.

The first program, established in 1948 and administered by a special state agency called the Medical School Loan Fund Board (MSLFB), was designed to recruit rural practitioners. Participating students received preferential admissions treatment at the University of Illinois School of Medicine, loans (having no forgiveness provisions), or both, if they agreed to serve as family practitioners for five years or more in rural areas. The second program, begun in 1970, provided grants to four private Illinois medical schools for admitting at least 20 Illinois residents each year. Based on the prior-contact hypothesis of location choice (i.e., that students entering medical school from Illinois are more likely than out-of-state entrants to practice in the state), the program was intended to increase the number of Illinois practitioners.[8]

Mattson et al. (1973) reviewed the performance of the MSLFB program in 1970. They compared the career decisions of program participants from 1948 through 1964 with those of two control-group samples. The first (urban) control group consisted of physicians who entered medical schools from Cook County. The second (rural) control group was made up of physicians who entered from other Illinois counties. The principal findings were that (1) MSLFB physicians were more likely than physicians in either of the two control groups to practice in Illinois; (2) 28 percent of the MSLFB physicians entered practice in rural areas in Illinois, in contrast with only 4 percent of the rural control group and none of the members of the urban control group; (3) nearly half of the MSLFB physicians entered general or family practice, as opposed to 20 percent of the rural control group physicians and 11 percent of those in the urban control group; and (4) MSLFB physicians represented almost half of the physicians entering practice in rural Illinois during the study period.

On the basis of these results, the MSLFB program was judged to be a success, and the number of first-year medical school places reserved for participants was increased from 10 to 24. However, Mattson et al. have questioned the effectiveness of the preferential admissions policy as the key feature of the state's physician location program. First, they noted that the participants given preferential treatment had an unusually high dropout rate due to academic failure. Second, they reported that the subgroup of participants best meeting the goals of the program were those who received loans without preferential admissions treatment.[9] Obviously, either or both of these circumstances may have been due to special characteristics of the applicant pools or applicant screening procedures. Still, they do suggest that preferential admissions policies may not be the most effective or efficient method of increasing rural physician supplies.

No firm evidence has been reported with respect to the performance of the second preferential admissions program in Illinois, but the state's projections of program costs were challenged in an unpublished paper by Dei Rossi (n.d.). The state assumed a 55 percent retention rate for in-state students placed at private schools. Contending that the estimate was much inflated, Dei Rossi proposed a lower figure of 29 percent derived from findings by Yett and Sloan (1974).[10] After adjusting the percentage slightly and applying it to the $19 million cost of the program, he estimated the expenses at $150,000 per retained physician and concluded that the program was grossly uneconomical.

In view of the difficulties of using average national retention rates to estimate physician retention rates for one state, it is impossible to say how telling Dei Rossi's criticism is. No data on the actual retention rates of the program have been published, making it impossible to determine, even retrospectively, whether the program was "too costly." This notwithstanding, Dei Rossi's argument does point up the types of considerations that should be taken into account in planning preferential admissions programs.

First, a successful outcome—the physician's locating in an area designated by the program—is a probabilistic phenomenon. That is, although the cost of the program (i.e., the subsidies paid to medical schools) are fixed, its outcomes are not. This, in turn, implies that a requisite for an efficient policy of this sort is a model that predicts physicians' location choices as accurately as possible, given the types of individual background traits that are used in admissions screening. If such a model cannot predict accurately—i.e., there is a large unexplained variation in location choices—there will be a large variance in the expected costs per successfully located physician. In this case, the policy will be vulnerable to the risk of high costs, and much more so than nearly all of the other types of policies discussed below.

It is also pertinent to ask whether some alternative policy can achieve the same results at a lower average cost. At present, the Illinois program pays about $16,000 in capitation grants to private medical schools for each in-state student graduated from a four-year program (Rosenthal 1980). Even if one assumes a 55 percent retention rate,[11] the average cost per retained graduate is nearly $30,000. The present value of the long-run benefits of retaining each additional practitioner may, in fact, exceed $30,000 for the state. If it does—and if no alternative policy would yield a higher present value of long-run benefits at the same cost —the retention program would be judged worthwhile in terms of conventional cost-benefit calculations. However, the large cost per "successful" location outcome makes it at least questionable whether this particular approach is really the most cost-effective means of retaining in-state practitioners. As was observed earlier, there have been almost no efforts to compare the cost effectiveness of alternative location policies. This is clearly an area where important evaluative research needs to be done.

Preceptorship Training

Preceptorship training, in which a medical student serves as an apprentice to a practicing physician, was a common method of teaching medicine up to the end of the nineteenth century. It was largely abandoned as the hospital became the primary teaching base. By the mid-1960s, fewer than three dozen preceptorship programs still existed (Steinwald and Steinwald 1975). Most of these—such as those at the Universities of Wisconsin and Kansas—were designed as training experiences for medical students rather than as methods of recruiting physicians for underserved areas (Bowers and Parkin 1957; Rising 1962). However, in the late 1960s and early 1970s, the possibilities for using preceptorships as a method of influencing physicians to locate in rural areas or inner cities began to be seriously considered. Additional programs were established, at least partly in the belief that they might persuade students to locate their future practices in areas like those of the preceptorship communities (Daugirdas 1971; Harrell 1973; Verby 1977; Onion 1978; Burke et al. 1979).

Nevertheless, it was federal funding that provided the major impetus for the revival of preceptorship training. The 1971 CHMTA authorized grants to medical schools to conduct rural preceptorships, and funding has been continued under the Public Health Service Act. The fact that preceptorship training represents a primarily passive influence on location decisions makes its impact difficult to assess. For most medical students it is simply an information-gathering experience. The experience may induce some students to opt for practice locations like the preceptorship area, but it may also have the opposite effect.

There are two sorts of empirical evidence on the effects of preceptorship training. The first comes from attitudinal studies, and the second from comparisons of the location choices of preceptorship participants and physicians in control groups. Large-sample studies tend to show that preceptorship training has at most a minor influence on location choices, although a few studies at individual medical schools suggest the contrary.

Using survey data on the practice location choices of approximately 3,400 graduates of medical schools in 1965, Steinwald and Steinwald (1975) found that urban-reared referral specialists were much more likely to locate in rural areas if they had participated in rural training (chiefly preceptorship) programs. On the other hand, there appeared to be no significant tendencies among rural-reared physicians or urban-reared primary care practitioners to choose rural locations as a result of participation in rural training programs. These results imply that rural training influences the location choices of at least some physicians, but the Steinwalds concluded that the influence is probably slight. In support of their interpretation, they noted that (1) only 5 percent of the program participants rated rural training as an important factor in their practice location decisions,[12] and (2) many of the participants (the number was not given) stated that they had decided on rural practice locations before attending medical school. They went on to argue that much of the observed association between rural training and rural practice location choices was due to self-selection—namely, that physicians predisposed toward rural locations were especially likely to enroll in the rural training programs.

Quenk (1976) studied 667 participants in preceptorships sponsored by the American Student Medical Association. She used regression analysis to predict the participants' preferred community sizes as functions of their background and personality traits and their subjective assessments of their preceptorships. The latter were defined as ordinal-valued variables measuring how well the preceptorships "clarified" the individual's community-size preference, specialty preference, and knowledge of health care delivery.

Regrettably, Quenk reported only the standardized beta coefficients on her explanatory variables (i.e., she did not present the regression coefficients or their standard errors). Moreover, only 59 of the individuals in her sample had actually begun to practice. Subject to these important limitations, the measure of how well the preceptorship clarified community-size preference ranked from second to sixth in numerical influence among 26 variables predicting preferences for various community sizes. It was most influential in predicting preferences for rural and small-city locations, and least influential in predicting preferences for large metropolitan areas. Because of her methodology, it is difficult to interpret these results. Still, they tend to indicate that students may be somewhat motivated to prefer rural practice locations insofar as they are affected at all by the preceptorship experience.

Another large-sample study by Applied Management Sciences (1978) sought to assess the effects of preceptorship training on the career preferences of 1,300 residents and medical students from the graduating classes of 1974 and 1977, respectively. Approximately two-thirds of the students and three-fifths of the residents who planned to practice in rural areas had taken rural preceptorships. By contrast, somewhat less than 50 percent of both groups who intended to practice in metropolitan areas had had preceptorship training. At first glance, these figures imply that rural preceptorships strongly encourage students' preferences for rural practice locations. However, as Barish (1979) noted in a summary of the study, its methodology neither ruled out self-selection of preceptorship programs by rural-oriented students nor provided estimates of the impact of preceptorship training on the participants' location preferences.

Aaron et al. (1980) studied the practice location choices of 2,600 practicing Kentucky physicians. Like authors of the previous studies, they found that the population of physicians' practice communities was closely correlated with the population of their community of upbringing. That is, physicians are more likely to locate their practices in towns of the same size as their places of upbringing than they are to select larger or smaller towns.[13]

Aaron et al. also compared the sizes of their respondents' practice communities with those of the towns where they had taken preceptorships, holding constant the effects of the sizes of communities of rearing. The size of practice community was positively related to preceptorship town size for all physicians, regardless of the sizes of the communities of upbringing. However, the relationship was strongest for physicians who preceptored in small towns. Among the physicians raised in large or medium-sized communities, those who took preceptorships in small towns were 65 to 80 percent more likely to choose small-town practice locations than those who preceptored in large or medium-sized communities. Even among the respondents raised in small towns, those who preceptored in small towns were 30 to 40 percent more likely to chose small-town practice locations than those who preceptored in large and medium-sized communities. While the methodology used by Aaron et al. did not totally eliminate the possibility that preceptorship self-selection by rural-oriented students may have been the source of their findings, it did control better than the others studies for one of the major sources of self-selection—rural upbringing. Thus, their work provides the most persuasive evidence to date that preceptorships, per se, actually influence location decisions.

Small-sample evaluations of preceptorship programs at individual medical schools have given largely negative results on this issue. Reviewing a program at the University of Utah, Harris and Bluhm (1977) found no significant differences between students' location preferences before and after they had taken their preceptorships. Likewise, Hale et al. (1979) found no changes in the location preferences of Dartmouth Medical School students after completion of their preceptorship training. Burket (1977) surveyed medical students and family practitioners in Kansas, and reported that two-thirds of each group considered their preceptorships to have had no effect on their location choices. Only about 10 percent of the physicians and 5 percent of the medical students characterized the preceptorships as "very important" influences on their location choices.

The most favorable small-sample findings on preceptorship programs were reported by Verby (1977). This study was drawn from the experience of the Minnesota Rural Redistribution Plan, which was established under state mandate at the University of Minnesota. Among the 31 program participants who had begun practice by 1977, Verby found that 21 had become rural family practitioners in Minnesota, and 6 had entered rural family practice in other states.[14]

The paucity and variability of the evaluative research on preceptorship programs make it difficult to judge the extent to which they are useful in attracting physicians into rural areas. Most of the results indicate they are not very effective in achieving that goal. Moreover, in cases where the programs are elective, measures of their success are likely to be biased upward by student self-selection. However, despite the generally negative findings, a few such programs appear to be more effective than others. Unfortunately, there is no solid research evidence on how the structure of a particular program affects its success rate. Such evidence would require carefully designed inter-program comparative studies.

Finally, it should be noted that no targets have ever been set for determining the success of preceptorships. Certainly, a program can be judged to be a failure if it has no (or a negative) impact on its participants' location choices, but, by the same token, it may be considered a success even if its success rate is low. The issue is whether it meets its goals in a cost-effective manner. Over a long period even a low success rate may be sufficient to remedy physician shortages in critical areas. Consequently, the low success rates reported in most of the research are not necessarily proof that preceptorships are inefficient policy tools. Furthermore, since the cost effectiveness of preceptorship training has not yet been studied, it is not presently possible to say whether such programs are more or less expensive methods of achieving given goals than other types of physician location policies.

Loan-Forgiveness Programs

Loans with forgiveness provisions are available to medical students through a variety of federal, state and other agencies. Although their specific conditions vary, the various loan-forgiveness programs exhibit certain basic characteristics. Students may borrow up to a maximum of $1,000 to $12,000 a year, depending on the program. If they later practice in localities designed by the lending agency as physician-shortage areas, a percentage of their debt is cancelled for each such year of service. The percentage of the debt principal which is "forgiven" for each year of service ranges from zero[15] to 100 percent, but is typically 20 to 30 percent. All programs allow the borrower to buy out of the forgiveness contract, but a physician who buys out must repay both the loan itself and accrued interest. Formerly, interest rates were set at low levels—until 1976, the federal rate was only 3 percent per year—but since the mid-1970s they have generally been from 5 to 10 percent.

The effectiveness of loan-forgiveness programs as a means of recruiting physicians for underserved areas has been examined by Mason (1971), the CONSAD Research Corporation (1973), and the U.S. General Accounting Office (GAO) (Comptroller General of the U.S. 1978b). Mason reviewed the experiences of 11 state programs established in 1960 or earlier. A total of nearly 1,100 of the program participants had entered practice at the time of his study (1970), 60 percent of them in the four states with the oldest programs. Mason found that (1) 60 percent of the participants in practice had obtained full or partial forgiveness of their loans through terms of service; (2) the extent of loan cancellation achieved through fulfillment of service commitments varied from 33 percent in Iowa to 98 percent in Kentucky; (3) in the three states for which data were available, about 75 percent of the physicians obtaining loan forgiveness remained in underserved areas after fulfilling their service commitments; and (4) only 2 percent of the participants defaulted on their loans.

On balance, Mason's results indicated that state loan-forgiveness programs were successful—albeit unevenly so—in attracting their participants into physician-shortage areas. The effects may not have been lasting, but if one multiplies the 60 percent forgiveness rate by the 75 percent long-term retention rate for the three-state subsample, this suggests that perhaps 45 percent of the participants remained permanently in shortage locations. On the other hand, some of the programs appeared to have been poorly funded or else not to have been very popular with medical students. Five states averaged five or fewer borrowers per year over the lifetimes of their programs, and only three states averaged more than 10. Consequently, state loan-forgiveness plans have not induced large numbers of physicians to locate in shortage areas.

CONSAD (1973) studied both federal loan-forgiveness programs and 10 of the 11 state programs investigated by Mason.[16] CONSAD limited the scope of its evaluation of the state programs to participants in the graduating classes of 1960–65 who were actively practicing in 1972. It also gave a markedly less favorable summary of the programs' performance than Mason's. Essentially, CONSAD reported that (1) only 42 percent of the total number of recipients repaid their loans with service in state-designated shortage areas, with the percentage by state ranging from zero to 83 percent; (2) only 17 percent of the participants were located in federally designated shortage areas in 1972, and half of these were in one state (Georgia); and (3) in 7 of the states' 14 medical schools, the average number of borrowers was less than one per year, and nearly a third of the borrowers came from only 2 of the 14 schools.

As CONSAD pointed out, these figures suggest that the measured success of loan-forgiveness programs depends on how shortage areas are defined. Moreover, the popularity and success rates of the programs varied enormously among medical schools. The study gave particular attention to the variability of success rates across states. It noted, for example, that the two states with the most liberal buy-out provisions, Kentucky and Illinois,[17] produced the largest percentages of participants who located in shortage areas (83 percent and 77 percent, respectively). CONSAD argued that if stringent buy-out conditions actually induce physicians to fulfill their service obligations, these two states should have had low success rates. It went on to suggest that unknown factors, over and above the stringency of buy-out conditions, accounted for the observed variation in program performance.[18]

CONSAD was even more critical of the federal loan-forgiveness program. First, it noted that 27 percent of the graduating classes of 1965 and 1966 across the nation had received federal loans with forgiveness provisions, as compared with an overall 4 percent participation rate for state programs. Second, it estimated that only 1 to 4 percent of the federal program recipients would obtain loan cancellation by practicing in physician shortage areas—as opposed to 17 percent of the states' loan recipients. Until the CHMTA of 1971, the federal program allowed a maximum of 15 percent of a loan to be forgiven for each year of practice in a designated shortage area. By contrast, a physician could buy out of the service by repaying the loan over a 10-year period at a 3 percent interest rate—a much more liberal stipulation than the penalties embodied in most state programs. Hence, CONSAD argued that the federal program was not only ineffective, but had probably attracted borrowers away from state programs where they might have been led by buy-out penalties to meet their service commitments.

Finally, noting that the loan-forgiveness participants appeared to account for only 10 to 15 percent of the new practitioners entering rural areas, CONSAD cited two further limitations on the effectiveness of the federal program. First, average medical student debts at the time of the study were only $5,000 to $6,000, a figure it said was too small to represent a significant incentive to move to a rural area in order to obtain forgiveness. CONSAD suggested that larger loans and commensurately more generous cancellation provisions would give physicians stronger motives to practice in shortage areas. It also presented evidence showing that state programs are subject to self-selection by loan recipients. In particular, data on 79 recipients located in federally designated shortage areas showed that 56 had graduated from high schools in towns with populations of less than 6,000. Moreover, among 98 recipients who had graduated from high school in towns with populations greater than 25,000, only 12 located in shortage areas. In view of the effects of small-town prior attachments on practice location choices, these figures indicate that many program participants who met their service commitments might have entered practice in rural communities even if they had not received forgiveness on their loans.

The study by the GAO dealt with the performance of the federal loan-forgiveness program under the CHMTA of 1971. Like CONSAD with respect to the 1965–70 program, the GAO was strongly critical of the later federal effort. It examined the practice location choices of 45,000 borrowers between 1973 and 1976, and augmented its data by a survey of about half of the 762 borrowers who had obtained loan cancellation by practicing in federally designated shortage areas. The GAO found that (1) less than 2 percent of the borrowers had repaid all or part of their debts by practicing in a shortage county; (2) 77 percent of the sample of physicians in shortage counties said they would have chosen the same locations without forgiveness of their loans; and (3) two-thirds of the sample were not even aware of the forgiveness provisions when they applied for and received their loans. On these grounds, the GAO concluded that the federal loan program had not significantly influenced physicians to locate in shortage areas. Indeed, it conjectured that the program had merely provided windfall gains to many recipients who had already planned to practice in such areas.

On balance, the three studies discussed here indicate that loan-forgiveness programs have not been especially influential in recruiting physicians for shortage areas. It seems questionable whether loan for-giveness itself is an effective policy tool, although—as CONSAD and the GAO both speculated—raising the amounts of loans might be a useful strategy.[19] Self-selection is apparently a major problem with the pro-grams. Indeed, it may be the explanation of why some states' programs appear to be successful. Screening loan applicants and providing them with counseling or assistance in choosing practice locations will almost certainly raise success rates, but it is unlikely to eliminate the self-selec-tion problem. No efforts have been made to estimate the cost effective-ness of loan-forgiveness programs, but if the dimensions of self-selection are anything like the GAO's estimate of 77 percent, the programs are probably an overly expensive method of attracting physicians into short-age areas.

The Hill-Burton Hospital Construction Act

The Hill-Burton Act, passed in 1946, provided federal subsidies for hospital construction. The act was intended to help offset the presumed tendency of market forces to concentrate health resources in affluent geo-graphic areas by supporting hospital construction in the poorer states. One aspect of its goals was to induce physicians to locate in poor and medically underserved areas. The contention was that since physicians prefer to settle near hospitals, they would locate in underserved areas if hospital facilities were made available in these areas. Some of the evi-dence presented in Chapters 4 and 7 indicates quite strongly that physi-cians do prefer locations near hospitals. However, other findings imply that the physician-hospital relationship is complex, and that, in rural areas where many physicians are general practitioners, the influence of hospital availability on physician location is weak. Not surprisingly, the results are mixed as to the effects of hospital construction on attracting physicians into poor, underserved areas.

Studies of the effects of the Hill-Burton program on physician loca-tion have been performed by Williams and Uzzell (1960), Durbin (1963), Pashigian (1973), Lave and Lave (1974), and Clark et al. (1980). Wil-liams and Uzzell reported on 42 rural hospitals built in Georgia between 1949 and 1956 with Hill-Burton funding. A survey conducted one year after each hospital began operation revealed that an average of 2.2 new physicians moved into each community—presumably attracted by the expansion of hospital availability. A follow-up survey five years later of 39 of the 42 hospitals showed that the new physicians tended to remain and were joined by a small number of others as well. Moreover, the smaller communities experienced a greater increase in the number of physicians per capita (chiefly general practitioners and surgeons) than the larger ones.

Although the Williams and Uzzell findings seem to demonstrate that the act met its objectives in Georgia, Durbin (1963) reached precisely the opposite conclusion in another small-sample study in Illinois. He compared six counties where hospitals subsidized by Hill-Burton funding were constructed between 1950 and 1960 with three rural counties where hospitals already existed in 1950 and three rural counties having no hospitals in 1950 and 1960. He found that physicians migrated out of all three groups of counties from 1950 to 1960, but that the rate of out-migration was highest in the group where hospitals had been built with Hill-Burton financing. The same six counties also lost more general practitioners than the other two groups, but attracted more specialists. On these grounds, Durbin contended that hospitals alone were a negligible factor in drawing physicians into rural areas.

The studies by Pashigian (1973) and Lave and Lave (1974) both employed regression analysis to test the effects of hospital facilities on the distribution of physicians among states. Using cross-sectional data for 1947 and 1969, Pashigian regressed the state physician-to-population ratio on the proportion of hospital beds financed by Hill-Burton funding, the volume of Hill-Burton funding per inpatient bed financed by the program, and a set of standardizing variables. Finding that the physician-to-population ratio was only weakly related to the two Hill-Burton variables, he inferred that the program had not significantly influenced the state-level distribution of physicians.

The Laves tested the program's effectiveness even less directly. They regressed the state physician-population ratio on only three explanatory variables: the number of hospital beds, per capita income, and the proportion of the population living in urban areas. The dependent variable was significantly positively associated with the number of hospital beds. This, they said, showed that Hill-Burton funding may have affected the state-level distribution of physicians.

In the most recent study, Clark et al. (1980) compared the interstate distributions of hospital beds and physicians in 1950 and 1970. In particular, they classified states into three groups by an index based on population, affluence and urbanization, hypothesizing that to the extent the Hill-Burton program succeeded, it should have reduced the disparity in hospital bed- and physician-population ratios between the groups of states over the period. They found, in fact, a significant movement toward equality in the per capita distribution of hospital beds, about two-thirds of which they credited to Hill-Burton subsidies. However, they found little indication that disparities in physician-population ratios were reduced. Indeed, the observed increases in hospital-bed–population ratios were not typically accompanied by increases in physician-population ratios. Clark et al. concluded that (1) Hill-Burton funding had no important impact on redistributing physicians into the least highly developed states; and (2) the act's premise that new hospital capacity would attract physicians into medically underserved areas was not correct.

Thus, among these five studies, three argued that the Hill-Burton program did not favorably influence the urban-rural location patterns of physicians. Moreover, one of the two positive assessments (by the Laves) merely tested the program's supposition that hospital capacity attracts physicians without testing the effects of the program itself. On balance, although the evidence cannot be called strong, it implies generally that Hill-Burton hospital construction subsidies did little to alleviate the urban-rural maldistribution of physicians.

The National Health Service Corps

The NHSC represents the largest federal effort to recruit physicians for practice in shortage areas. It was created by the Emergency Health Personnel Act of 1970. Its objective (which evolved in the early 1970s) is to set up primary care practices in those physician-shortage areas where they have a reasonable chance of surviving without permanent subsidies.[20] The program's start-up subsidies are of two kinds. First, funding is provided to qualifying communities and state agencies to enable them to buy or rent medical equipment and facilities. Second, physician and allied health manpower are furnished to staff the practice sites for predesignated lengths of time. Eligible communities must be situated in federally specified physician-shortage areas. Subject to federal monitoring, operation of NHSC sites is left to the communities themselves.

Physicians and other health professionals are recruited for NHSC sites through a system of scholarships that were initiated in 1972, and are similar to loans with forgiveness provisions. A medical student who participates in the program receives a fixed amount per month,[21] tuition, and a lump sum covering reasonable educational costs for up to four years of undergraduate medical education. For each year of scholarship support, the student is obliged to spend one year of service at an NHSC site after completing residency. Penalties for buying out of the service obligation are steep,[22] and few participants seem to have bought out. As a result, a large and growing number of physicians have completed their training and become available for NHSC service. According to estimates by the GAO, the number increased from 190 in fiscal 1977 to nearly 1,100 in fiscal 1980 (Comptroller General of the U.S. 1978b), and the

AMA (1980) has reported that the number of medical students receiving NHSC scholarships rose to 1,300 in 1979. NHSC physicians have the freedom to select their sites, and—with the exception of those who elect the private practice option—they are paid salaries by the federal government during their terms of service. Thus, the NHSC is the first large-scale program to provide primary care in shortage areas by federally employed physicians, even though this characteristic was incidental to its main purpose.

The NHSC has encountered a number of administrative and related problems. Although most appear to be easily correctable, they have prompted criticism of the program. As summarized by Rosenblatt and Moscovice (1980), the major difficulties are: (1) a fragmentation of control over the program, which has inhibited administrative efficiency; (2) a failure to limit the supply of scholarship recipients so that it matches the demand for NHSC physicians; (3) unclear or changing definitions of physician-shortage areas and, as a consequence, ambiguous forecasts of the number of physicians necessary to staff NHSC sites; and (4) indications that NHSC physicians are underutilized—apparently because of low rates of demand for their services.[23] These problems notwithstanding, the ultimate success of the NHSC will depend upon the degree to which it actually attracts physicians into shortage communities, and the extent to which these physicians remain there after completing their terms of service.

One study by Family Health Care (1977) examined the retention rates of NHSC physicians during the early years of the program (1974–76). Using attitudinal data and physician background traits, the study compared the program's "leavers" (physicians leaving their sites after two years) and "stayers" (those who remained as NHSC officers or private practitioners). The results showed that (1) only 25 percent of the physicians remained at their sites after two years; (2) less than 10 percent planned to remain permanently at their sites; (3) depending on the sample year, 30 to 40 percent of the physicians had been raised in rural areas —more than twice the percentage for medical students as a whole; (4) stayers exhibited much stronger preferences for rural practice than leavers; and (5) half of the leavers departed to resume their residency training.

Thus, the NHSC physicians in the study sample appear to have constituted two groups. One group consisted of physicians who already had a desire to practice in rural areas, while the other consisted of those for whom NHSC service was a kind of intermediate career stage. The participants claimed that idealism played only a small part in their decisions to accept service in the Corps. Indeed, most reported that they had joined in order to experience professional growth or to try out rural family practice. In many if not most instances, simple financial need may have motivated medical students to accept the NHSC's scholarships. Moreover, regardless of their motives for participating, approximately one-quarter of the sample said they had made up their minds to return to residency training even before they had begun their service.

Another, generally negative, assessment of the NHSC's early performance was made by the GAO, who contended that recruiting policies were responsible for the program's low retention rate (Comptroller General of the U.S. 1978b). Through July 1976, the GAO found that only 42 of the approximately 800 participants serving in the Corps had remained, or were planning to remain, at the sites. Like Family Health Care, it reported that most physicians left to continue their residencies, and it suggested that a deferment of service until the end of residency training might raise retention rates. In fact, the CHMTA of 1976 authorized the PHS to give such deferments, but it has not yet been determined whether they have reduced the retention problem.

The GAO further criticized the NHSC for failing to staff large numbers of sites. At the close of 1975, it said, 261 of the 497 approved sites had never been staffed, and 62 percent of the unstaffed sites had gone without physicians from one to four years. Although the GAO observed that the unstaffed sites were the most remote and least desirable practice locations, it argued that the NHSC had a responsibility to place physicians in them.

In this connection, Woolf et al. (1981) compared the 1977 socioeconomic characteristics of counties in which staffed and "never-staffed" NHSC sites were located. They found no significant differences between the two groups of counties in terms of population density, degree of urbanization, population growth rates, number of hospital beds, inpatient days per capita, and per capita government spending on medical care. However, they did find that counties with never-staffed sites were markedly poorer than those with with staffed sites, and had fewer physicians per capita, fewer white-collar workers, and lower average educational levels. Observing that most of these indicators of low community economic development have been described as deterring physicians from settling in such areas, they speculated that the NHSC will continue to have staffing problems at some of its sites.

Four other studies have investigated the NHSC's physician retention rate or its success in establishing self-sufficient medical practices. Woolf (1978) reported that—like the communities that succeed in attracting NHSC physicians—those with the highest retention rates tend to be relatively well developed economically. Rosenblatt and Moscovice (1978a, 1978b) drew a similar inference about sites in the Pacific Northwest. They found that physicians who remained in NHSC communities

were most likely to be family practitioners who had finished their residencies. The most important factors relating to the success or failure of
the individual practices they studied were community size and the presence of hospital facilities. In particular, they identified two requisites for
a practice to become profitable and self-sufficient: (1) a minimum population of 4,000 to 5,000, and (2) the presence of at least a few inpatient
beds.[24] Geomet (1979) obtained rather different results at NHSC sites in
the Northeast and West. It found that practices becoming independent of
NHSC support were generally not profitable. Therefore, physicians who
remained in NHSC communities beyond their terms of service evidently
did so for nonpecuniary reasons. Geomet observed that the "successful"
but unprofitable practices were in geographic areas preferred by physicians because of climate and other life-style considerations. This indicates that, at least in some instances, NHSC physicians are willing to
trade off pecuniary income for the psychic benefits of practicing in certain underserved communities.

The evidence on the performance of the NHSC is inconclusive. On
the one hand, the program certainly has recruited sizable numbers of
physicians to practice temporarily in medically underserved communities. However, it is questionable to what extent the NHSC is meeting its
basic objective of establishing self-sufficient primary care practices over
the long run. Recent data indicate that the physician retention rate is rising (Scheffler et al. 1979), but whether the new trend is a long-run phenomenon remains to be seen.

The studies discussed here emphasize the two characteristics that
are essential if the program is to be successful in meeting its stated goals.
First, physicians selected for the Corps should have some likelihood of
remaining at NHSC sites. However, restricting applicants to those with
definite preferences to remain, even if it could be done, would be waste-
ful of the scholarship aid, since it would amount to rewarding the recipients for doing what they had already decided to do. Nevertheless, the
high defection rate in the early years of the program by physicians who
returned—and who had always intended to return—to their graduate
medical education was certainly not consistent with the program's goals.
Some type of applicant screening to eliminate those with weak preferences for shortage-area practices may well be necessary for the program's
success.

Second, not all physician-shortage communities are capable of supporting viable medical practices. This has been demonstrated by the ina-
bility of many NHSC sites to attract volunteers, to fully utilize the services of those they do attract, and to develop profitable, ongoing
practices. While some physicians may select and remain in shortage
communities primarily for nonpecuniary reasons, even they require a

minimum economic base to support their practices. Accordingly, realistic targets need to be set with respect to what NHSC can actually do in seeking to alleviate local area physician shortages.

Policymakers and administrators recognize the program's recruitment, staffing, and retention problems, and progress has been made toward solving them. However, it is likely to be at least several more years before we will know whether these steps have been sufficient. According to some projections, the NHSC's "need" for physicians may be as high as 15,000 by 1990—amounting to a quarter or more of each new medical school graduating class. Recent cutbacks in NHSC funding make it highly improbable that the projected "need" will be met.

Since its inception in 1970, the NHSC has undergone a continuous evolution in terms of its size and scope. Some authorities have argued that the program has never been able to reconcile its goals of providing physicians to shortage areas and establishing self-sufficient medical practices in those areas. To the extent that the first goal dominates the second, they argue, the NHSC has been transformed into a system of government-provided medical care for communities that would otherwise be excluded from the marketplace for physicians.

Decentralized Medical Education

As we have seen, the premise underlying the supposed locational effects of preceptorships is that physicians will develop a positive attitude toward rural practice when they are placed in rural training locations away from the urban, hospital-based medical educational environment. Much the same rationale has been advanced in support of decentralizing medical education. Although there is certainly diversity among the existing decentralized educational programs, their broad objective is to transfer students or residents out of the traditional environment in the belief that they will form attachments to their new training locations or to nearby communities.

The best-known decentralized program is the WAMI program, which was created with federal funding in 1971 by the states of Washington, Alaska, Montana, and Idaho. Its major purposes are to increase the number of medical graduates from the four states (especially the last three, which have no medical schools of their own), and to increase the number of rural primary care practitioners in the four-state area (Schwarz and Flahault 1978; Schwarz 1979). The program is operated through the University of Washington School of Medicine in Seattle.

The essential features of the WAMI program are as follows. Students admitted from Alaska, Montana, and Idaho take their first medical school year in the basic sciences at universities in their home states. At the end of this year they transfer to the University of Washington, which provides the rest of their medical education. At the end of the second year, all students are required to enroll in a specialty pathway such as the family physician pathway discussed above. Students are required to take hospital clerkships in the basic specialties, but they may also elect six-week to six-month "community clerkships" (i.e., preceptorships) at clinics in various towns and cities within the four-state area. Furthermore, residents at the University of Washington can take their graduate training in the same community clinics where the clerkships are provided. Thus, WAMI graduates who complete their residencies at the University have as many as three exposures to community sites away from the medical school: during their first year of training, during their community clerkship, and during their residency training.

The WAMI program employs a combination of policy tools, of which decentralized education is only one. The undergraduate curriculum entails a large proportion of elective course work with an optional emphasis on family medicine, and applicants to the program from rural areas are given preferential admissions status (Schwarz 1979). Moreover, as of 1979, only nine WAMI participants had finished their training in both the undergraduate and graduate phases of the program. These factors all make it difficult to judge the effectiveness of the WAMI's decentralized training feature as a policy device.

Schwarz (1979) compared the practice locations of 80 residents who had rotated through WAMI's community clinics with those of other University of Washington residents trained in the traditional way. Although only a few of the former were undergraduate participants in WAMI, 35 percent of them chose practice locations in towns with populations of less than 10,000. By contrast, only 14 percent of the traditionally trained residents chose practice towns of that size. This could, of course, indicate either that decentralized residency training leads to rural practice locations, or that the "community-trained" residents chose the WAMI route because they had already decided to practice in small towns.

Other studies of the possible influence of decentralized training on physician location have generated similar findings. For example, Royce (1972) traced the practice locations of 515 practitioners who were on the house staff of a rural Pennsylvania hospital between 1930 and 1965. He found that 19 percent had located within 100 miles of the hospital, and that 42 percent were living in Pennsylvania or New York. Among the former, two-thirds had selected practice communities of less than 25,000 people, and among the latter, more than 50 percent had settled in small towns. Conceding that many of his study subjects might have chosen the rural hospital for their graduate service because they planned to become rural practitioners, Royce nevertheless interpreted his results as supporting the view that rural graduate training leads physicians to choose rural practice communities.

Stefanu et al. (1980) studied family practitioners who had served residencies during 1975–79 at a Fort Worth hospital affiliated with the nearby Texas Southwestern Medical School at Dallas. The residency program was designed as a preparation for rural practice. Despite the fact that it was given in a large city, two-thirds of its graduates located their practices in towns of less than 25,000 people. Stefanu et al. compared this fraction favorably with the 53 percent of all new U.S. family practitioners who, they reported, began practice in towns of similar size in 1977. They interpreted this comparison as showing that rural-oriented residency programs can be used to recruit primary care physicians into rural communities, even if they are not themselves located in rural areas. An alternative interpretation, of course, is that these results lend even greater credence to the view that graduate training programs oriented toward basic practice attract larger proportions of applicants who are predisposed toward rural areas.

A large-scale federal effort to support decentralized medical education—the Area Health Education Center (AHEC) program—was designed at least partly to promote rural practice. Established by the CHMTA of 1971, it envisioned the extension of medical schools' services to the remote parts of states. Among other things, the program is meant to provide undergraduate and graduate medical education in rural areas, to enable rural practitioners to take continuing education courses, and to set up referral relationships between rural practitioners and the specialty departments of medical schools. Thus, the program involves both decentralizing medical education and reducing the professional isolation of rural practitioners, which has sometimes been cited as a barrier to rural practice. Eleven medical schools were initially chosen as AHECs, but the program has not yet been evaluated in terms of its impact on intrastate distributions of physicians.

On balance, it is still an open question whether decentralized training really influences physicians who would not otherwise be so inclined to locate in rural areas. Although none of the available findings suggest that overall such programs discourage the choice of rural practice, the fact that similar results have been achieved by family practice residency programs that do not involve direct exposure to rural practice conditions indicates that such programs tend to attract participants with prior rural practice preferences. While it is undoubtedly useful to reinforce these preferences, it is not clear that decentralized training as such changes physicians' location tastes.[25] Thus, it is questionable that such programs could contribute in a major way toward the solution of the physician maldistribution problem.

Community Recruitment of Physicians

It has long been advocated that underserved communities desiring the services of physicians should make greater efforts on their own behalf to attract practitioners. Typically, the kinds of policies recommended consist of furnishing physician candidates with information about the town's attractiveness and life-style, and offering them various forms of subsidies (e.g., Fein 1956; Charles 1971). Several studies have shown that community-based recruitment efforts can be moderately to highly successful.

Marr (1972) described a program established by the Jackson County (Michigan) Medical Society, which he said recruited 12 new physicians into the county in four years. The techniques used were almost exclusively promotional. The Medical Society began a small public relations campaign, sent descriptions of the county to interested physicians, and offered help in finding them housing, office space, and personnel.

Brierly (1973) reported on a subsidy-oriented program used by the community of Grover, North Carolina. Grover advertised for new practitioners, offering to rent clinic facilities to them at $1 per year, furnish them with rent-free housing, and provide income guarantees covering the first five years of practice. Interestingly, the plan failed initially because the town sought to recruit only one physician. Four practitioners accepted the town's offer in succession, but each left because of the long work hours and the responsibility of being the town's only physician. However, the town eventually solved its problems by recruiting two physicians who were able to share work loads and practice coverage.

In 1956, the Sears-Roebuck Foundation began a community-based physician recruitment project called the Community Medical Assistance Program (CMAP). CMAP's premise was that towns could successfully attract physicians if they had adequate medical facilities to offer. Accordingly, the foundation entered into agreements with 253 rural communities whereby the towns constructed medical clinics and the foundation provided technical assistance (including architectural plans), an advisory staff, and help in recruiting physicians. The foundation also supported the introduction of preceptorships in the towns. Clinics were actually built in 165 of the communities, but the foundation judged CMAP a failure and discontinued it in 1970.

However, Kane et al. (1975) reviewed CMAP's achievements as of the mid-1970s and concluded that the program had been highly successful. They found that 132 of the towns where clinics were built still had physicians. However, there was a high rate of physician turnover, the median length of stay being just over two years. Nevertheless, the towns had physicians an average of 80 percent of the time after the clinics were constructed. Thus, despite the high turnover rate, Kane et al. reported that the CMAP had created a large number of viable medical practices in rural communities.

Two studies, by Korman and Feldman (1977) and Jones (1978), analyzed income guarantees as instruments for attracting physicians into rural areas. The former study surveyed 78 physicians (including FMGs) who moved into three rural upstate New York counties between 1971 and 1975. It found that about half of the physicians had received income guarantees through local community groups. The guarantees were judged to be the most important element in the location decisions of the physicians who received them, although the physicians as a whole rated factors such as family and friendship ties with the area as other important considerations. About 10 percent of the total sample later left the area, but it is not known how many of the leavers were recipients of guarantees.

In a study of the Fort Worth, Texas, family practitioner residency program discussed earlier, Jones (1978) surveyed 16 physicians who participated in the program in 1976. They ranked income low among their location considerations, and personal and professional factors—e.g., the area's topography and access to group practice—the highest. Even so, 9 of the 16 selected communities where they received guaranteed salaries, and 4 others chose towns where they were given short-term income subsidies. These results indicate that the assurance of a minimal or stable income is an effective community recruitment device.

Although the small number of available studies hardly "prove" that community-based physician recruitment is cost-effective, they do suggest that it deserves greater attention. Unfortunately, little is known about unsuccessful community recruitment projects. Such information would be quite useful in helping to determine what the ingredients of a generally successful program are likely to be. The findings discussed here show that some type of subsidy—e.g., a direct income guarantee or the provision of office or clinical facilities—is probably essential.[26] The advantage of this approach is that the community can tailor the expenditure it is willing to make to its particular demand for physicians. The disadvantage is that it may not be well enough organized politically to carry on a concerted recruitment campaign, or may be too poor to support a physician on a long-term basis. Moreover, at present, indications are that the NHSC has largely supplanted community-sponsored recruitment projects (e.g., Lewis 1978). Given the large-scale federal effort to draw physicians into rural towns, the communities themselves have little incentive to finance independent programs.

Neighborhood Health Centers

The Neighborhood Health Center (NHC) program was established in 1966 primarily to provide health services to the urban poor. Commensurate in size with the NHSC, the program was first administered by the Office of Economic Opportunity, but was moved to DHEW in 1973. Originally, it was intended that NHCs—like NHSC sites—would become independent of direct federal assistance. This requirement has since been relaxed, although the centers are expected to earn as much revenue as possible from third-party payers, principally Medicaid. In 1978, there were 112 operating NHCs serving approximately 900,000 persons (Comptroller General of the U.S. 1978a).

The NHC program has been the subject of controversy almost from its beginning. While some centers appear to have been successful (e.g., Orso 1979), it has been claimed that many are inefficient and overstaffed, and that they do not always serve the needy (Comptroller General of the U.S. 1978a). The program was not intended primarily as a means of attracting physicians into poor, urban areas. Indeed, perhaps significantly, the NHC program has rarely been mentioned as a policy tool for recruiting physicians permanently into inner cities.

The evidence on the locational effects of the NHC program is sparse. According to a study by Tilson (1973a), a disproportionate number of NHC physicians in the early 1970s were blacks, women, and FMGs.[27] They also included large numbers of primary care physicians who were not board-certified.

Like the NHSC, the NHC program has had a high physician turnover rate, despite average salaries comparable with the net earnings of private practitioners. Tilson (1973b) reported that half of the participating physicians left the program after two years, and that nearly three-quarters left after three or fewer years. Not surprisingly, the physicians who stayed the longest received the highest salaries or had outside employment. In addition, they tended to be black, board-certified, and older than their colleagues. However, Paxton et al. (1975) found a generally different set of characteristics of stayers in a case study of the Denver NHC. They reported that physicians' prior experience, board certification, and marital status were unrelated to their propensity to remain beyond the first term of employment. The stayers were older than the leavers and were more likely to be women, to have had residency training, and to have moved into the Denver area from other locations.

In effect, the NHC program evolved into a health care delivery system subsidized by the federal government. In 1978, the GAO estimated that the average NHC had been in existence continuously for five years (Comptroller General of the U.S. 1978a). Thus, the program succeeded in maintaining medical practices—albeit not individual physicians—in medically underserved inner-city areas. Possibly the most critical testimony with respect to the problems inherent in recruiting inner-city physicians is the fact that it was impossible for all NHCs to become self-sufficient. Furthermore, the NHC turnover rate indicates that practitioners cannot be attracted on a long-term basis to many urban shortage areas even with the promise of assured and reasonably high salaries.

Group Practice Subsidies

The attitudinal findings described in Chapter 3 show that many physicians say they prefer to locate where they can join group practices. Groups provide collegial contact and the sharing of practice coverage. Thus, the establishment of group practices is thought to encourage physicians to locate in underserved areas. However, as discussed in Chapter 7, the behavioral evidence on this point is neither ample nor conclusive.

Two programs—one in Kentucky, the other funded by The Robert Wood Johnson Foundation—have sought to recruit rural practitioners by providing financial support for rural group practices. Regrettably, the effectiveness of neither program has been evaluated. Clearly, the success of this approach depends on two conditions: (1) the degree to which rural areas can support two-physician or larger practices, and (2) the importance of practice set-up costs as a barrier to the entry of new groups. The first condition cannot be changed by outside funding unless the funding is in the form of a permanent guarantee. Also, unless set-up costs are large, temporary subsidies are not likely to be effective. As is true for most other kinds of physician recruitment policies, group practice subsidies may be effective in certain communities, but they have not been widely employed for this purpose.

Scholarships

A number of programs offer scholarships to medical students or graduates with the objective of recruiting physicians into underserved areas. The one administered by National Medical Fellowships (NMF) has been described by Reitzes and Elkhanialy (1976).

The NMF program was established in 1946. It was meant to assist black medical students and graduates, and its ultimate goal was to improve medical services to black and other minority communities. Reitzes and Elkhanialy reported that it was more successful in helping the physicians (e.g., in obtaining board certification) than it was in helping black communities obtain physician services. After comparing NMF fellows with a control group of other black physicians, they found that only 55 percent of the former, but 76 percent of the latter, served exclusively black patient populations.[28] But they did not determine whether the difference was due to the type of physician selected for NMF aid or to the nature of the program itself.[29]

SUMMARY

All of the policies examined in this chapter were founded either explicitly or implicitly on the belief that, left on their own, the markets for physicians' services do not yield a socially optimal allocation of physician manpower. Many different reasons have been given for supposing that the markets for physicians' services do not function efficiently, but most programs to redistribute physicians among specialties and practice locations have been based on two in particular.

First, the medical education system which admits, trains, and produces physicians is not a collection of profit-motivated firms. Although a government or not-for-profit entity may be sensitive to market demands for its output, it is not the case—as it is with private firms—that failing to be responsive will jeopardize its chances for survival. Indeed, giving precedence to market demands over such factors as political considerations or donor concerns, is more likely to jeopardize the survival of such entities. Thus, since all medical schools are governmental or not-for-profit, they need not formulate their admissions policies or design their mix of training programs in response to market signals.

If medical schools were profit-seeking firms, they would almost certainly have responded differently in terms of pricing and output strategies than they did to the decades of excess demands for medical training.[30] By the same token, the substantial increase in enrollments associated with the federal program of subsidies to medical schools shows that they are not immune to financial incentives. Unfortunately, no estimates have been made of the responsiveness of medical schools to such incentives. Accordingly, it is an open question how responsive medical schools would be to tying government subsidies more closely to changes in admissions-mix and curricular policies designed to affect the specialty and locational distribution of graduates.

Second, it is widely held that physicians themselves are, in fact, relatively unresponsive to market opportunities. That is, it is often contended that physicians' career decisions are dominated by nonpecuniary rather than pecuniary motives—at least at the current high levels of pecuniary rewards in most fields and locations. The implication is that the typical physician experiences large utility losses by selecting "unattractive" specialties such as many of the primary care fields or unattractive locations such as rural and inner-city areas. Thus, the extra money income required to induce the typical physician to make relatively unattractive choices—that is, to compensate him or her for lower psychic income—is presumably large. In those cases where the required compensatory incomes are quite large, the supplies of physicians' services will not be forthcoming in the amounts consumers desire at prices they are willing and able to pay. It is in this sense that "shortages" of primary care physicians or shortages of all physicians occur in certain areas. Most physician manpower programs—especially those affecting practice location—have sought to persuade some physicians to make what they consider to be relatively unattractive career choices by offering them compensatory income that normally functioning private markets would not provide.

In preceding chapters we argued that the content of medical training is probably not an especially strong factor influencing physicians' career decisions. Nor is it clear that physicians are as insensitive to pecuniary income opportunities as many experts contend. Even so, a reasonable strong prima facie case can be made for government intervention in physician manpower markets along the lines just described. Structural imperfections that prevent some markets from functioning normally and the existence of "merit goods"—socially adequate amounts of which will not be produced even when markets do function normally—are both widely accepted justifications for government intervention to modify private market behavior.

What is troubling in this instance is that almost none of the specialty and location policies for which evaluative evidence is moderately abundant seem to work very well. There are, of course, exceptions. Moreover, the success of a program may depend more on its administration than on its underlying rationale. The loan-forgiveness programs represent a case in point. The general conclusion of most studies of loan-forgiveness programs is that they must offer substantial incentives to medical students coupled with large buy-out penalties. The recruiting success of the NHSC—which embodies both of these features—tends to substantiate that judgment. Additionally, it has been found that an integrated policy combining two or more mutually reinforcing programs has a better chance of success than one program alone. The two examples of such integrated policies—the Illinois preferential admissions/loan-forgiveness program and the WAMI program—would seem to bear out this conclusion as well.

Nevertheless, it is at least questionable whether most specialty and location policies have had any significant causative or lasting effects on the career decisions of physicians. For example, a U.S. DHEW (1976) position paper observed that "[a]lthough . . . studies have identified a number of concerns affecting the location choices of health professionals, there is no single factor amenable to influence either by educational institutions or by the government." This may be an excessively pessimistic assessment of policy prospects, but it is an understandable reaction to frustrating policy experiences.

Why is it that policies to influence physicians' specialty and location choices do not seem to work as well as expected? At least part of the explanation lies in the weaknesses of their underlying premises. An effective policy must alter the causal structure of physicians' career choices. However, as we have emphasized, the causes of physicians' career choices are still not well understood. Statistical correlations, anecdotal testimony (even by physicians), and plausible theories are not enough. Programs such as rural preceptorships, hospital construction, and group practice subsidies are based more on attitudinal evidence and conventional wisdom than they are on evidence from rigorous evaluation studies. As a result, some programs to alter the distribution of physicians may be grounded on false or only partly correct premises.

It also seems to be the case that the advocates of some policies may have expected too much from them. Policymakers have tried to effect rapid and drastic revisions in the supply and composition of new physicians. In some instances, programs to achieve these ends have clearly been poorly organized and carried out on too massive a scale. The federal effort to expand the supply of physicians—which began in 1971 and all but ended a few years later—is a good illustration. The effort succeeded, but its effects are not easily reversible. Indeed, it is now claimed that they threaten to produce a large "oversupply" of physicians in the next decade.

As a practical matter, it is doubtful whether government policy can alleviate primary care physician shortages in every community desiring practitioners. There are two basic alternatives. One is to persuade private physicians to locate in areas of greatest need. The other is to permanently supply such areas with medical services via government-employed physicians. Nearly all of the programs we have discussed fall into the first of these two categories. For their success, it is essential that the shortage communities ultimately be capable of sustaining private practitioners. However, the available evidence indicates that this is often impossible. A policy designed to expose physicians to medically underserved areas is bound to fail—or only partly succeed—if it ignores economic realities. Accordingly, the limitations of physician redistribution policy should be more realistically appraised before any new initiatives are undertaken or established ones are continued.

Another dimension of policy targets also needs to be reconsidered. Eschewing cost-benefit analysis, objectives have typically been set in the form of loosely specified quotas. That is, a program is judged successful if a sufficiently large percentage of the physicians to which it is addressed make the desired career choices, or if a sufficiently large number of "shortage" positions (e.g., in the primary care fields or in underserved communities) become filled. As a consequence, most assessments of these policies have been based primarily on subjective judgments with respect to both the targets and the degree to which the programs achieved the targets. Indeed lacking the kind of evidence we prefer on programmatic costs and benefits, we have used this approach more extensively than we would have liked.

However, it should also be emphasized that the "success rates" of policies to ameliorate physician maldistribution have often been measured against overly high standards. For example, on a year-to-year basis, loan-forgiveness programs and preceptorships seem to have marginal impacts on physicians' location and specialty choices—or significant impacts only under some incompletely understood circumstances. If such programs actually alter the career decisions of only a small fraction of physicians in any given year, should they be considered failures? The answer is yes if policy is aimed at the immediate remediation of physician maldistribution problems. On the other hand, a low success rate can produce satisfactory results over a long time horizon. As was true in the case of the physician "shortage," policymakers may have tried to bring about too rapid a correction of physician maldistribution problems. The dangers of this approach are overcommitment and disorganization, the disregard of long-run solutions, and—when results are not quickly forthcoming—disenchantment with the possibility of remedying the problems.

Both the quantity and the quality of the evaluative evidence on physician redistribution policy leave much to be desired. Almost no efforts have been made to esimate program costs per successfully placed physician, let alone to compare the costs of alternative programs. Many of the findings are of the descriptive, case-study type. Program evaluations are often performed by the operating agencies or their current or former employees. Standardizing for participant self-selection is a pervasive methodological problem, and one which almost no study has handled adequately.

The state of the evaluative research in this area is itself a reflection of the difficulty of the problem. As long as the benefits of physicians' services cannot be readily measured, it will be difficult to tell whether any program generates benefits that exceed its costs. In turn, this situation invites researchers to substitute evaluation standards based on the program's administrative objectives for standards derived from social welfare considerations.

The role of the federal government in supporting policy evaluations further enhances the use of administrative targets. The agencies that administer federal physician manpower programs are often required by Congress to conduct or sponsor assessments of their effectiveness. In these assessments, "effectiveness" is commonly measured in terms of the degree to which the programs meet their mandated goals. Such assessments have yielded useful—and sometimes the most significant—information about policy performance. But in following this approach, the agencies have not sufficiently encouraged the researchers who perform the assessments to question the underlying premises of the programs or their targets, nor have they promoted interprogram comparisons or experiments with cost-benefit analysis.

In view of the hundreds of millions of dollars that have been spent on physician redistribution policy, it cannot but impress an observer how little has been spent on policy evaluation. Most programs to influence physicians' specialty and location choices have (or soon will have) accumulated considerable operating experience. It is greatly to be hoped that this experience—whether positive or negative—will not go unreported and unevaluated. Whatever new directions physician manpower policy may take in the future, the lessons of the 1970s deserve to become known.

NOTES

1. See Bloom and Peterson (1979) for a discussion of these views.
2. The U.S. Department of Health, Education, and Welfare (1973) reported that only 60 of more than 75,000 borrowers had actually obtained loan cancellations by the end of fiscal 1971.
3. Simon and Shriver (1964) also remarked that nearly one-fifth of the students originally preferring psychiatry later switched to other fields. This finding tends to weaken their conclusion still further.
4. Silberstein and Scott (1978) reported that about 80 percent of all U.S. and Canadian medical schools had such programs in 1975, but they did not present a figure for U.S. medical schools alone.
5. See Chapter 4.
6. Anecdotal reports of a shortage of positions in internal medicine during 1977 support this view. They suggest that there were large new demands for programs in the field even before the federal efforts to promote them.
7. A few states or medical schools have considered preferential admissions policies as a means of influencing the intrastate distribution of physicians (e.g., Fulton et al. 1980), but so far the idea has been little more than a proposal (Edwards 1974; Moradiellos and Athelstan 1979). The state of Kentucky has reportedly ordered its medical schools to consider rural upbringing and applicants' career preferences in its admissions ratings (Hadley 1980), and

Northwestern began a minority recruitment program at least partly in the belief that minority physicians are more likely than white physicians to locate
in underserved neighborhoods (Daugirdas 1971).

8. Fifteen other states have similar programs (Rosenthal 1980).

9. Among this subgroup, 95 percent graduated, two-thirds were practicing in Illinois in 1970, and 35 percent were practicing in rural areas.

10. Yett and Sloan found that 29 percent of all specialists who entered practice in
1966 did so in states where their previous contact consisted only of birth and
attending medical school.

11. As of 1975, the retention rate for graduates of the University of Illinois College of Medicine was 40 percent for the classes of 1950–69. This may be a
more accurate figure than the 55 percent used in this illustration.

12. Similar negative results have been reported by Heald et al. (1974), Cooper et
al. (1975), and Coleman (1976), all using the same data base. A comparable
finding was also obtained by Schwartz and Cantwell (1976) in a study of approximately 2,000 1960 medical graduates who had taken preceptorships.
Only one-sixth of this group claimed that the preceptorship programs had influenced their practice location decisions in either direction.

13. Also see Chapter 3 on this point.

14. No efforts have yet been made to evaluate the federally supported preceptorship programs. A report by the U.S. General Accounting Office (GAO) indicated that, as of 1976, it was too soon to determine the effectiveness of the
programs (Comptroller General of the U.S. 1978b). The GAO noted that although an unusually large percentage (67 percent) of participants were entering primary care residencies, only 48 of the many thousands of participants
had started practice. Among the 48, seven had located in government-desig-
nated physician-shortage areas.

15. States such as Ohio provide forgiveness only for interest and not for the loan
principal.

16. The Mississippi program was excluded because it was terminated in the mid-
1960s.

17. Technically, the Illinois program offered no forgiveness provisions for either
loan payments or interest. However, physicians buying out of their service
contracts were required to pay a higher interest rate than those who met their
service obligations.

18. As indicated above, the Illinois program was operated by the MSLFB, and
was coupled with a preferential admissions policy for students reared in rural
areas. It has been suggested that the success of the program in Kentucky was
due to an extensive screening, counseling, and placement service provided to
loan applicants (Hadley 1980). In light of its effectiveness, other states such
as Florida and South Carolina chose to use the Kentucky model (Barrett
1978; Fulton et al. 1980).

19. The HPEAA of 1976 introduced a new loan program along these lines. Called
the Health Education Assistance Loan (HEAL) Program, it permits students
to borrow up to $10,000 per year and $50,000 in total. A ceiling interest rate
of 12 percent (plus 2 percent for insurance) was established for repayment,

and loans can be cancelled at the rate of $10,000 per year for service in the NHSC or a designated shortage area. The old program, known as the Health Professions Student Loan (HPSL) Program, was substantially modified. It was restricted to students with "exceptional financial need," and its amounts were limited to $2,500 per year plus tuition. Up to 85 percent of the HPSL loans can be cancelled by service in a designated shortage area. No evaluations of the HEAL Program have been reported to date.

20. See Rosenblatt and Moscovice (1980) for a brief history and discussion of the structure of the program.

21. In 1980, the amount was $453 per month for a 12-month year, and it has been raised annually to meet increases in living costs.

22. Under the HPEAA of 1976, physicians buying out of their obligations must repay three times the total amount of their scholarships within one year at the maximum prevailing interest rate.

23. The GAO reported that NHSC physicians average 49 percent fewer patient visits per hour than general and family practitioners in private practice in nonmetropolitan areas. It suggested that the program overestimated the need for physicians at many sites, and that patients often had access to medical care in nearby communities (Comptroller General of the U.S. 1978b).

24. Rosenblatt and Moscovice (1978a) indicated that retention rates were also favorably influenced by the existence of group practices. They have also reported evidence that nurse practitioners' practices could succeed in towns with populations of less than 4,000 and no hospital facilities (1978b).

25. Howard (1980), for example, reporting on a pediatrics residency program in rural Kentucky, found that the participants who later located in small towns were almost exclusively those who had been raised in small towns. The short duration of the rotation (one month) makes this particular case atypical of decentralized programs in general, but the results indicate that other factors are probably more important than training location as influences on practice location choices.

26. The experience of the NHSC—which has not been uniformly effective in attracting physicians into rural areas—indicates that income guarantees are not always effective. Nevertheless, in the case of the NHSC it can be argued that federal salaries are not high enough to persuade physicians to locate in "unattractive" communities.

27. Blacks, women, and FMGs represented 17, 20, and 22 percent respectively, of all NHC physicians up to 1971. Their respective percentages in the overall 1971 physician population were 2, 7, and 15.

28. About 90 percent of each group served black or mixed black and white patient clienteles, and about 40 percent of each group treated patients primarily from low-income classes.

29. During one of its phases, the program was directed toward clinical and research training at the graduate level. This may have stimulated recipients to choose specialties or practice settings leading them out of minority communities. Unfortunately, no specialty or employment breakdowns were given (except for medical school appointments), and thus it is impossible to resolve the question from the evidence presented.

30. The notion that medical schools are largely (if not wholly) insulated from pressures to produce physicians in conformity with social needs or demands has been advanced by many authorities. See, for example, Mick (1978).

NINE

Conclusion

In this final chapter it is fitting to stop and ask what all the studies of physicians' career choices have taught us. Physicians are a class of highly trained professionals who are vital to the nation's welfare. Do we know enough about how they select specialties within medicine and how they decide where to locate their practices? The past 20 years have seen the establishment of many programs to influence the ways that physicians choose fields and places to practice. These programs were motivated by the premise that some consumer populations—chiefly, those in isolated rural areas and inner cities—were underserved by physicians, and by the conviction that the population at large received too little primary care. According to evaluative studies, the results of these programs are mixed. Do we now know enough about physicians' behavior to design better and more effective programs? Beyond that, and in view of the promised physician surpluses for the next decade or two, do we need a public policy to influence or regulate the functional distribution of new physicians? Might such a policy even create new social problems, however narrowly it is targeted? While there is room for reasonable observers to disagree about the answers to these questions, certain general conclusions can be drawn.

THE STATE OF KNOWLEDGE ABOUT PHYSICIANS' CAREER CHOICES

In the sense that we can accurately forecast physicians' career choices, it can be said that we know a great deal about how they are made. Because of the "pipeline" effect—that is, the long duration of medical education—accurate predictions of the total supply of new physicians for the next decade and longer are well within current capabilities. Although the number of medical school applicants leveled off at about 36,000 in the late 1970s and early 1980s (Sherman 1982), it is still considerably larger than the number of first-year positions. Hence, with minor adjustments for attrition rates and the lengths of residency training, the numbers of physicians who will enter practice at future dates are essentially translations of the current numbers of first-year medical students. Adding in the numbers trained in foreign medical schools is slightly trickier, but given the tightening of immigration restrictions in the late 1970s, the figures are sure to decline substantially in the next decade.

Except for the upward shift in medical students' preferences for primary care that occurred around 1970, the specialty distributions of medical school graduates have remained remarkably stable in the recent past. Similarly, states' retention rates of their medical graduates generally show little variation over time. At the intrastate level, the strongest single predictor of the number of physicians in an area is the size of the area's population. As a result, moderately accurate forecasts of the proportional distributions of new physicians by specialty, state location, and (to a lesser extent) intrastate location can be made by using time trends of specialty choices, state retention rates, and population concentrations. Applying these proportional estimates to the expected numbers of physicians entering practice gives us fairly reliable and simply derived predictions of the functional distribution of new physicians. It is not necessarily the most sophisticated or accurate technique, but it can be implemented with a minimal amount of information.

In the past 10 years, considerable progress has also been made in the ability to predict the career choices of individual physicians. According to recent statistical studies, the individual's choice of a specialty can be estimated with a 50 percent or greater chance of success if the classification of fields is not too greatly disaggregated. Other findings suggest that the choice of a state of practice or size of practice community can be predicted at least equally well. Unfortunately, the most reliable forecasts of individuals' specialty choices seem to require fairly detailed information on their personality traits, and there is no firm consensus as yet about which traits are the best predictors of specialty preferences. The main problem in forecasting practice location choices is that the choices are closely correlated with physicians' histories of prior contact, including contact during graduate training. Hence, accurate forecasts cannot be made until after physicians have entered residency training or shortly before they begin practice. Nevertheless, by the late 1970s the state of the art had reached the point where some authorities proposed incorporating predictive models of career choice into medical schools' admissions procedures. Such models, they contended, could be used if needed to select applicants with the highest probabilities of entering primary care practice in physician-shortage areas.

At the conceptual level, a general theory of physicians' career choices has emerged which contains three subtheories or behavioral hypotheses. The first of them, which might be called the "experiential" hypothesis, maintains that physicians' learning experiences during medical education are the major forces acting on their career decisions. Under this hypothesis, the physician's choice of specialty is determined largely by the character of his or her medical school and graduate training environment. The principal locational version of the hypothesis holds that physicians develop attachments to places where they have lived, especially to the states and communities where they received their medical education. It argues that these attachments lead physicians to locate their practices in areas of prior personal contact or in communities resembling those areas.

The second subtheory can be called a "nonexperiential" or "taste" hypothesis. It states that students enter the medical education system with established preferences for patient contact, professional activities and status, life-styles, geographic areas (e.g., as a result of prior contact), and other work or leisure characteristics associated with different specialties and practice locations. Once in the system, they select the fields and locations they most prefer from the set of alternatives made available to them. The educational environment may well influence ultimate career decisions by providing or precluding specialty and locational alternatives, but the hypothesis itself stresses the effects of the background and personality traits that physicians bring with them when they first enter medical schools.

The third subtheory is economic. It argues that, other things equal, physicians choose specialties and places to practice that will maximize the present value of their lifetime earnings. The "other things equal" proviso applies mainly to the factors just cited—learning experiences and nonpecuniary preferences for practice and living conditions. Given these factors, the hypothesis contends, physicians select the fields and practice locations which yield them the highest incomes over their productive lives.

The three subtheories are not, of course, mutually exclusive, even though much of the early research tended to treat them as competing rather than complementary explanations of physicians' behavior. This tendency has all but disappeared from recent studies, but there are still reasons for asking which of the three best or most plausibly accounts for the patterns of career choice we observe. For one thing, they imply somewhat different mechanisms underlying the functional distribution of physicians. The experiential hypothesis, for example, asserts that the underlying mechanism is the character, scope, and emphasis of medical education. The nonexperiential hypothesis implies that it is the nature of the medical school admissions process, and the distribution of personality and background traits among medical school applicants. The economic hypothesis holds that the mechanism is the price system for medical care, which, inter alia, determines physicians' income levels by specialty and geographic location.

The three hypotheses also yield rather different implications concerning the persistence of specialty or locational maldistributions of physician manpower. Under both the experiential and nonexperiential subtheories, the medical education system is primarily responsible for the distribution of physicians by specialty and location. Thus, unless medical educators are responsive to society's wishes for physicians, they have no incentives to design their teaching and admissions policies so as to provide adequate numbers of new practitioners in desired (e.g., primary care) fields or desired (e.g., underserved) practice locations. Until the late 1970s, considerable criticism of the medical education system focused on precisely this issue: that medical educators sought to recruit and train scientist-physicians who overpopulated the referral specialties and were ill equipped by their training to settle in rural or inner-city communities. Moreover, so the argument went, the educational system contained no inherent controls for reversing the process. As long as it defined its model graduate as the scientist-physician, there was little chance of altering the functional distribution of new practitioners. Public policies had to be implemented which would change the kinds of students admitted into the system or the ways in which they were trained.

By contrast, traditional economic theory tells us that maldistributions of physicians tend to be short-run phenomena, and that the marketplace tends to correct them in the long run. In principle (we will have more to say about this shortly), competition for patients reduces fee levels and physician net incomes in fields or at locations where there are "surpluses" of physicians. Hence, new—and possibly even established—practitioners are induced to choose other, higher-paying specialties and locations instead. In this way, the price system reallocates physician manpower away from "surplus" specialties and locations and into other specialties and locations where there are relative shortages. We need to emphasize, however, that these are theoretical propositions. The traditional economic hypothesis does not necessarily guarantee that the supplies of physician labor will be sufficient to meet consumers' medical "needs" (or what one believes those medical "needs" to be), and in this sense it does not foreclose the possibility of long-run physician maldistributions. Even in the long run, supplies are forthcoming only in the amounts that communities, subpopulations of consumers, or consumers as a group are willing and able to pay for. In addition, and regardless of whether the market mechanism works smoothly, it may take an unacceptably long time to reallocate physician labor in conformity with society's demands. As a consequence, medical economists may take a more conservative view of the urgency for policy intervention than others, but they would not generally deny that remedial actions can be warranted.

If, for whatever reason, we decide that policies for correcting a physician maldistribution are justified, we again need to fall back on the three basic subtheories of physicians' career choices. Among the types of policies discussed in Chapter 8, those intended to revise the structure of the training environment—by introducing new curricula, preceptorships, changes in training locations, primary care residency programs, efforts to upgrade the status of family medicine, and the like—are all essentially derived from the experiential hypothesis. Policies that would alter admissions standards so as to favor entrants with (what are presumed to be) given specialty or locational preferences are logical implications of the nonexperiential subtheory. Policies that offer pecuniary inducements to physicians for selecting particular locations or fields—loan-forgiveness programs, fellowships, the National Health Service Corps, practice start-up subsidies, and so forth—are based primarily on the economic hypothesis of physicians' career choices.

To design a mix of programs for redistributing physicians, then, we need to assign weights to the three hypotheses corresponding to their probable validities. Restructuring medical teaching to favor particular fields is hardly an efficient policy if the educational environment has only a marginal impact on most physicians' specialty choices. There is little point in revising and disrupting admissions programs if the preferences for specialties or locations that physicians acquire before medical school have only a slight influence on their final career decisions. And offering pecuniary rewards for socially desirable career choices is likely to be an ineffective or very costly strategy if, in fact, physicians are insensitive to differences in lifetime earnings opportunities among their career alternatives.

These theoretical and policy considerations give us a variety of motives for going beyond a general explanation of physicians' career decision making. The qualitative factors acting on these decisions can be considered well known, but what can we say about their quantitative importance? Which types of factors, experiential, nonexperiential, and economic, appear to have the greatest influence on physicians' career choices?

Cross-sectional studies have shown that the educational environment does affect physicians' perceptions of their professional roles, and their attitudes toward medicine and medical practice. Yet there is very little compelling evidence that educational experiences significantly alter specialty choices. If, to put the matter another way, we were to randomly assign identical medical students to different medical schools and educational pathways, it is not clear that their choices of specialties would be radically different from one another. Obviously, this may mean only that differences in teaching environments are too small (despite outward appearances) to have major effects on specialty choices. Beliefs about medical practice, whether promoted by medical educators or not, may easily exist apart from particular teaching environments. For example, even in a clinically oriented medical school, students are likely to be aware of the low professional status accorded to general medicine, and, if status is an important element in their specialty choices, they might well select referral fields regardless of curricula or faculty encouragement to do otherwise.

Indeed, the strongest support for the experiential hypothesis is probably historical. The trend toward specialization during most of this century occurred during times when medical schools sought to raise the scientific foundations of their teaching programs. Moreover, the trend accelerated from the 1950s up to the 1970s when medical schools received large federal subsidies for biomedical research, and research itself became an important medical school product. Yet however much these facts suggest a cause-effect relationship, it is also notable that large numbers of physicians switched from general to specialty practice long after they had completed their medical training. Thus, there are grounds for believing that the trend toward specialization was not simply a consequence of increasingly specialized teaching. An equally plausible argument is that specialization was a natural response to technological progress in medicine, a phenomenon with self-evident counterparts in engineering and the other increasingly specialized applied sciences. In addition, the first marked reversal of the trend toward specialization— the upsurge in interest in primary care practice among medical students in the early 1970s—occurred without large-scale encouragement for primary care practice among medical educators. In this case, the apparent cause was the social upheavals of the 1960s, and it seems to have had little connection with new educational policies. This is not to say that the educational environment has had no historical impact on physicians' specialty preferences, but the effects themselves were almost certainly commingled with those of forces outside the direct control of the educational system.

The principal experiential theory of physician location choice—the prior-contact hypothesis—is, as we have said, a successful predictor of practice location choices. What is less well known is the degree to which prior contact and area attachments cause the selection of locations, or for which types of physicians these factors are influential. Several studies have shown that some physicians decide on their practice locations at early career stages, perhaps before medical school, and it has been contended that later types of area contact are sometimes the effects, rather than the causes, of practice location choices. In other words, physicians may select either medical schools or residency hospital locations because they have already decided to practice in the same areas. It remains to be determined whether we can identify the numbers and types of physicians who make late location decisions, and for whom attachments to medical school and residency training areas are important locational desiderata.

Of the three basic subtheories of physicians' career choices, the least well supported by existing empirical evidence is the economic hypothesis. As a whole, the evidence indicates that physicians are not very sensitive to income differentials across specialties or practice locations. Essentially, this means that large disparities in physicians' long-run earnings levels can exist between specialties and types of practice locations without causing significant shifts in physician manpower from the lower-paying to the higher-paying career alternatives. It also means that financial inducements to physicians to persuade them to enter unpreferred fields or practice locations must be large in order to have material or long-lasting effects. At least superficially, the ambiguous record of policies employing such inducements seems to bear this conclusion out.

Nevertheless, judgments as to the strength of physicians' economic motivation must be viewed as tentative. Research results tend to be scanty (particularly regarding specialty choices) and conflicting, due in no small part to the inherent difficulties of measuring lifetime earnings opportunities. Relatively little work has been done on changes in specialties and locations after physicians begin practice, when, we can surmise, they are more immediately confronted by pecuniary incentives than they are during their medical education. Moreover, to say that physicians are insensitive to earnings opportunities runs the risk of overgeneralizing and ignoring income effects altogether. For example, low earnings opportunities are undoubtedly a major barrier to physician entry in poor or thinly populated areas—and more so for specialists than generalists. Another possibility is that physicians engage in some form of "income-satisficing" behavior when they select specialties and locations. That is, they may restrict their choices to those yielding minimally satisfactory long-run incomes, and be relatively insensitive to earnings differences among the alternatives that pass this screening test. This and other questions concerning physicians' economic motives are only beginning to be explored in the literature.

For the most part, the best-documented explanation of physicians' career choices is given by the nonexperiential theory. Perhaps one reason for this is the attention the theory has received and the ease with which it can be tested. In some instances, of course, the influence of preferences is difficult to separate from that of pecuniary motives or learning experiences. As one illustration, the historical tendency of older medical students to enter general practice is less likely the result of "innate" preferences for general practice than it is a response to lifetime earnings opportunities. The disproportionate propensity of rural-reared physicians to select rural practice locations can be ascribed either to tastes for rural living or to favorable early contact with rural areas. And it is not clear whether women have traditionally avoided the surgical fields because of "feminine" specialty preferences, the time demands of marriage and child rearing, or informal barriers within the educational system.

Regardless of these kinds of qualifications, however, physicians' tastes for specialties and locations—reflected in their background and personality traits—seem to affect their career decisions more than either pecuniary considerations or learning experiences. As a result, it is reasonable to believe that historical trends in the functional distribution of physicians are significantly (if not exclusively) due to the types of medical students who were accepted into the educational system. On the basis of many research findings, there are even grounds for arguing that the shortages of rural, inner-city, and primary care practitioners during the 1960s and 1970s would have been much smaller than they were had more rural-reared, older, less academically qualified, minority, and women applicants been admitted into the educational system. This is not necessarily to claim that admissions committees were perverse or unfair. If discrimination against women and minorities ever officially existed, it ended by 1970, and after that time many schools actively sought to recruit both female and minority applicants. There were (and are) few incentives for schools to favor rural applicants, and discrimination against older and less academically qualified applicants was motivated by policies to control dropout rates.

All that notwithstanding, it is evident that admissions standards in the 1950s and 1960s did not favor the types of applicants with the greatest likelihood of selecting the primary care fields or underserved areas. Nor did they succeed in attracting applicants whose background traits, researchers tell us, are associated with these kinds of career choices. Admissions standards were designed largely to enroll future scientist-physicians, and to assure that accepted applicants would survive the rigors of an increasingly demanding and specialized educational process.

In this way, admissions standards were an integral part of the trend toward specialization.

If the "gatekeeping" function of admissions committees contributed to the physician maldistribution, is that function also responsible for what is widely regarded as an end (or an approaching end) to the maldistribution? Probably not. To be sure, the entry of large numbers of women into medical schools should increase the proportion of pediatricians in the physician stock, and it appears that the entry of more minority students will eventually increase the supply of physicians to minority populations. In addition, a few medical schools have experimented with admissions-variance programs to recruit applicants with supposed preferences for rural or inner-city practice. However, the major change in new physicians' specialty choices since 1970—the shift toward family practice and primary care generally—had no palpable connection with admissions policies. Some still controversial research showing that the supply of rural practitioners is growing attributes that growth to the overall growth of physician supply and market forces, and not to the screening effects of admissions committees.[1] Finally, despite the revision of entrance tests and a recognition that admissions screening does influence the distribution of medical students' career preferences, there is no real indication that current admissions criteria differ much from those of the 1950s and 1960s.

Thus, although the preponderance of findings implies that a physician redistribution policy should begin with admissions standards, there are limits to what such a policy can do. It cannot control the social forces that encourage physicians to make certain kinds of career choices, and it cannot change the economic conditions physicians face, or believe they will face, when they enter practice. There are practical obstacles as well. Medical schools as a group are unlikely to react warmly to proposals for departures from Flexnerian admissions standards. If they actually do reduce the competence or quality of new physicians, then one can legitimately debate the wisdom of using them to promote particular specialty or locational distributions. In addition, there are legal and ethical questions as to the degree to which procedures can be based on such applicant traits as race, ethnic background, or religion.[2]

Moreover, even though enough is known of physicians' background characteristics to design criteria that will tend to admit students with high probabilities of choosing primary care or rural practice, it is not yet clear that candidates for other types of shortage fields or locations can be so easily identified. For example, in a 1981 study, the Graduate Medical Education National Advisory Committee (GMENAC) predicted shortages of physicians by 1990 in some of the pediatric subspecialties, psychiatry, emergency medicine, preventive medicine, and anesthesiology

(GMENAC 1981c). At present, it is not possible to select medical school applicants whose background and personality traits make them exceptionally likely to choose these fields.

The rationale for a physician distribution policy based chiefly on admissions standards is therefore persuasive but not overwhelming. The effectiveness of such a policy cannot be estimated very accurately because we have no large-scale experiments to draw evidence from, and its practical limitations are a further drawback. Realistically speaking, it is hard to believe that admissions standards will become a routine tool in redistribution policies, at least in the near future, and this appears to leave us with the same mix of policy strategies that we now have. If the recruitment of participants is a measure of their success, many existing redistribution programs seem to work. However, the real questions are whether participation rates merely reflect self-selection by students or physicians already planning to enter shortage fields or locations, and, if not, whether the programs have lasting impacts on career choices. The direct and indirect evidence on these points remains equivocal.

THE THEORY OF SUPPLIER-INDUCED DEMAND AND ITS IMPLICATIONS

The massive growth of physician supply since the early 1970s has, of course, all but ended public pressures to increase the number of new practitioners. In 1978 an influential study by the Institute of Medicine (1978) called for the stabilization of medical school enrollments, and two years later GMENAC (1980c) recommended ceilings on medical school class sizes and a halt to the construction of new medical schools. Then, in 1980 the federal government's expansionist physician manpower programs came to an official close with the expiration of the Health Professions Educational Assistance Act of 1976. Pressures on the federal budget clearly contributed to the demise of these programs, but it was equally evident that spending to enlarge the supply of new physicians was no longer necessary.

As yet there is no visible consensus supporting a reduction in medical school capacity. Nevertheless, many observers view the expected oversupply of physicians with alarm, partly because of a new economic theory of physician behavior put forward by health economists in the early 1970s. Known variously as the theory of "supplier-induced" (or "physician-induced") demand and the "target income" theory, it is usually credited to empirical work by Feldstein (1970) and Newhouse (1970). Mainly, it argues that physicians' pricing and output behavior has highly inflationary implications for health care expenditures in the face of growing practitioner supplies. After nearly two decades of rapid price and expenditure inflation in the health care sector, this alone is justification for concern about an increasing supply of physicians. If the theory is true, one can have serious reservations about any program to remedy physician "shortages" unless the program can be quickly and effectively shut down when its goals are achieved. Even then, a policy to correct a narrowly defined shortage may involve a trade-off in terms of its consequences for expenditure inflation.

However, the theory also has an important direct implication for the distribution of physicians by specialty and location. That is, it implies that physicians are able to resist the economic pressures to leave overpopulated fields or locations, which means that maldistributions of physician manpower tend to be self-perpetuating. By the same token, redistribution programs are likely to be ineffective because physicians have no strong income incentives to participate in them. If physicians are able to enter their preferred specialties or practice locations without income penalties, there is little chance that they will participate in programs that induce them to choose other specialties or locations instead.

Briefly, the theory of supplier-induced demand is based on three axioms. First, it holds that consumers are typically poorly informed about the types and quantities of medical services necessary for their well-being. Thus, by virtue of consumer ignorance physicians occupy "agency relationships" with their patients, in which they recommend or order medical services in addition to providing them. Second, the theory claims that physicians attempt to realize or maintain certain "target" net incomes. The targets have rarely been defined very precisely, but they can be thought of as the net incomes physicians plan to earn, believe they should earn, or in some way find satisfactory (e.g., vis-à-vis the net incomes they believe their peers earn). Third, the theory contends that any factor that depresses physicians' net incomes below the target levels motivates them to try to reachieve the target levels by prescribing unnecessary services, raising their fees, or both. They are able to generate demands or raise their fees, the theory tells us, because of their power to order services, in combination with consumers' ignorance of alternative prices, treatment regimens, and the quality of care given by other providers.

Given an increase in the market supply of physicians, the consequences of supplier-induced demand are straightforward. The increase reduces the number of patients per physician, lowers physicians' gross income, and lowers their net income as well. When net income falls below the target level, physicians begin to generate demands, raise their fees, or both. Hence, the results are rises in utilization and expenditures for the market as a whole and on a per-patient or per capita basis, and possibly a rise in physicians' fee levels. Since some of the new demands are likely to be for inpatient care, supplier-induced demand tends to raise hospital utilization rates and expenditures, and (depending on hospitals' pricing behavior) it may also raise the prices of hospital care.

These consequences can be compared with those of the standard or neoclassical market theory to which we alluded in the preceding section. Under the standard theory, a rise in the market supply of practitioners also reduces the number of patients per physician. But in this case physicians are forced to compete with one another in price in order to retain their clienteles, and the result is a fall in market fee levels without demand generation. Now assuming the decline in fee levels is translated into lower out-of-pocket costs to patients, it should increase per capita and market utilization rates—just as the supplier-induced-demand theory predicts. However, the effects on expenditures depend on the individual and market price elasticities of demand for medical care. Expenditures rise, remain constant, or decrease in response to a fall in out-of-pocket prices according to whether (individual or market) demands are price-elastic, unit-price-elastic, or price-inelastic. In fact, most, if not all, of the research on the demands for medical services shows that demands are price-inelastic (e.g., Newhouse 1981; Kimbell and Yett 1974). Thus, under the standard market theory the most probable result of an increase in the supply of physicians is a decline in per capita and market spending on physicians' services.[3]

To summarize these observations, we have three points for contrasting the standard market and supplier-induced demand theories when the supply of physicians increases. First, fee levels fall under the standard theory, but the change in fees is indeterminate under the inducement theory. Second, both theories predict a rise in per capita and market utilization rates after the increase. Third, the standard theory predicts a decline in expenditures on physicians' services (if demand is price-inelastic), whereas the inducement theory predicts a rise. The last point is the critical one. If the inducement theory is true, it means that real spending on physicians' services grows proportionately with the number of practitioners in a market, and the proportionality factor is equal to physicians' average target level of gross income.[4]

The ramifications of the inducement theory for the distribution of physicians are now clear as well. As we have indicated, the standard market theory holds that the price of physicians' time falls as the supply of practitioners in a market rises. Accordingly, the price system tends, albeit slowly and imperfectly, to reallocate physicians away from fields and locations where there are relative surpluses of manpower and toward other fields and locations where there are relative deficits. The theory of supplier-induced demand denies that any such reallocation takes place, and claims, in effect, that the price system does not work. Physicians in surplus fields and locations are able to generate sufficient demands or raise their fees sufficiently to achieve their net income targets, and they are thereby able to deflect economic pressures which would ordinarily lead them to choose or switch to alternatives.

Consequently, from the perspectives of containing medical care costs or correcting a physician maldistribution, it makes a difference whether we believe the theory of supplier-induced demand. The early tests of the theory focused on relationships between area physician-population ratios and utilization rates for physicians' services. It was usually asserted—falsely, as we have indicated—that positive partial correlations between physician densities and per capita utilization rates were prima facie evidence of demand generation. Many authors who employed the test did find such positive partial correlations (Fuchs and Kramer 1972; Newhouse and Phelps 1974, 1976; Holahan 1975; May 1975; Davis and Reynolds 1975; Wennberg and Gittleson 1975; Fuchs 1978), although, perhaps surprisingly, a few negative correlations were reported as well (Kimbell and Barros 1978; Held and Manheim 1980).

It was not until 1978 that Reinhardt (1978) pointed out the theoretical ambiguity of utilization tests, and showed that both the inducement and standard-market theories imply a rise in utilization when the supply of physicians increases. Instead, along the lines given above, he suggested that an inconclusive test might be based on relationships between fee levels and physician density. If fee levels remained constant or rose as the physician-population ratio increased, it would conform with predictions of the inducement theory, but not with those of the standard theory. On the other hand, negative partial correlations between market or individual practitioners' fees and physician density would be consistent with either the standard or inducement theories, inasmuch as physicians may reduce their fees in response to new competition (and still generate demands) even if the inducement theory is valid.

Unfortunately, empirical tests involving the relationships between fee levels and physician density have also proved equivocal. While some authors have reported positive partial correlations (Huang and Koropecky 1973; Newhouse and Phelps 1974, 1976; Redisch et al. 1977; Kimbell and Barros 1978), about an equal number have obtained negative partial correlations (Steinwald and Sloan 1974; Sloan 1976a, 1982; Hadley and Lee 1978; Paringer 1980). The results could be interpreted as showing that physicians induce demands at some times or in some places, but we obviously cannot ignore the possibility that they were produced by the vagaries of model specifications and data.

Most other efforts to resolve the demand-inducement issue have been just as frustrating. One problem hampering their progress is the limited number of theoretical models that might tell us how to measure target net incomes, under what conditions physicians elect to generate demands, and whether demand creation is likely to take the form of fee increases or the ordering of unneeded services. Virtually all existing mathematical models yield a high level of indeterminacy about physicians' pricing and output behavior and very few testable propositions (Evans 1974, 1976; Sloan and Feldman 1978; Sweeney 1982). It has even been argued that the theory is inherently untestable by ordinary methods.[5] In some instances authors have returned to the original formulations of the theory, criticized them, and hinted that they were too eagerly pursued by other researchers. For example, in his seminal paper Feldstein (1970) obtained a positively sloped demand function for physicians' services from a time series of aggregate national data. Rather than rejecting the result as intrinsically implausible (since it meant that the quantity of services demanded increases as fees rise), he suggested that it was due to demand creation by physicians. But Hixson and Mocniak (1980) noted that the model lacked a supply function, and hence that the price-quantity relationship was underidentified.[6] After adding a supply function and reestimating the model, they found their estimated demand function to be negatively sloped in price, just as the standard market theory predicts. On those grounds, they claimed their finding refuted Feldstein's hypothesis that physicians generate demands for their services.

Despite their inventiveness, the most recent attempts to test the inducement hypothesis have either rejected it or reported ambivalent conclusions. Pauly and Satterthwaite (1980, 1981) proposed a variant of the standard market model which implies—as the inducement theory may—that fee levels rise in response to an increase in physician supply. They argued that increasing physician concentration in a market raises the time and travel costs consumers must incur to search for low-priced practitioners (inasmuch as there are more providers to be investigated). As a consequence, the extent and accuracy of consumers' price information decline, and physicians are thereby able to raise their fees with diminished risks of losing patients to competitors. In effect, their pricing behavior becomes more—not less—monopolistic as the market supply of physicians increases. Pauly and Satterthwaite then tested their "increasing monopoly" theory against the inducement theory using fee, physician supply, and other data from a sample of SMSAs. Although they refused to reject the inducement hypothesis outright, they contended that their own model provided an equally good or better explanation of actual fee behavior.

Sweeney (1982) reviewed the inducement theory and concluded that it gave no determinate, testable propositions regarding physician

demand generation. Instead, he designed a statistical procedure for estimating the levels of physicians' target net incomes and applied it to 1975
data for a group of U.S. cities. According to his estimates, physicians had
less than a 50-50 chance of realizing their income targets in roughly two-
thirds of the cities. Since the inducement theory states that physicians
can always achieve their income targets when they attempt to do so,
Sweeney argued that his findings failed to support it and that it did not
account for prevailing forms of physician pricing.

Using another approach, Yett et al. (1982) fitted a physician-
specific supply and demand model to data from two Blue Shield Plans.
In one part of their analyses they tested the effects of rising physician-
population ratios on physicians' average revenue functions. Under the
inducement theory, physicians should shift their average revenue functions outward ("create demands") as the area physician-population ratio
rises. But in one of the two plans, estimates of the model indicated that
the shift was inward—contradicting the theory—while in the other the
evidence was unclear. Hence, the results, like Sweeney's, seem to cast
doubt on the theory's ability to explain physicians' general pricing and
output behavior.

Pauly (1980) and Hay and Leahy (1982) employed still another
strategy for testing the existence of supplier-induced demand. They proposed that medically sophisticated or well-informed consumers ought to
be more resistant to demand inducement than consumers who are medically unsophisticated or poorly informed. Among other things, Pauly
studied physician utilization rates among subpopulations of different
educational attainment. For the least well educated persons he found
that utilization increased with area physician densities, precisely as the
inducement theory claims. However, for the most highly educated persons, utilization rates declined significantly as physician density rose.
This last result has no plausible explanation under either the inducement
theory or the standard market hypothesis. Hay and Leahy compared
physician utilization rates between samples of individuals from two
types of households. In the first sample, described as "well informed,"
the households contained at least one health care professional who could
presumably judge whether a condition required medical care. In the second, described as "less well informed," the households contained no
health professionals. Hay and Leahy contended that the first sample
should exhibit a lower rate of demand for physicians' services than the
second if the inducement theory is valid. But they found that utilization
rates were actually higher among the "well informed" consumers than
among the "less well informed" consumers, and they consequently rejected the thesis that physicians create unnecessary demands for medical
care.

In spite of its implications for the distribution of physicians, the theory of supplier-induced demand has never been directly tested in models of physician specialty or location choice. Indeed, it is difficult to conceive of a persuasive test in the context of such models. Newhouse et al. (1982b) addressed the question indirectly by citing supplier-induced demand as one of several possible reasons for the market's failure to equalize the geographic distribution of physicians. But, as we have indicated, they found evidence that increasing numbers of physicians are locating in relatively underserved rural communities, and they dismissed the notion that demand inducement is a significant impediment to the workings of geographic markets.

If we consider this large and varied body of findings as a whole, it is fair to say that the theory of supplier-induced demand remains a provocative but unproven hypothesis. Nearly all of the evidence purporting to confirm it is consistent with standard market theory, and recent tests give reason for being skeptical about its validity. Our own feeling is that demand inducement presents no immediate threat to the goal of health care cost containment. Nor does it appear to be a factor that must be reckoned with in analyzing or predicting physicians' specialty and location choices. At least for the present, it ought not to be used to justify actions for curtailing the supply of new physicians, or to introduce new approaches for physician distribution policy.

On the other hand, none of the evidence demonstrates that physicians cannot generate demands, and no one would seriously argue that demand creation never occurs. The growth of physician supply expected over the next decade should provide important new data for examining the inducement theory. Because of the theory's importance for physician manpower policy, and because the conditions under which demand generation is profitable to physicians should become more prevalent, additional theoretical and empirical work on the issue must be encouraged.

PHYSICIAN SUPPLIES AND EXPANSIONIST POLICY: SOME CLOSING REMARKS

Throughout this book we have spoken freely—perhaps too freely— of physician "shortages" and "surpluses." We have done so mostly to cite popular perceptions or authoritative views of the physician supply issue. Even so, it is worthwhile to remember that judgments as to whether there are too many, too few, or just enough doctors are all normative at bottom. We can, like GMENAC, employ elaborate methodologies to compute the "need" for physicians, but even the most sophisticated calculations are no better than our judgment of what constitutes an adequate supply. One problem, of course, is that expert medical opinion can disagree about the needs for physicians. We might all concede that one primary care physician for a community of 100,000 is inadequate, and that one physician per capita is excessive. With little or no effort, we might also narrow very considerably the interval between what we believe are inadequate and excessive supplies. However, it does not follow that the range can be delimited to a point where a consensus standard is obvious. Indeed, it may be impossible for reasonable authorities to produce a standard of adequate supply that is beyond medical disagreement.

But that is not really all there is. Suppose a medical standard of adequate supply can be developed and the actual supply of physicians falls below the standard. Then if the actual supply is increased, expenditures must be incurred to train more physicians or to attract them into "shortage" areas and specialties. Thus, the next question is: what is the social opportunity cost of meeting the standard of adequate physician supply? In other words, what must be given up in the way of alternative spending, public or private, to provide society with a medically adequate supply of physicians? The question has been all too infrequently addressed in formal evaluations of the "needs" for physicians, and it is not primarily an issue for medical experts to decide. One can, for example, suggest that the funding to train more doctors, which was first authorized in the 1960s, might have been equally well (or even better) spent if it had been devoted effectively to job training for the poor, rebuilding slums, or even the pursuit of global peace. We do not argue that the funding was wasted, but simply that other welfare goals exist besides increasing the supply of physicians. The lesson has been brought home to us by the federal and state budget crises of the late 1970s and early 1980s, and it seems destined to become a permanent aspect of physician manpower policy. What we conceive to be an adequate supply of physicians—that is, what we are willing to do about correcting a "shortage" or "maldistribution" of physician manpower—depends on the competing demands for tax dollars.

An economic technique for evaluating the adequacy of physician supply does exist, at least in principle. Economists tend to measure the adequacy of replaceable resources by measuring the resource owners' earnings. For example, if, after standardizing for differences in educational investments, skill requirements, and the like, earnings in one occupation are higher than they are in others, one ordinarily concludes that resources in the first occupation are in short supply, in the sense that a larger labor force could be absorbed into the occupation without special pecuniary inducements to raise employment. Applying the theorem to physicians, it means that physician supply is in balance with demands when lifetime earnings in medicine are equal to those in comparable professions. By implication, we should test the adequacy of physician supply by comparing the lifetime earnings with those of persons in other fields having closely similar educational, skill, and job requirements.

As we indicated in Chapter 6, a few efforts have been made to estimate lifetime earnings in medicine, and to determine whether physicians derive monopoly rents or excess profits (i.e., premia over that they could earn in other professions). Unfortunately, they are generally too imprecise and too out-of-date to give reliable impressions of the current adequacy of physician supply. For practical purposes, then, empirical economics has not yet provided us with market-oriented guidelines for what constitutes a surplus or shortage of physicians.[7]

There is no reason to suppose that, given sufficient data, earnings-based evaluations of physician-supply balances could not be generated as readily as the widely used requirements-supply estimates. Still, many authorities would deny that market measures have a central place in physician manpower policy on the grounds that access to health care is a right rather than a matter to be determined by the marketplace. If we accept that premise, we cannot necessarily argue that there are enough physicians, even if earnings in medicine are competitive with those in other professions. Indeed, if we accept it, there is no longer room for economic debate as to the adequacy of physician supplies. We can only ask ourselves whether the right to health care takes precedence over other social rights or goals that are also costly to provide.

Directly or indirectly, the "rights" theory of health care seems to underlie the continuing (if, perhaps, abating) pressures to correct the maldistribution of physician manpower. But its effects, for better or worse, are to force us into the realm of subjective judgment regarding what ought to be done about rectifying the maldistribution; to remove the market mechanism from consideration; and to leave decisions about the size and costs of policies to the political process.

Political decisions related to physician manpower policy are by no means to be avoided, and, in fact, probably cannot be avoided. Nevertheless, physician manpower decisions have sometimes occurred in an atmosphere of near crisis where polemics and acrimonious disputes have had as much (or more) influence as thoughtful reasoning. The result is that decisions are made under conditions characterized by a high degree of uncertainty, both as to the needs for policy and its outcomes. Much of what we have written in this book emphasizes that there is, in fact, a lot of uncertainty about policies to increase physician supplies. But the inherent ambiguities have often been compounded by hurried policymaking, which has led to massive, hard-to-reverse programs with long-lasting consequences.

In most circumstances where we cannot accurately predict results or where we cannot define objectives very precisely, the efficient strategy is to begin on a small scale, monitor the policy's outcomes, learn by trial and error, and adapt the program as rapidly as possible to planning mistakes and unexpected events. The physician manpower expansion policies of the 1960s and early 1970s violated nearly all of these axioms.

Arguably, the physician "shortage" of the 1950s and 1960s was not as great as was popularly believed, and it is equally unclear whether it would have worsened dramatically over time. Hence, one can at least debate the wisdom of instituting so large a program to remedy the shortage. Medical schools responded to the capitation incentives embodied in the program much more powerfully and lastingly than was anticipated, and, at the same time the federal government initiated the program, many states had already legislated their own funding for new medical schools. The huge growth in the number of female medical students was not predicted, even though it came about partly as a result of federal affirmative action policies. The significant shift in medical students' preferences for primary care was also unforeseen, and even the slowdown in the national birthrate, which has reduced the future need for physicians, does not seem to have been taken into account in governmental planning. To add to that, foreign-trained physicians were allowed to immigrate into the country in large numbers until well into the 1970s.

The expansionist policy has undoubtedly achieved its objectives, and in this way it can be called strikingly successful. Moreover, by producing such a large increase in the total supply of practitioners, it may have had some effect in ameliorating geographic and specialty shortfalls of physicians. Nevertheless, it lacked explicit targets, coordination, and the flexibility to deal with unexpected events, and it largely failed to consider the long-run impact on the medical education system. It is especially noteworthy that no detailed, authoritative studies of physician requirements preceded the development of the policy; instead, they appeared a decade later with the publication of the GMENAC reports. If we take the best available estimates of physician requirements and supply forecasts, the result is that the expansionist policy greatly overshot its mark, with consequences that will probably reach into the next century.

Are those consequences bad? If we believe the supplier-induced demand theory, the answer is an unqualified "yes." In fact, we may consider ourselves lucky that, as yet, so little evidence has confirmed the theory. But even setting the theory aside, the expansionist policy may well have led to some net social losses. For one thing, medical school teaching capacity was almost certainly overbuilt, and the excessive public monies invested in medical education have been lost for other desirable social uses. In a lesser sense, the end of federal funding has also produced at least a temporary disruption of medical education. Schools and students were forced to find financial support from other sources, calls for the closure of some marginal institutions began to appear, and the system itself seemed to be struggling to reestablish its priorities.

Yet by and large it is still much too soon to evaluate the net gains or losses of physician expansionism. As some of the research we have cited indicates, the growth of physician supply and commensurately more price competition among doctors may lower the secular trend of fee inflation. It may also enable both the government and private health insurance carriers to promulgate new types of reimbursement that are less remunerative to physicians, but less inflationary as well. But there remain other questions whose answers cannot be so readily conjectured. For example, there is no way of telling whether, at some future time, the medical profession may lobby for restrictions on the number of new graduates. And if it does, there is no way of knowing whether public policy will resist the proposals, or endorse them as a means of phasing out excess medical school capacity.

It is also unclear whether there will be a restoration of the trend toward specialization. If the Flexnerian tradition is not dead, medical schools may easily return to it with the decline in financial support for primary care training and diminishing demands for new primary care practitioners. The upsurge in medical students' preferences for primary care may have been temporary, and even if it is not, competition among physicians may provide incentives for new practitioners to specialize as a way of differentiating their services.

With respect to other issues, it is just very difficult to say how conditions in medical education and medical practice will interact with the increase in physician supply. The entry of large, for-profit corporations into the medical care industry, federal and state efforts to reduce spending on Medicare and Medicaid, the health maintenance organization movement, the rising costs of medical education, and the various financial pressures on teaching hospitals are only some of the factors that significantly affect how and where physicians organize their practices. And the impacts of these factors on physicians' incomes, modes of practice, specialties, and locations may not become evident for a decade or more.[8]

In short, the environment of medical education and medical practice is probably as uncertain today as it was in the 1960s—although for different reasons. If we take the cautious view, the implication is that no precipitous changes should be forced on the medical education system until the outlook becomes clearer. Among other things, this means that we ought not to initiate programs for reducing the supply of physicians hastily, and we ought to keep open policy options for adjusting the specialty and location distributions of new graduates to meet public demands. The real danger at this point comes less from the threat of benign neglect of the medical education system than from the potential for over-reacting to the surplus of physicians.

With some exceptions, past programs to remedy specialty and geo-graphic shortages of physicians have been of the small-scale type. We have reservations about their effectiveness, but it may be a virtue that most have been conducted experimentally and without large commit-ments of public resources. We see no overwhelming reasons to dismantle them, but, by the same token, it is hard to argue that support for them ought to be increased. There are no important indications that primary care physicians are in short supply, or that the situation in any field is critical enough to justify corrective action. While it is apparent that many communities and areas continue to have low physician-population ratios, a preeminent and now generally recognized problem is that such areas may be too poor or too sparsely populated to support full-time phy-sicians without subsidizing them. Broadly speaking, the intent of most physician location programs is to induce practitioners to settle perma-nently or semipermanently in underserved areas without subsidies, and it seems to us doubtful whether this is generally a realistic goal.

But if the times are not ripe for bold new policies, they are certainly opportune for reinvestigating the research issues we have discussed in this book. It is unfortunate that research issues sometimes occupy policy-makers' attention only as long as immediate political demands mandate, and we hope that the fading concerns about physician shortages do not also signal an end to research. Theoretically and empirically, many of the questions involving physicians' specialty and location decisions have not been resolved. The next years ought to be a period for designing and evaluating alternative models of society's needs for physicians, for as-sessing the programs of the 1970s, and for conducting long-term basic re-search on the causes of physicians' career choices. Aside from contribut-ing to our overall understanding of the medical care system, such a plan would give us far more precise tools for dealing with physician man-power imbalances than we had in the 1960s.

NOTES

1. See Schwartz et al. (1980) and Newhouse et al. (1982a, 1982b, 1982c). The ar-gument is that the overall expansion of supply reduces the ratio of population to physicians in urban communities, where physicians tend to settle first, and thereby also reduces earnings opportunities in those communities. As a conse-quence, some new and established practitioners are led to locate (or relocate) in rural communities where population-physician ratios and earnings oppor-tunities are higher.

2. The issue was raised in the recent court case of *Allen Bakke vs. the Regents of the University of California.* Bakke, a white, applied to and was rejected by the University of California Medical School at Davis in 1973 and 1974. Thereafter, he sued the University, charging that he was academically qualified to enter the Davis medical school and that he had been rejected only because of the school's preferential minority admissions program which restricted entry by white applicants. The case was decided by the U.S. Supreme Court in 1978. The Court agreed that Bakke had been rejected solely because of his race, found that Davis had set aside positions for nonwhite applicants, and declared that the University had violated Bakke's constitutional rights under the Fourteenth Amendment. (Bakke was subsequently admitted to Davis.) However, by a five-to-four vote the Court refused to declare minority preferential admissions programs unconstitutional per se. Its ruling has been interpreted as stating only that quota systems for nonwhite applicants, rather than affirmative action admissions programs in general, are unconstitutional.

   When the University argued its case before the California Supreme Court in 1976, it defended the Davis admissions program partly on the grounds that minority physicians tend more than whites to settle in minority communities and to serve minority populations. The California court dismissed the argument, saying that medical schools had no constitutional authority to produce physicians for any given racial or ethnic groups. Although the University did not pursue the issue with the U.S. Supreme Court, the California Supreme Court's opinion raises doubt as to how far medical schools can go in modifying their admissions policies to change the locational or specialty distributions of their graduates.

3. The effect on expenditures for hospital services is indeterminate. Assuming substitutability between the demands for inpatient and outpatient care, the decline in net or out-of-pocket prices for physicians' services should tend to lower hospital utilization and expenditures on hospital services. That is, patients should tend to consume more physicians' services and fewer hospital services. However, if hospitals were to respond to the fall in utilization rates by raising their charges—a not unlikely event if their average costs rose—the price inelasticity of demands for hospital services could result in a rise in hospital expenditures.

4. Some of the empirical implications of supplier-induced demand and the standard theory can be found in recent papers by Davis (1982) and Rodgers (1981). Adopting the inducement theory, Davis first regressed a number of measures of health care utilization and expenditures on the aggregate physician-population ratios in 202 DHHS "health service areas" for 1978. Using the estimated relationships, she then projected the national levels of utilization and expenditures for 1990 using GMENAC's prediction of the national physician-population ratio in that year. Among other things, her forecasts showed a 2 percent rise in hospital admissions per capita between 1978 and 1990, a 10 percent rise in hospital costs per admission, and a 9 percent rise in the per-beneficiary costs of the Medicare program. All told, the forecasts indicated a $52 billion increase in the deflated costs of the Medicare program

from 1978 to 1990, due solely (under the inducement hypothesis) to the expected increase in the number of physicians.

Rodgers based his projections on a macroeconometric model by Hixson (1979), which was derived from the standard economic theory of markets. According to his calculations, we can expect a 5 percent decline in the real prices of physicians' services between 1980 and 1990 due to the expected increase in physician supply. But we can also expect a 35 percent increase in the national utilization rate for physicians' services and a 27 percent increase in expenditures on those services. In addition, expenditures on hospital services should rise by 39 percent, and total national spending on physicians' and hospital services (unadjusted for general inflation) should increase by $98 billion annually. Even if we assume a relatively modest general inflation rate of 4 percent per year, Rodgers's estimate of the increase in health care expenditures seems somewhat lower than Davis's.

Because forecasts tend to be sensitive to model specifications, these two sets of figures should probably be regarded as illustrative rather than the last word. For example, Hixson obtained estimates of the demands for physicians' services that were price-elastic, unlike most of the other results reported in the literature. This accounts for Rodgers's prediction of a rise in spending on physicians' services following the decline in fee levels. All the same, it serves to emphasize that differences in expenditure projections between the inducement and standard theories depend on the latter's estimate of the price elasticity of demand. The standard theory does not unambiguously predict a decline in spending on physicians' services when physician supply increases.

5. Most of the challenges have been theoretical, but tests of the hypothesis also face empirical problems. For instance, comparisons of utilization rates and fee levels between physician-rich and physician-poor areas can be distorted for reasons having nothing to do with demand inducement. As we showed in Chapter 7, physicians tend to locate in communities where demand is strong —that is, where the population consists of heavy users of services, fee levels are already high, and so forth. Patients in physician-poor areas may go to physician-rich areas for treatment, thereby raising demands for services in the latter areas and reducing them in the former. There may be higher levels of service quality in physician-rich communities, lower travel and time costs of obtaining services (leading to higher rates of demand), or simply different standards of medical care and higher service intensities. Any or all of these factors could produce positive but misleading correlations between physician concentration and fee levels or utilization rates. See Sloan and Feldman (1978) and Yett (1978) for a further discussion.

6. That is, the estimated relationship between price and quantity commingled the effects of supply and demand. If the quantity of physicians' services supplied increases as the price rises, it would tend to be manifested in a positive association between utilization and price. This clearly biases the estimated price-quantity correlation upward, and can lead to the conclusion that quantity demanded is positively correlated with price. Hixson and Mocniak suggested that Feldstein's result was more the consequence of this kind of bias

than of physician demand creation. See Ramsey (1980) for some other methodological criticisms of the early work.

7. Nevertheless, it is of passing interest to observe that, according to AMA data, physicians' real net incomes fell slightly during the decade 1970–80 (Goldfarb 1981). While this does not tell us whether physicians earn excess profits, it suggests that lifetime earnings may have begun to decline in the face of increasing supply. In work cited above, Davis (1982) and Rodgers (1981) also obtained results showing that physicians' real net incomes are likely to continue falling to 1990.

8. See Ginzberg et al. (1981) for some speculations about the impact of growing physician supplies.

References

AAMC. 1959. "Datagram: Type of Practice Planned." *Journal of Medical Education* 34 (November):1108–9.

_____. 1975a. *Medical School Admissions Requirements, 1976–77: U.S.A. and Canada.* Washington, D.C.: Association of American Medical Colleges.

_____. 1975b. *Postdoctorals Vs. Non-Postdoctorals: Career Performance Differentials within Academic Medicine.* DHEW Publication No. (HRA) 75-73. Washington, D.C.: U.S. Department of Health, Education, and Welfare, April.

Aaron, P.R.; Somes, G.W.; Marx, M.B.; and Cooper, J.K. 1980. "Relationship between Traits of Kentucky Physicians and Their Practice Areas." *Inquiry* 17 (Summer):128–36.

Adams, R.E. 1962. "Intern Education and the Intern Market." *Journal of Medical Education* 37 (May):446–53.

Aiken, L.H.; Lewis, C.E.; Craig, J.; Mendenhall, R.C.; Blendon, R.J.; and Rogers, D.E. 1979. "The Contribution of Specialists to the Delivery of Primary Care: A New Perspective." *New England Journal of Medicine* 300 (June 14): 1363–70.

Alpert, J.J. 1975. "Graduate Education for Primary Care: Problems and Issues." *Journal of Medical Education* 50 (December, Part 2):123–28.

AMA. 1967. "Medical Education in the United States." *Journal of the American Medical Association* 202 (November 20):725–832.

_____. 1968. "Medical Education in the United States, 1967–1968." *Journal of the American Medical Association* 206 (November 25):1987–2105.

_____. 1970. "Medical Education in the United States." *Journal of the American Medical Association* 214 (November 23):1483–1549.

_____. 1971. "Medical Education in the United States, 1970–1971." *Journal of the American Medical Association* 218 (November 22):1199–1316.

_____. 1972. "Medical Education in the United States, 1971–1972." *Journal of the American Medical Association* 222 (November 20):961–1048.

_____. 1973. "Medical Education in the United States, 1972–1973." *Journal of the American Medical Association* 226 (November 19):893–1023.

_____. 1974. *Medical Licensure Statistics for 1973*. Chicago: American Medical Association.

_____. 1976. "Medical Education in the United States, 1975–1976." *Journal of the American Medical Association* 236 (December 27):2935–3082.

_____. 1977. *"Physician Distribution and Medical Licensure in the U.S., 1976*. Chicago: American Medical Association.

_____. 1980. "Medical Education in the United States, 1978–1979." *Journal of the American Medical Association* 243 (March 7):835–989.

_____, Council on Medical Education. 1966. *The Graduate Education of Physicians: The Report of the Citizens' Commission on Graduate Medical Education*. Chicago: American Medical Association.

American Medical Association. See AMA.

Anderson, R.B.W. 1974. "A Markov Chains Model of Medical Specialty Choice." *Journal of Mathematical Sociology* 3 (July):259–74.

_____. 1975. "Choosing a Medical Specialty: A Critique of Literature in the Light of 'Curious Findings'." *Journal of Health and Social Behavior* 16 (June):152–62.

Applied Management Sciences. 1978. *An Assessment of the Influence of Medical Preceptorships and Other Factors on Career Choice and Medical Education of Physicians*. Final Report on Contract No. HRA-231-76-00040. Silver Spring, Md.: Applied Management Sciences.

Aronson, J.M.; Baumann, R.J.: and Aronson, S.S. 1965. "Students Select a Medical School." *Journal of Medical Education* 40 (February):155–60.

Association of American Medical Colleges. See AAMC.

Auster, R.D., and Oaxaca, R.L. 1981. "Identification of Supplier Induced Demand in the Health Care Sector." *Journal of Human Resources* 16 (Summer):327–42.

Balfe, B.E.; Lorant, J.H.; and Todd, C., eds. 1971. *Reference Data on the Profile of Medical Practice*. Chicago: American Medical Association.

Balinsky, W.L. 1974. "Distribution of Young Medical Students from Western New York." *Medical Care* 12 (May):437–44.

Ball, D.S., and Wilson, J.W. 1968. "Community Health Facilities and Services: the Manpower Dimensions." *American Journal of Agricultural Economics* 50 (December):1208–21.

Barish, A.M. 1979. "The Influence of Primary Care Preceptorships and Other Factors on Physicians' Career Choices." *Public Health Reports* 94 (January–February):36–47.

Barrett, P.C. 1978. "Health Professions Education in the State University System." *Journal of the Florida Medical Association* 65 (June):446–49.

Bartlett, J.W. 1967. "Medical School and Career Performance of Medical Students with Low MCAT Scores." *Journal of Medical Education* 42 (March):231-37.

Becker, G.S. 1963. *Human Capital.* New York: National Bureau of Economic Research.

———. 1975. *Human Capital,* 2d ed. New York: National Bureau of Economic Research and Columbia University Press.

Becker, H.S., and Geer, B. 1975. "The Fate of Idealism in Medical School." In *Medical Behavioral Science,* ed. T. Millon. Philadelphia: W.B. Saunders and Company.

———; Hughes, E.C.; and Strauss, H.L. 1961. *Boys in White: Student Culture in Medical School.* Chicago: University of Chicago Press.

Becker, P.; Hartz, A.; and Cuttler, J. 1979. "Time Trends in the Association of a Rural or Urban Background with Physician Location." *Journal of Medical Education* 54 (July):544–50.

Beiser, H.R., and Allender, J.S. 1964. "Personality Factors Influencing Medical School Achievement." *Journal of Medical Education* 39 (February):175–80.

Beloff, J.S.; Korper, M.; and Weinerman, E.R. 1970. "Medical Student Response to a Program for Teaching Comprehensive Care." *Journal of Medical Education* 45 (December):1047–59.

Benham, L.; Maurize, A.; and Reder, M.W. 1968. "Migration, Location, and Remuneration of Medical Personnel: Physicians and Dentists." *Review of Economics and Statistics* 50 (August):332–47.

Beran, R.L. 1979. "The Rise and Fall of Three-Year Medical School Programs." *Journal of Medical Education* 54 (March):248–49.

Berman, B.U. 1979. "Three-Year Programs in Medical and Dental Schools: An Appraisal." *Public Health Reports* 94 (January-February):85–87.

Best, W.R.; Diekema, A.J.; Fisher, L.A.; and Smith, N.E. 1971. "Multivariate Predictors in Selecting Medical Students." *Journal of Medical Education* 56 (January):42–50.

Bible, B.L. 1970. "Physicians' Views of Medical Practice in Nonmetropolitan Communities." *Public Health Reports* 85 (January):11–17.

Bidese, C.M., and Danais, D.G. 1982. *Physician Characteristics and Distribution in the U.S., 1981 Edition.* Chicago: American Medical Association.

Blair, R.J. 1975. "A Multivariate Analysis of Factors Influencing the Location and Distribution of Physicians in the Northeast U.S." Master's thesis, Pennsylvania State University.

Blau, P.M.; Gustad, J.W.; Jessor, R.; Parnes, H.S.; and Wilcox, R.C. 1956. "Occupational Choice: A Conceptual Framework." *Industrial and Labor Relations Review* 9 (July):531–43.

Bloom, B.S., and Peterson, O.L. 1979. "Physician Manpower Expansionism: A Policy Review." *Annals of Internal Medicine* 90 (February):249–56.

Bloom, S.W. 1971. "The Medical School as a Social System." *Milbank Memorial Fund Quarterly* 49 (April, Part 2):1–191.

———. 1979. "Socialization for the Physician's Role: A Review of Some Contributions of Research to Theory." In *Becoming a Physician: Development of*

Values and Attitudes in Medicine, ed. E.C. Shapiro and L.M. Lowenstein. Cambridge, Mass.: Ballinger.

Bodel, P.T., and Short, E.M. 1972. "Women in Medicine: Views from a Medical School." *Clinical Research* 20 (February):125–29.

Boskin, M.J. 1974. "A Conditional Logit Model of Occupational Choice." *Journal of Political Economy* 82 (March-April):389–98.

Boverman, H. 1965. "Senior Student Career Choices in Retrospect." *Journal of Medical Education* 40 (February):161–65.

Bowers, J.Z. 1968. "Special Problems of Women Medical Students." *Journal of Medical Education* 43 (May):532–37.

———, and Parkin, R.C. 1957. "The Wisconsin Preceptor Program—A 30 Year Experiment in Medical Education." *Journal of Medical Education* 32 (September):610–12.

Brandt, E.N.; Holmstrom, F.; and Fitzsimmons, E.L. 1979. "A Study of UTMB Graduates: 1967–1976." *Texas Medicine* 75 (June):54–58.

Breed, J.E. 1970. "The Plans of Our Doctors in Training (Part 1)." *Illinois Medical Journal* 85 (January):11–17.

Breisch, W.F. 1970. "Impact of Medical School Characteristics on Location of Physician Practice." *Journal of Medical Education* 45 (December):1068–70.

Brierly, C. 1973. "It Worked in Grover and It's Worth a Try." *Prism* (May):4–8.

Brown, E.R. 1979. *Rockefeller Medicine Men: Medicine and Capitalism in America.* Berkeley, Calif.: University of California Press.

———. 1980. "He Who Pays The Piper: Foundations, the Medical Profession, and Medical Education Reform." *International Journal of Health Services* 10:71–88.

Brown, L.A., and Belcher, J.C. 1966. "Residential Mobility of Physicians in Georgia." *Rural Sociology* 31 (December):439–48.

Bruhn, J.G., and Parsons, D.A. 1964. "Medical Student Attitudes toward Four Medical Specialties." *Journal of Medical Education* 49 (January):40–49.

———. 1965. "Attitudes toward Medical Specialties: Two Follow-Up Studies." *Journal of Medical Education* 40 (March):273–80.

Bucher, R., and Stelling, J.G. 1977. *Becoming Professional.* Beverly Hills, Calif.: Sage Publications.

Burke, W.M.; Eckhert, N.L.; Hays, C.W.; Mansell, E.; Deuschle, K.W.; and Fulmer, H.S. 1979. "An Evaluation of the Undergraduate Medical Curriculum: The Kentucky Experiment in Community Medicine." *Journal of the American Medical Association* 241 (June 22):2726–30.

Burket, G.E. 1977. "Rural Manpower: A Different Perspective as Viewed by the Kansas Physician and Senior Medical Student." *Journal of the Kansas Medical Society* 78 (November):475–77.

Busch, L., and Dale, C. 1978. "The Changing Distribution of Physicians." *Socio-Economic Planning Sciences* 12: 167–76.

Butter, I. 1976. *Foreign Medical Graduates: A Comparative Study of State Licensure Policies.* DHEW Publication No. (HRA) 77-3166. Washington, D.C.: U.S. Department of Health, Education, and Welfare, June.

————, and Schaffner, R. 1971. "Foreign Medical Graduates and Equal Access to Medical Care." *Medical Care* 9 (March–April):136–43.

Buzek, J., and McNamara, M. 1968. "A Partial Solution to the Manpower Problem." *Journal of Medical Education* 43 (November):1197–99.

Cain, A.S., and Bowen, L.G. 1961. "A Study of the Full-Time Medical School Faculty Member." *Journal of Medical Education* 36 (October):1433–48.

Calahan, D.; Collette, P.; and Hilmar, N.A. 1957. "Career Interests and Expectations of U.S. Medical Students." *Journal of Medical Education* 32 (July):557–63.

California Medical Association, Bureau of Research and Planning. 1976. *The 1975 Survey of Attitudes of Medical Students and Recent Graduates.* February. (Processed.)

Campbell, J.A. 1964. "The Internship: Origins, Evolution, and Confusion." *Journal of the American Medical Association* 189 (July 27):273–78.

Canning, C.; Kane, R.; and Gray, R. 1974. "Attitudes and Electives: Predicting Enrollment and Measuring Effects." *Journal of Medical Education* 49 (October):986–88.

Cantwell, J.R., ed. 1976. *Reference Data on Profile of Medical Practice, 1975–76 Edition.* Chicago: American Medical Association.

Caplovitz, D. 1961. "Reanalysis of 1958 Institute Data Pertaining to the Internship." *Journal of Medical Education* 36 (April, Part 2):68–81.

Carline, J.D.; Cullen, T.J.; Dohner, C.W.; Schwartz, M.R.; and Zinser, E.A. 1980. "Career Preferences of First- and Second-Year Medical Students: The WAMI Experience." *Journal of Medical Education* 55 (August):682–91.

Carnegie Commission on Higher Education. 1970. *Higher Education and the Nation's Health—Policies for Medical and Dental Education.* New York: McGraw-Hill.

Carnegie Council on Policy Studies in Higher Education. 1976. *Progress and Problems in Medical and Dental Education.* San Francisco: Jossey-Bass Publishers.

Carter, G.M.; Chu, D.S.; Koehler, J.E.; Slighton, R.L.; and Williams, A.P. 1974. *Federal Manpower Legislation and the Academic Health Centers: An Interim Report.* Publication No. R-1464-HEW. Santa Monica, Calif.: Rand Corporation.

Cartwright, L.K. 1972. "Personality Differences in Male and Female Medical Students." *Psychiatry in Medicine* 3 (July):212–18

Cauthen, J.B.; Adams, R.L.; De La Rosa, R.; Meyer, G.G.; and Holcomb J. 1980. "Medical Students and Family Practice: A Prospective Study." *Texas Medicine* 76 (July):57–60.

Champion, D.J., and Olsen, D.B. 1971. "Physician Behavior in Southern Appalachia: Some Recruitment Factors." *Journal of Health and Social Behavior* 12 (September):245–52.

Charles, E.D. 1971. "Analysis of Policies Designed to Aid Rural Communities Recruit Physicians: A Case Study of Alabama." Ph.D. dissertation, University of Alabama.

Child, C.G. 1964. "Assets and Liabilities of the University Hospital Internship." *Journal of the American Medical Association* 189 (July 27):294–98.

Chipman, M.L.; Clarke, G.G.; and Steiner, J.W. 1969. "Career Choice within Medicine: A Study of One Graduating Class at the University of Toronto." *Canadian Medical Association Journal* 101 (November 29):34–39.

Chyatte, S.B., and Slater, S.B. 1971. "Medical Student Training in Rehabilitation and Career Choice Selection." *Archives of Physician Medicine and Rehabilitation* 52 (July):306–10.

Clark, L.J.; Field, M.J.; Koontz, T.L.; and Koontz, V.L. 1980. "The Impact of Hill-Burton: An Analysis of Hospital Bed and Physician Distribution in the United States, 1950–1970." *Medical Care* 18 (May):532–50.

Clute, K.F. 1963. *The General Practitioner: A Study of Medical Education and Practice in Ontario and Nova Scotia.* Toronto: University of Toronto Press.

Coggeshall, L.T. 1965. *Planning for Medical Progress through Education.* Evanston, Ill.: Association of American Medical Colleges.

Cohen, E.D., and Korper, S.P. 1976a. "Women in Medicine: A Survey of Professional Activities, Career Interruptions, and Conflict Resolutions, Part I." *Connecticut Medicine* 40 (February):103–10.

_____. 1976b. "Women in Medicine: A Survey of Professional Activities, Career Interruptions, and Conflict Resolutions, Part II." *Connecticut Medicine* 40 (March):195–200.

Coker, R.E.; Back, K.W.; Donnelly, T.G.; and Miller, N. 1960. "Patterns of Influence: Medical School Faculty Members and the Values and Specialty Interests of Medical Students." *Journal of Medical Education* 35 (June):518–27.

Coker, R.E.; Kosa, J.; and Back, J.W. 1966. "Medical Students' Attitudes toward Public Health." *Milbank Memorial Fund Quarterly* 44 (April, Part 1):155–80.

Coleman, S. 1976. *Physician Distribution and Rural Access to Medical Services.* Publication No. R-1887-HEW. Santa Monica, Calif. Rand Corporation, April.

Collins, F., and Roessler, R. 1975. "Intellectual and Attitudinal Characteristics of Medical Students Selecting Family Practice." *Journal of Family Practice* 2 (December):431–32.

Comptroller General of the United States. 1978a. *Are Neighborhood Health Centers Providing Services Efficiently to the Most Needy?* Publication No. HRD-77-124. Washington, D.C.: U.S. General Accounting Office, June 20.

_____. 1978b. *Progress and Problems in Improving the Availability of Primary Care Providers in Underserved Areas.* Publication No. HRD-77-135. Washington, D.C.: U.S. General Accounting Office, August 22.

Comroe, J.H. 1962. "The Effect of Research Emphasis on Facilities and Support of the Medical School." *Journal of Medical Education* 37 (December, Part 2):123–203.

Conger, J.J., and Fitz, R.H. 1963. "Prediction of Success in Medical School." *Journal of Medical Education* 38 (November):943–46.

CONSAD Research Corporation. 1973. *An Evaluation of the Effectiveness of Loan Forgiveness as an Incentive for Health Practitioners to Locate in Medically Underserved Areas.* DHEW Publication No. DHEW-OS-73-68. Washington, D.C.; U.S. Department of Health, Education, and Welfare.

Coombs, R.H., and Boyle, B.P. 1971. "The Transition to Medical School: Expectations Versus Realities." In *Psychological Aspects of Medical Training*, ed. R.H. Coombs and C.E. Vincent. Springfield, Ill.: Charles C. Thomas.

Cooper, J.K.; Heald, K.; Samuels, M.; and Coleman, S. 1975. "Rural or Urban Practice: Factors Influencing the Location Decision of Primary Care Physicians." *Inquiry* 12 (March):18–25.

Cordes, S.M. 1978. "Factors Influencing the Location of Rural General Practitioners." *Western Journal of Medicine* 128 (January):75–80.

Crawford, R.L., and McCormack, R.C. 1971. "Reasons Physicians Leave Primary Care Practice." *Journal of Medical Education* 46 (April):263–68.

Crowley, A.E., ed. 1975a. *Medical Education in the United States, 1973–1974.* Chicago: American Medical Association.

———, ed. 1975b. "Medical Education in the United States, 1974–1975." *Journal of the American Medical Association* 234 (December 29):1325–1432.

Cuca, J.M. 1977. "Career Choices of the 1976 Graduates of U.S. Medical Schools." Washington, D.C.: Association of American Medical Colleges, March. (Processed.)

———; Sakakenny, L.A.; and Johnson, D.G. 1976. *The Medical School Admissions Process: A Review of the Literature, 1955–76.* Washington, D.C.: Association of American Medical Colleges.

Cullison, S.; Reid, C.; and Colwill, J.M. 1976a. "Medical School Admissions, Specialty Selection, and Distribution of Physicians." *Journal of the American Medical Association* 235 (February 2):502–5.

———. 1976b. "The Rural-Urban Distribution of Medical School Applicants." *Journal of Medical Education* 51 (January):47–49.

Curran, J.A. 1959. "Internships and Residencies: Historical Backgrounds and Current Trends." *Journal of Medical Education* 34 (September):873–84.

Daugirdas, J.T. 1971. "The Urban Doctors Program." *Journal of the American Medical Association* 218 (November 22):1197–98.

Davidson, L.R. 1979. "Choice by Constraint: The Selection and Function of Specialties among Women Physicians-in-Training." *Journal of Health Politics, Policy, and Law* 4 (Summer):200–220.

Davies, B.M., and Mowbray, R.M. 1968. "Medical Students: Personality and Academic Achievement." *British Journal of Medical Education* 2 (September):195–99.

Davis, K. 1982. "Implications of an Expanding Supply of Physicians: Evidence from a Cross-Sectional Analysis." *Johns Hopkins Medical Journal* 150 (February):55–64.

———, and Reynolds, R. 1975. "Medicare and the Utilization of Health Care Services by the Elderly," *Journal of Human Resources* 10 (Summer):361–77.

Dei Rossi, J.A. n.d. "Physician Location Choice and State Policy: A Case Study." Santa Barbara, Calif.: Interplan Corporation. (Processed.)

D'Elia, G., and Johnson, I. 1980. "Women Physicians in a Nonmetropolitan Area." *Journal of Medical Education* 55 (July):580–88.

Deuschle, K.W. 1969. "A University's Response to Demands for Care: Community Medicine at Kentucky." *Journal of Medical Education* 44 (September):755–61.

Dewey, D. 1973. *Where the Doctors Have Gone: The Changing Distribution of Private Practice Physicians in the Chicago Metropolitan Area, 1950–70.* Chicago: Illinois Regional Medical Program, Chicago Regional Hospital Study.

Dinkel, R.M. 1946. "Factors Underlying the Location of Physicians within Indiana." *American Sociological Review* 11 (February):16–25.

Diseker, R.A., and Chappell, J.A. 1976. "Relative Importance of Variables in Determination of Practice Location: A Pilot Study." *Social Science & Medicine* 10 (November/December):559–63.

Donovan, J.C.; Salzman, L.F.; and Allen, P.Z. 1972. "Studies in Medical Education: The Role of Cognitive and Psychological Characteristics as Career Choice Correlates." *American Journal of Obstetrics and Gynecology* (October 15):461–68.

Dorsey, J.L. 1969. "Physician Distribution in Boston and Brookline, 1940 and 1961." *Medical Care* 7 (November-December):429–40.

Dougherty, L.A. 1970. *The Supply of Physicians in the State of Arkansas.* Santa Monica, Calif.: Rand Corporation.

Dube, W.F., and Johnson, D.G. 1974. "Study of U.S. Medical School Applicants, 1972–73." *Journal of Medical Education* 49 (September):849–69.

_____. 1975. "Study of U.S. Medical School Applicants, 1973–74." *Journal of Medical Education* 50 (November):1015–32.

Dube, W.F.; Stritter, F.T.; and Nelson, B.C. 1971. "Study of U.S. Medical School Applicants, 1970–71." *Journal of Medical Education* 46 (October):837–57.

Durbin, R.L. 1963. "Do New Hospitals Attract New Doctors?" *Modern Hospital* 100 (June):98–102.

Dyckman, Z. 1976. *Study of Physicians' Income in the Pre-Medicare Period—1965.* HEW Publication No. (SSA) 76-11932. Washington, D.C.: U.S. Government Printing Office.

Dykman, R.A., and Stalnaker, J.M. 1957. "Survey of Women Physicians Graduating from Medical School 1925–1940." *Journal of Medical Education* 32 (March, Part 2):3–38.

Eagleson, B.K., and Tobolic, T. 1978. "A Survey of Students Who Chose Family Practice Residencies." *Journal of Family Practice* 6 (January):111–18.

Edwards, C.C. 1974. "A Candid Look at Health Manpower Problems." *Journal of Medical Education* 49 (January):19–26.

Egger, R.L. 1978. "Family Medicine: Where Do We Stand After Five Years?" *Delaware Medical Journal* 50 (March):147–52.

Elesh, D., and Schollaert, P.T. 1972. "Race and Urban Medicine: Factors Affecting the Distribution of Physicians in Chicago." *Journal of Health and Social Behavior* 13 (September):236–50.

Ernst, R.L.; Greenlees, J.S.; and Yett, D.E. 1978. "U.S. and Foreign Medical Graduates: Comparison of Initial Career Choices." Paper presented at a Joint Session of the American Economic Association and the Health Economics Research Association, Chicago, August 30.

Eron, L.D. 1955. "Effect of Medical Education on Medical Students' Attitudes." *Journal of Medical Education* 30 (October):559–66.

Evans, J.P. 1970. "Notes on the Foreign Medical Graduate Problem in North America." *British Journal of Medical Education* 4 (September):249–51.

Evans, R.G. 1974. "Supplier-Induced Demand: Some Empirical Evidence and Implications." In *The Economics of Health and Medical Care*, ed. M. Perlman. London: Macmillan.

―――. 1976. "Beyond the Medical Marketplace: Expenditure, Utilization, and Pricing of Insured Health Care in Canada." In *The Role of Health Insurance in the Health Services Sector*, ed. R.N. Rosett. New York: National Bureau of Economic Research.

Evashwick, C.J. 1976. "The Role of Group Practice in the Distribution of Physicians in Nonmetropolitan Areas." *Medical Care* 14 (October):808–23.

Family Health Care. 1977. "Retention of National Health Service Corps Physicians in Health Manpower Shortage Areas." Report on Contract No. 282-76-0439 for the Bureau of Health Manpower, U.S. Department of Health, Education, and Welfare, February.

Fein, R. 1956. "Factors Influencing the Location of North Carolina General Practitioners: A Study in Physician Distribution." Ph.D. dissertation, Johns Hopkins University.

―――. 1967. *The Doctor Shortage: An Economic Diagnosis.* Washington, D.C.: The Brookings Institution.

―――, and Weber, G.I. 1971. *Financing Medical Education.* New York: McGraw-Hill.

Feldman, R. 1979. "A Model of Physician Location and Pricing Behavior." In *Research in Health Economics*, ed. R.M. Scheffler. Greenwich, Conn.: JAI Press.

Feldstein, M.S. 1970. "The Rising Price of Physicians' Services." *Review of Economics and Statistics* 52 (May):121–33.

Feldstein, P.J. 1971. "Prepaid Group Practice: An Analysis and Review." Ann Arbor, Mich.: School of Public Health, University of Michigan. (Processed.)

Fishman, D.B., and Zimet, C.N. 1972. "Specialty Choice and Beliefs about Specialties among Freshman Medical Students." *Journal of Medical Education* 47 (July):524–33.

―――. 1973. "Freshman Medical Students and Specialty Choice." *Colorado School of Medicine Quarterly* 15 (Fall):6–8.

Fredericks, M.A., and Mundy, P. 1967. "The Relationship Between Social Class, Average Grade in College, Medical School Admission Test Scores, and Academic Achievement of Students in a Medical School." *Journal of Medical Education* 42 (February):126–33.

Freeman, R.B. 1971. *The Market for College-Trained Manpower.* Cambridge, Mass.: Harvard University Press.

―――. 1975a. "Legal 'Cobwebs': A Recursive Model of the Market for New Lawyers." *Review of Economics and Statistics* 57 (May):171–80.

―――. 1975b. "Supply and Salary Adjustments to the Changing Science Manpower Market: Physics, 1948–73." *American Economic Review* 45 (March) 27–39.

Friedman, M. and Kuznets, S. 1945. *Income from Independent Professional Practice.* New York: National Bureau of Economic Research.

Fruen, M.A., and Cantwell, J.R. 1982. "Geographic Distribution of Physicians: Past Trends and Future Influences." *Inquiry* 19 (Spring):44–50.

Fruen, M.A.; Rothman, A.I.; and Steiner, J.W. 1974. "Comparison of Characteristics of Male and Female Medical Student Applicants." *Journal of Medical Education* 49 (February):137–45.

Fuchs, V.R. 1978. "The Supply of Surgeons and the Demand for Operations." *Journal of Human Resources* 13 (Winter, Supplement):35–56.

_____, and Kramer, M.J. 1972. *Determinants of Expenditures for Physicians' Services in the United States, 1948-1968.* DHEW Publication No. (HSM) 73-3013. Rockville, Md.: U.S. Department of Health, Education, and Welfare.

Fulton, G.P.; Syiek, J.A.; Evans, C.W.; and Mayes, C.R. 1980. "Strategies for a Statewide Approach to Improving Geographic Distribution of Health Professionals." *Journal of Medical Education* 55 (October):865–71.

Funkenstein, D.H. 1966. "Current Changes in Education Affecting Medical School Admissions and Curriculum Planning." *Journal of Medical Education* 40 (May):401–23.

_____. 1971. "Medical Students, Medical Schools, and Society during Three Eras." In *Psychosocial Aspects of Medical Training,* ed. R.H. Coombs and C.E. Vincent. Springfield, Ill.: Charles C. Thomas.

_____. 1978. *Medical Students, Medical Schools, and Society during Five Eras.* Cambridge, Mass.: Ballinger.

Gabel, J.R., and Redish, M.A. 1979. "Alternative Physician Payment Methods: Incentives, Efficiency, and National Health Insurance." *Milbank Memorial Fund Quarterly/Health and Society* 57 (Spring):38–59.

Garfield, S.L., and Wolpin, M. 1961. "MCAT Scores and Continuation in Medical School." *Journal of Medical Education* 36 (August):888–91.

Gee, H.H., and Schumacher, C.F. 1961. "Some Characteristics of 1958–59 Interns and Internships." *Journal of Medical Education* 36 (April, Part 2):34–60.

Geertsma, R.H., and Chapman, J.E. 1966. "Progress through Medical School." *Journal of Medical Education* 41 (August):772–79.

Geertsma, R.H., and Grinols, D.R. 1972. "Specialty Choice in Medicine." *Journal of Medical Education* 47 (July):509–17.

Geomet. 1979. *Comparative Evaluation of NHSC and Appalachian Regional Commission Sites.* Washington, D.C.: U.S. Department of Health, Education, and Welfare.

Geyman, J.P. 1979. "Graduate Education in Family Practice: A Ten-Year View." *Journal of Family Practice* 9 (May):859–71.

Giacalone, J.J., and Hudson, J.I. 1977. "Primary Care Education Trends in U.S. Medical Schools and Teaching Hospitals." *Journal of Medical Education* 52 (December):971–81.

Ginzberg, E.; Brann, E.; Hiestand, D.; and Ostow, M. 1981. "The Expanding Physician Supply and Health Policy: The Clouded Outlook." *Milbank Memorial Fund Quarterly/Health and Society* 59 (Fall):508–41.

Ginzberg, E.; Ginzberg, S.W.; Axelrod, S.; and Herma, J.L. 1951. *Occupational Choice: An Approach to a General Theory.* New York: Columbia University Press.

Glandon, G.L. and Shapiro, R.J. 1980. *Profile of Medical Practice, 1980.* Chicago: American Medical Association.

Glaser, W.A. 1959. "Internship Appointments of Medical Students." *Administrative Science Quarterly* 4 (December):337–56.

GMENAC. 1981a. *Geographic Distribution Technical Panel, vol. 3.* DHHS Publication No. (HRA) 81-651. Washington, D.C.: U.S. Government Printing Office, April.

———. 1981b. *Nonphysician Health Care Provider Technical Panel, vol. 6.* DHHS Publication No. 81-656. Washington, D.C.: U.S. Government Printing Office, April.

———. 1981c. *Summary Report, vol. 1.* DHHS Publication No. (HRA) 81-651. Washington, D.C.: U.S. Government Printing Office, April.

Gober, P., and Gordon, R.J. 1980. "Intraurban Physician Location: A Case Study of Phoenix." *Social Science & Medicine* 14D (December):407–17.

Goldblatt, A.; Goodman, L.W.; Mick, S.S.; and Stevens, R. 1975. "Licensure, Competence, and Manpower Distribution: A Follow-up Study of Foreign Medical Graduates." *New England Journal of Medicine* 292 (January 16):3–7.

Goldfarb, D.L. 1981. "Trends in Physicians' Incomes, Expenses, and Fees: 1970-1980." In *Profile of Medical Practice 1981*, ed. D.L. Goldfarb. Chicago: American Medical Association.

Goodman, L.J. 1976. "Physician Distribution by Regional, State, County, and Metropolitan Areas." In *Physician Distribution and Medical Licensure in the U.S., 1975.* Chicago: American Medical Assocation.

———; Bennett, E.H.; and Odem, R.J. 1976. *Group Medical Practice in the U.S., 1975.* Chicago: American Medical Association.

Goodman, L.J., and Mason, H.R. 1976. *Physician Distribution and Medical Licensure in the U.S., 1975, Part 1.* Chicago: American Medical Association.

Gordon, T.L. 1978. "1975 Medical School Graduates Entering Family Practice Residencies." *Journal of Medical Education* 53 (November):939–42.

Gough, H.G. 1967. "Nonintellectual Factors in the Selection and Evaluation of Medical Students." *Journal of Medical Education* 42 (July):642–50.

———. 1971. "The Recruitment and Selection of Medical Students." In *Psychological Aspects of Medical Training*, ed. R.H. Coombs and C.E. Vincent. Springfield, Ill.: Charles C. Thomas.

———. 1975. "Specialty Preferences of Physicians and Medical Students." *Journal of Medical Education* 50 (June):581–88.

———. 1978. "Some Predictive Implications of Premedical Scientific Competence and Preferences." *Journal of Medical Education* 53 (April):291–99.

———, and Ducker, D.G. 1977. "Social Class in Relation to Medical School Performance and Choice of Specialty." *Journal of Psychology* 96 (May):31–43.

Gough, H.G., and Hall, W.B. 1964. "Prediction of Performance in Medical School from the California Psychological Inventory." *Journal of Applied Psychology* 48 (August):218–26.

_____. 1975a. "An Attempt to Predict Graduation from Medical School." *Journal of Medical Education* 50 (October):940–50.

_____. 1975b. "The Prediction of Academic and Clinical Performance in Medical School." *Research in Higher Education* 3:301–12.

_____. 1978. "Medical School Graduates Who Leave California: A Study at the University of California, San Francisco." *Western Journal of Medicine* 128 (January):81–84.

Graduate Medical Education National Advisory Committee. See GMENAC.

Graettinger, J.S. 1976. "Graduate Medical Education Viewed from the National Intern and Resident Matching Program." *Journal of Medical Education* 51 (September):703–15.

_____. 1978. "The Residency Matching Program." *Archives of Otolaryngology* 104 (November):615–19.

_____. 1979. "Results of the NRMP for 1979." *Journal of Medical Education* 54 (April):347–49.

Graves, J., ed. 1973. *The Future of Medical Education.* Durham, N.C.: Duke University Press.

Gray, L.C. 1977. "The Geographic and Functional Distribution of Black Physicians: Some Research and Policy Implications." *American Journal of Public Health* 67 (June):519–26.

Greenwood, M.J. 1975. "Research on Internal Migration in the United States: A Survey." *Journal of Economic Literature* 13 (June):397–433.

Guzick, D.S., and Jahiel, R.I. 1976. "Distribution of Private Practice Offices of Physicians with Specified Characteristics among Urban Neighborhoods." *Medical Care* 14 (June):469–88.

Hadley, J. 1975. "Models of Physicians' Specialty and Location Choices." Ph.D. dissertation, Yale University.

_____. 1977. "An Empirical Model of Medical Specialty Choice." *Inquiry* 14 (December):384–401.

_____. 1979. "A Disaggregated Model of Medical Specialty Choice." In *Research in Health Economics,* ed. R.M. Scheffler. Greenwich, Conn.: JAI Press.

_____. 1980. "State and Local Financing Options." *Medical Education Financing: Policy Analyses and Options for the 1980s,* ed. J. Hadley. New York: Prodist.

_____, and Lee, R. 1978. "Physicians' Price and Output Decisions: Theory and Evidence." Final Report on Contract No. 600-76-0054 with the Social Security Administration, U.S. Department of Health, Education, and Welfare. Washington, D.C.: The Urban Institute.

Hadley, J., and Levenson, M. 1980. "Institutional Support for Medical Schools and Teaching Hospitals." *Medical Education Financing: Policy Analyses and Options for the 1980s,* ed. J. Hadley. New York: Prodist.

Hale, F.A.; McConnochie, K.M.; Chapman, R.J.; and Whiting, R.D. 1979. "The Impact of a Required Preceptorship on Senior Medical Students." *Journal of Medical Education* 54 (May):396–401.

Haley, H.B.; Juan, I.R.; and Paiva, R.E.A. 1971. "MCAT Scores in Relation to Personality Measures and Biographical Variables." *Journal of Medical Education* 46 (November):947–58.

Hall, T.D. 1976. "The Behavior of Medical Schools as Non-Profit Firms." Ph.D. dissertation, University of California, Los Angeles.

Hambleton, J.W. 1971. "Determinants of Geographic Differences in the Supply of Physicians' Services." Ph.D. dissertation, University of Wisconsin, Madison.

————. 1972. "Foreign Medical Graduates and the Doctor Shortage," *Inquiry* 9 (December):68–72.

Harrell, G.T. 1973. "Training in a Small Town for Rural Practice." *Journal of the American Medical Association* 225 (August 27):1103–5.

Harris, D.L., and Bluhm, H.P. 1977. "An Evaluation of Primary Care Preceptorships." *Journal of Family Practice* 5 (October):577–79.

Hassinger, E.W. 1963. "Background and Community Orientation of Rural Physicians Compared with Metropolitan Physicians in Missouri." Research Bulletin No. 822. Columbia, Mo.: University of Missouri College of Agriculture. (Processed.)

Haug, J.N. 1975. "A Review of Women in Surgery." *Bulletin of the American College of Surgeons* 60 (September):21–23.

————, and Roback, G.A. 1968. *Distribution of Physicians, Hospitals, and Hospital Beds in the U.S., 1967.* Chicago: American Medical Association.

————. 1970. *Distribution of Physicians, Hospitals, and Hospital Beds in the U.S., 1969,* vol. 1. Chicago: American Medical Association.

————, and Martin, B.C. 1971. *Distribution of Physicians in the United States, 1970.* Chicago: American Medical Association.

Haug, M.R.; Lavin, B.; and Breslau, N. 1980. "Practice Location Preferences at Entry to Medical School." *Journal of Medical Education* 55 (April):333–38.

Hay, J. 1980. "Occupational Choice and Occupational Earnings: Selectivity Bias in a Simultaneous Logit-OLS Model." Ph.D dissertation, Yale University.

————. 1981. "Selectivity Bias in a Simultaneous Logit-OLS Model: Physician Specialty Choice and Specialty Income." University of Connecticut Health Center, Farmington, Conn. (Processed.)

————, and Leahy, M.J. 1982. "Physician-Induced Demand: An Empirical Analysis of the Consumer Information Gap." *Journal of Health Economics* 1 (December):231–44.

Haynes, M.A. 1969. "Distribution of Black Physicians in the United States, 1967." *Journal of the American Medical Association* 210 (October 6):93–95.

Heald, K.A.; Cooper, J.K.; and Coleman, S. 1974. *An Analysis of Two Surveys of Recent Medical School Graduates.* Publication No. R-1477-HEW. Santa Monica, Calif.: Rand Corporation.

Heine, R.W. 1960. "The Internship: Factors in Choice and Level of Satisfaction." *Journal of Medical Education* 35 (May):404–8.

Held, M.L., and Zimet, C.N. 1975. "A Longitudinal Study of Medical Specialty Choice and Certainty Level." *Journal of Medical Education* 50 (November):1044–51.

Held, P.J. 1972. "The Migration of the 1955–65 Graduates of American Medical Schools." Ph.D. dissertation, University of California, Berkeley.

———, and Manheim, L.M. 1980. "The Effect of Local Physician Supply on the Treatment of Hypertension in Quebec." *The Target Income Hypothesis and Related Issues in Health Manpower Policy.* DHEW Publication No. (HRA) 80-27. Washington, D.C.: U.S. Department of Health, Education, and Welfare.

Hensher, D.A., and Johnson, L.W. 1981. *Applied Discrete Choice Modelling.* New York: John Wiley and Sons.

Herman, M.W., and Veloski, J. 1977. "Family Medicine and Primary Care: Trends and Student Characteristics." *Journal of Medical Education* 55 (February):99–105.

Herrmann, T.J. 1972. "Influence of an 'All Elective' Fourth Year on Career Goal Selection." *Journal of Medical Education* 57 (July):518–23.

———. 1973. "A New Trend in Career Interests among University of Michigan Medical Students." *Journal of Medical Education* 47 (May):451–53.

Hixson, J.S. 1979. "A Simultaneous Equation Time-Series Model of the Market for Physicians' Services." In *Profile of Medical Practice, 1979,* ed. J.C. Gaffney and G.L. Glandon. Chicago: American Medical Association.

———, and Mocniak, N. 1980. "The Aggregate Supplies and Demands of Physician and Dental Services." In *The Target Income Hypothesis and Related Issues in Health Manpower Policy.* DHEW Publication No. (HRA) 80-27. Washington, D.C.: U.S. Department of Health, Education, and Welfare, January.

Holahan, J. 1975. "Physician Availability, Medical Care Reimbursement, and Delivery of Physician Services: Some Evidence from the Medicaid Program." *Journal of Human Resources* 10 (Summer):378–402.

Holden, W.D. 1969. "The Evolutionary Functions of American Specialty Boards." *Journal of Medical Education* 54 (September):819–28.

———. 1970. "Specialty Board Certification as a Measure of Professional Competence." *Journal of the American Medical Association* 213 (August 10):1016–18.

———, and Levit, E.J. 1978. "Migration of Physicians from One Specialty to Another: A Longitudinal Study of U.S. Medical School Graduates." *Journal of the American Medical Association* 249 (January 16):205–9.

Holen, A.S. 1965. "Effects of Professional Licensing Arrangements on Interstate Labor Mobility and Resource Allocation." *Journal of Political Economy* 73 (October):492–98.

Howard, J.P. 1980. "Community Project in Pediatrics: An Effort to Influence Physician Distribution." *Journal of the Kentucky Medical Association* 78 (September):551–53.

Huang, L., and Koropecky, O. 1973. "The Effects of the Medicare Method of Reimbursement on Physicians' Fees and on Beneficiaries' Utilization." In *A Report on the Results of the Study of Methods of Reimbursement for Physicians' Services under Medicare.* SS Publication No. 92-73 (10-73). Washington, D.C.: U.S. Department of Health, Education, and Welfare.

Hunter, R.C.A. 1965. "Some Factors Affecting Undergraduate Academic Achievement." *Canadian Medical Association Journal* 92 (April 3):732–36.

Hutchins, E.B. 1961. "Factors Affecting the Choice of an Internship." *Journal of Medical Education* 36 (April, Part 2):60–68.

———. 1962. "The Student and His Environment." *Journal of Medical Education* 37 (January, Part 2):67–82.

———. 1964. "The AAMC Longitudinal Study: Implications for Medical Education." *Journal of Medical Education* 39 (March):265–77.

———. 1965. "The AAMC Study of Medical Student Attrition: School Characteristics and Dropout Rate." *Journal of Medical Education* 60 (October):921–27.

———, and Gee, H.H. 1961. "The Study of Applicants, 1959–60." *Journal of Medical Education* 36 (April):289–304.

Ingersoll, R.S., and Graves, G.O. 1965. "Predictability of Success in the First Year of Medical School." *Journal of Medical Education* 60 (April, Part 1):351–63.

Institute of Medicine. 1974. *Costs of Education in the Health Professions: Report of a Study, Parts I and II.* DHEW Publication No. (HRA) 74-32. Washington, D.C.: U.S. Department of Health, Education, and Welfare, January.

———. 1978. *A Manpower Policy for Primary Health Care.* Washington, D.C.: National Academy of Sciences, May.

Jacoby, I. 1979. "Impact of the Health Professions Educational Assistance Act on Specialty Distribution Among First-Year Residents." *Public Health Reports* 94 (January-February):22–30.

———. 1981. "Graduate Medical Education: Its Impact on Specialty Distribution." *Journal of the American Medical Association* 245 (March 13):1046–51.

Jason, H. 1970. "The Relevance of Medical Education to Medical Practice." *Journal of the American Medical Association* 212 (June 22):2092–95.

Johnson, D.G., and Hutchins, E.B. 1966. "Doctor or Dropout? A Study of Medical Student Attrition." *Journal of Medical Education* 41 (December): 1099–1269.

———; Smith, V.C.; and Tarnoff, S.L. 1975. "Recruitment and Progress of Minority Medical School Entrants, 1970–72." *Journal of Medical Education* 50 (July):713–55.

Johnson, S.E.; Baeumler, W.L.; and Carter, R.E. 1973. "The Family Physician: A Comparative Study of Minnesota and Wisconsin Family Physicians Practicing in Rural and Urban Communities." *Minnesota Medicine* 36 (August):713–18.

Johnston, J. 1972. *Eonometric Methods*, (2d ed.) New York: McGraw-Hill.

Jones, C.B. 1978. "Community Recruitment of Family Physicians from Family Practice Residencies." *Texas Medicine* 74 (March):74–79.

Joroff, S., and Navarro, V. 1971. "Medical Manpower: A Multivariate Analysis of the Distribution of Physicians in Urban United States." *Medical Care* 9 (September-October):428–38.

Juan, I.R., and Haley, H.B. 1970. "High and Low Levels of Dogmatism in Relation to Personality, Intellectual, and Environmental Characteristics of Medical Students." *Psychological Reports* 26 (April):535–44.

Jussim, J. and Muller, C. 1975. "Medical Education for Women: How Good an Investment?" *Journal of Medical Education* 50 (June):571–80.

Kane, R.L.; Warnick, R.; Proctor, P.H.; Olsen, D.M.; and Gourley, D. 1975. "Mail Order Medicine: An Analysis of the Sears Roebuck Foundation's Community Medical Assistance Program." *Journal of the American Medical Association* 232 (June 9):1023–27.

Kaplan, D., and Plotz, C.M. 1974. "A Controlled Analysis of Medical Students in a Family Practice Program." *Journal of Medical Education* 49 (February):154–57.

Kaplan, H.I. 1971. "Woman Physicians." *New Physician* 20 (January):11–19.

Kaplan, R.S., and Leinhardt, S. 1973. "Determinants of Physician Office Location." *Medical Care* 11 (September-October):406–15.

Kehrer, B.H. 1974. "Factors Affecting the Incomes of Men and Women Physicians: An Exploratory Analysis." Paper presented at the Annual Meetings of the Southern Economic Association, Atlanta, Ga., November 15.

———. 1976. "Factors Affecting the Incomes of Men and Women Physicians: An Exploratory Analysis." *Journal of Human Resources* 11 (Fall):526–45.

Kendall, P.L. 1965. *The Relationship Between Medical Educators and Medical Practitioners.* Evanston, Ill.: Association of American Medical Colleges.

———. 1971. "Medical Specialization: Trends and Contributing Factors." In *Psychological Aspects of Medical Training*, ed. R.H. Coombs and C.E. Vincent. Springfield, Ill.: Charles C. Thomas.

Kessel, R.A. 1958. "Price Discrimination in Medicine." *Journal of Law and Economics* 1 (October):20–53.

———. 1970. "The AMA and the Supply of Physicians." *Law and Contemporary Problems* 35 (Spring): 267–83.

———. 1974. "The Role of Organized Medicine in Determining Our Health Care System." In *The U.S. Medical Care Industry: The Economist's Point of View*, ed. J.C. Morreale. Ann Arbor, Mich.: Graduate School of Business Administration, University of Michigan.

Kettel, L.J.; Dinham, S.M.; Drach, G.W.; and Barbee, R.A. 1979. "Arizona's Three-Year Medical Curriculum: A Postmortem." *Journal of Medical Education* 54 (March):210–16.

Kimbell, L.J., and Barros, L.L. 1978. *Statistical Hypothesis Testing of the MAB Health Systems Data Base.* Final Report on Contract No. HRA-231-77-0128 with the U.S. Department of Health, Education, and Welfare. Santa Monica, Calif.: Technology Service Corporation.

Kimbell, L.J.; and Lorant, J.H. 1977. "Physician Productivity and Returns to Scale." *Health Services Research* 12 (Winter):367–79.

Kimbell, L.J.; and Yett, D.E. 1974. "An Evaluation of Policy Related Research on the Effects of Alternative Health Care Reimbursement Systems." Final Report on NSF Grant No. GI-39344. Los Angeles: Human Resources Research Center, University of Southern California. (Processed.)

Kimberly, J.R., and Counte, M.A. 1978. "Issues in Family Practice: Medical Student and Practicing Physician Perspectives." *Medical Care* 16 (March): 214–25.

Korman, L., and Feldman, H.A. 1977. "A Study of the Recruitment of Physicians into Three Northern New York Counties." *Journal of Medical Education* 52 (April):308–15.

Korman, M.; Stubblefield, R.L.; and Martin, L.W. 1968. "Patterns of Success in Medical School and Their Correlates." *Journal of Medical Education* 43 (March):405–11.

Knobel, R.J. 1973. "Placement of Foreign-Trained Physicians in U.S. Medical Residencies." *Medical Care* 11 (May-June):224–39.

Knowles, J.H. 1965. "The Role of the Hospital: The Ambulatory Clinic." *Bulletin of the New York Academy of Medicine* 40 (January):625–57.

Kosa, J.D. 1969. "The Medical Student: His Career and Religion," *Hospital Progress* 50 (April):51–53.

⸻, and Coker, R.E. 1965. "The Female Physician in Public Health: Conflict and Reconciliation of the Sex and Professional Roles." *Sociology and Social Research* 49 (April):294–305.

⸻; Greenberg, B.G.; and Donnelly, T.G. 1966. "The Transiency of Physicians in Public Health: Study of a Cost Factor in Institutional Work." *Milbank Memorial Fund Quarterly* 54 (April, Part 2):229–58.

Kosa, J.D.; Greenberg, B.G.; and Coker, R.E. 1966. "The Novice Physician in the Local Public Health Service: A Study of Continuities in the Patterns of Recruitment." *Milbank Memorial Fund Quarterly* 54 (April, Part 1):214–28.

Kraus, A.S.; Botterell, E.H.; Einarson, D.W.; and Thompson, M.G. 1971. "Initial Career Plans and Subsequent Family Practice," *Journal of Medical Education* 46 (October):826–30.

Kritzer, H., and Zimet, C.N. 1967. "A Retrospective View of Medical Specialty Choice." *Journal of Medical Education* 42 (January):47–58.

Langwell, K.M. 1980a. "Career Paths of First-Year Resident Physicians: A Seven-Year Study." *Journal of Medical Education* 55 (November):897–905.

⸻. 1980b. "Real Returns to Career Decisions: The Physician's Specialty and Location Choices." *Journal of Human Resources* 15 (Winter):278–86.

⸻. 1981. "Factors Affecting the Incomes of Men and Women Physicians: Further Explorations." *Journal of Human Resources* 17 (Spring):261–75.

⸻, and Budde, N.W. 1978. "Urban-Rural Differences in General and Family Practices: An Examination of Location Choice Incentives." In *Reference Data on Socioeconomic Issues of Health, 1978,* ed. J.L. Warner and J.R. Leopold. Chicago: American Medical Association.

Last, J.M.; Martin, F.M.; and Stanley, G.R. 1967. "Academic Record and Subsequent Career." *Proceedings of the Royal Society of Medicine* 60 (August):21–24.

Latham, R.J. 1973. "Operating Expenditures and Sponsored Research at U.S. Medical Schools: Comment." *Journal of Human Resources* 8 (Fall):519–22.

Lave, J.R., and Lave, L.B. 1974. *The Hospital Construction Act: An Evaluation of the Hill-Burton Program, 1948–73.* Washington, D.C.: American Enterprise Institute for Public Policy Research.

Lawlor, A.C. and Reid, J.T. 1981. "Hierarchical Patterns in the Location of Physician Specialists among Counties." *Inquiry* 18 (Spring):79–90.

Lee, M.W., and Wallace, R.L. 1970. "Demand, Supply, and the Distribution of Physicians." Studies in Health Care, Report No. 5. Columbia, Mo.: Department of Community Health and Medical Practice, University of Missouri. (Processed.)

Lee, R.H. 1980. "Regional Physician Supply and Graduate Medical Education." *Health Policy and Education* 1 (December):351–66.

Leffler, K. 1975. "Quality, Search, and Licensure." Ph.D. dissertation, University of California, Los Angeles.

Leserman, J. 1980. "Changes in the Professional Orientation of Medical Students: A Follow-Up Study." *Journal of Medical Education* 55 (May):415–22.

Levine, A. 1976. "Educational and Occupational Choice: A Synthesis of Literature from Sociology and Psychology." *Journal of Consumer Research* 2 (March):276–89.

Levine, D.M., and Bonito, A.J. 1974. "Impact of Clinical Training on Attitudes of Medical Students: Self-Perpetuating Barrier to Change in the System." *British Journal of Medical Education* 8 (March):13–16.

Levit, E.J.; Schumacher, C.F.; and Hubbard, J.P. 1963. "The Effect of Characteristics of Hospitals in Relation to the Caliber of Interns Obtained and the Competence of Interns After One Year of Training." *Journal of Medical Education* 38 (November):909–19.

———. 1964. "The Internship: An Evaluation of Input and Output." *Journal of the American Medical Association* 189 (July 27):299–305.

Levitt, L.P. 1966. "The Personality of the Medical Student: A Brief Historical Review and Contemporary Psychiatric Study." *Chicago Medical School Quarterly* 25 (Winter):201–14.

Lewis, C.S. 1978. "Physician Manpower in Oklahoma in 1978." *Oklahoma State Medical Association Journal* 71 (December):468–75.

Lieberson, S. 1958. "Ethnic Groups and the Practice of Medicine." *American Sociological Review* 23 (October):542–49.

Lief, H.I. 1971. "Personality Characteristics of Medical Students." In *Psychological Aspects of Medical Training*, ed. R.H. Coombs and C.E. Vincent. Springfield, Ill.: Charles C. Thomas.

Lief, V.F.; Lief, H.I.; and Young, K.M. 1965. "Academic Success: Intelligence and Personality. *Journal of Medical Education* 40 (February):114–24.

Lienke, R.I. 1970. "The Family Practice Model in Health Education." *Journal of the American Medical Association* 212 (June 22):2097–2101.

Lindsay, C.M. 1973. "Real Returns to Medical Education." *Journal of Human Resources* 8 (Summer):331–48.

———. 1976. "More Real Returns to Medical Education." *Journal of Human Resources* 11 (Winter):127–30.

Linn, B.S., and Zeppa, R. 1980. "Career Preference of Medical Students and Their Attitudes about Themselves and Medical Specialists." *Psychological Reports* 46 (April):349–50.

Little, J.M.; Little, H.H.; and Novick, M.R. 1960. "A Study of the Medical School Admission Test in Relation to Academic Difficulties in Medical School." *Journal of Medical Education* 35 (March):264–72.

Littlemeyer, M.H. 1969. "Medical School Admissions Requirements and Curricula." In *Preparation for the Study of Medicine*, ed. R.G. Page and M.H. Littlemeyer. Chicago: University of Chicago Press.

Livingston, P.B., and Zimet, C.N. 1965 "Death Anxiety, Authoritarianism, and the Choice of Specialty in Medical Students." *Journal of Nervous and Mental Disease* 140 (March):222–30.

Lloyd, S.M.; Johnson, D.G.; and Mann, M.M. 1978. "Survey of Graduates of a Traditionally Black College of Medicine." *Journal of Medical Education* 53 (August):640–50.

Lockett, B.A., and Williams, K.N. 1974. *Foreign Medical Graduates and Physician Manpower in the United States.* DHEW Publication No. (HRA) 74-30. Washington, D.C.: U.S. Department of Health, Education, and Welfare, February.

Long, M.D. 1980. "Specialty Choice of Black Medical School Graduates." *Journal of Medical Education* 55 (May):409–14.

Longnecker, D.P. 1975. "Practice Objectives and Goals: A Survey of Family Practice Residents." *Journal of Family Practice* 2 (October):347–51.

Lopate, C. 1968. *Women in Medicine.* Baltimore: Johns Hopkins Press.

Lyden, F.J.; Geiger, H.J.; and Peterson, O.L. 1968. *The Training of Good Physicians.* Cambridge, Mass.: Harvard University Press.

Lyman, R.W. 1976. "Public Rights and Private Responsibilities: A University Viewpoint." *Journal of Medical Education* 51 (January):7–13.

———. 1980. "Economic Models for Probabilistic Choice among Products." *Journal of Business* 53 (July, Part 2):S13–S29.

McGrath, E., and Zimet, C.N. 1977. "Female and Male Medical Students: Differences in Specialty Choice Selection and Personality." *Journal of Medical Education* 52 (April):293–300.

McShane, M.G. 1977. *An Empirical Classification of U.S. Medical Schools by Institutional Dimensions.* DHEW Publication No. (HRA) 77-55. Washington, D.C.: U.S. Department of Health, Education, and Welfare.

Mahoney, A.R. 1973. "Factors Affecting Physicians' Choice of Group or Independent Practice." *Inquiry* 10 (June):9–18.

Malinvaud, E. 1970. *Statistical Methods of Econometrics*, 2d ed. Amsterdam: North-Holland.

Maloney, J.V. 1970. "A Report on the Role of Economic Motivation in the Performance of Medical School Faculty." *Surgery* 67 (July):1–19.

Malt, R.A., and Grillo, H.C. 1969. "Prospective Interns' View of the Model Surgeon." *Journal of Medical Education* 44 (February):141–44.

Mantovani, R.E.; Gordon, T.L.; and Johnson, D.G. 1976. *Medical Student Indebtedness and Career Plans, 1974–75.* DHEW Publication No. (HRA) 77-21. Washington, D.C.: U.S. Government Printing Office, September.

Marden, P.G. 1966. "Demographic and Ecological Analysis of the Distribution of Physicians in Metropolitan America, 1960." *American Journal of Sociology* 72 (November):290–300.

Marr, J. 1972. "Trying to Recruit New Doctors for Your Community? Take Some Hints from Jackson." *Health Manpower for Michigan* 4 (Spring):1.

Marshall, C.L.; Hassanein, K.; Hassanein, R.; and Marshall, C. 1971. "Principal Components Analysis of the Distribution of Physicians, Dentists, and Osteopaths in a Midwestern State." *American Journal of Public Health* 61 (August):1556–64.

Martin, B.C. 1975. *Medical School Alumni*. Rockville, Md.: Aspen Systems.

Martin, E.D.; Moffat, R.E.; Falter, R.T.; and Walker, J.D. 1968. "Where Graduates Go. The University of Kansas School of Medicine: A Study of the Profile of 959 Graduates and Factors Which Influenced the Geographic Distribution." *Journal of the Kansas Medical Society* 69 (March):84–89.

Mason, H.R. 1971. "Effectiveness of Student Aid Programs Tied to a Service Commitment." *Journal of Medical Education* 46 (July):575–83.

———. 1975. "Medical School, Residency, and Eventual Practice Location: Toward a Rationale for State Support of Medical Education." *Journal of the American Medical Association* 233 (July 7):49–52.

Matlack, D.R. 1972. "Changes and Trends in Medical Education." *Journal of Medical Education* 47 (August):612–19.

Matteson, M.T., and Smith, S.V. 1977. "Selection of Medical Specialties: Preferences versus Choices." *Journal of Medical Education* 52 (July):548–54.

Matthews, M.R. 1970. "The Training and Practice of Women Physicians: A Case Study." *Journal of Medical Education* 45 (December):1016–24.

Mattson, D.E.; Stehr, D.E.; and Will, R.E. 1973. "Evaluation of a Program Designed to Produce Rural Physicians." *Journal of Medical Education* 48 (April): 323–31.

Maurice, W.L.; Klonoff, H.; Miles, J.E.; and Krell, R. 1975. "Medical Student Change during a Psychiatry Clerkship: Evaluation of a Program." *Journal of Medical Education* 50 (February):181–89.

Maurizi, A. 1969. *Economic Essays on the Dental Profession*. Iowa City, Iowa: College of Business Administration, University of Iowa.

May, J.J. 1975. "Utilization of Health Services and the Availability of Resources." In *Equity in Health Services: Empirical Analyses in Social Policy*, eds. R. Andersen et al. Cambridge, Mass.: Ballinger.

Mechanic, David. 1974. *The Character of the Medical Marketplace and Its Failures in the Delivery of Medical Services*. Madison, Wis.: Center for Medical Sociology and Health Services Research/Health Economics Research Center, University of Wisconsin-Madison. (Processed.)

Mennemeyer, S.T. 1978. "Really Great Returns to Medical Education?" *Journal of Human Resources* 13 (Winter):75–90.

Meyer, G.C.; Adams, R.L.; and Holcomb, J. 1976. "Preferences for Family Practice among Entering Medical Students." *Texas Medicine* 72 (March):86–90.

Mick, S.S. 1978. "Understanding the Persistence of Human Resource Problems in Health." *Milbank Memorial Fund Quarterly/Health and Society* 61 (Fall):463–99.

Miller, A.E.; Miller, M.G.; and Adelman, J. 1978. "The Changing Urban-Suburban Distribution of Medical Practice in Large American Metropolitan Areas." *Medical Care* 16 (October):799–818.

Miller, N.; Coker, R.E.; Greenberg, B.G.; and McConnell, F.S. 1966. "Toward a Typology of Public Health Careers." *Milbank Memorial Fund Quarterly* 44 (April, Part 1):200–212.

Miller, N.; Coker, R.E.; McConnell, F.S.; Greenberg, B.G.; and Back, K.W. 1966. "A Comparison of Career Patterns of Public Health Physicians and Other Medical Specialists." *Milbank Memorial Fund Quarterly* 44 (April, Part 1):181–99.

Millis, J.S. 1969. "Graduate Medical Education Revisited." *Journal of Medical Education* 44 (September):734–36.

Mitchell, W.D. 1975. "Medical Student Career Choice: A Conceptualization." *Social Science & Medicine* 9 (November-December):641–53.

Monk, M.A., and Terris, M. 1956. "Factors in Student Choice of General or Specialty Practice." *New England Journal of Medicine* 255 (December 13):1135–40.

Monk, M.A., and Thomas, C.B. 1970. "Characteristics of Male Medical Students Related to Their Subsequent Careers." *Johns Hopkins Medical Journal* 127 (November):254–72.

———. 1973. "Personal and Social Factors Related to Medical Specialty Practice." *Johns Hopkins Medical Journal* 133 (July):19–29.

Moradiellos, D.P., and Athelstan, G.T. 1979. "Selection of Medical Students to Meet Physician Manpower Needs." *Public Health Reports* 94 (January-February):16–21.

Morgan, B.C. 1971. "Admission of Women into Medical Schools in the United States: Current Status." *Woman Physican* 26 (June):305–9.

Morgan, T.E., and Jones, D.D. 1976. *Trends and Dimensions of Biomedical and Behavioral Research Funding in Academic Medical Centers.* Washington, D.C.: Association of American Medical Colleges.

Motto, J.A. 1965. "Background Data of Significance to Medical School Performance." *Journal of Medical Education* 40 (February):98–113.

Mowbray, R.M., and Davies, B. 1971. "Personality Factors in Choice of Medical Specialty." *British Journal of Medical Education* 5 (June):110–17.

Mumford, E. 1970. *Interns, From Students to Physicians.* Cambridge, Mass.: Harvard University Press.

Myers, I.B., and Davis, J.A. 1964. "Relation of Medical Students' Psychological Type to Their Specialties Twelve Years Later." Paper presented at the Annual Meeting of the American Psychological Association, Los Angeles, Calif., September 4–9.

Nerlove, M., and Press, S.J. 1973. *Univariate and Multivariate Log-Linear and Logistic Models.* Publication no. R-1306-EDA/NIH. Santa Monica, Calif.: Rand Corporation.

Newhouse, J.P. 1970. "A Model of Physician Pricing." *Southern Economic Journal* 37 (October):174–83.

———. 1981. "The Demand for Medical Services: A Retrospect and Prospect." In *Health, Economics, and Health Economics,* ed. J. van der Gaag and M. Perlman. Amsterdam: North-Holland.

_____, and Marquis, M.S. 1978. "The Norms Hypothesis and the Demand for Medical Care." *Journal of Human Resources* 13 (Supplement):159–82.

Newhouse, J.P., and Phelps, C.E. 1974. "Price and Income Elasticities for Medical Care." In *The Economics of Health and Medical Care*, ed. M. Perlman. New York: John Wiley and Sons.

_____. 1976. "New Estimates of Price and Income Elasticities of Medical Care Services." In *The Role of Health Insurance in the Health Services Sector*, ed. R.N. Rosett. New York: National Bureau of Economic Research.

_____, and Marquis, M.S. 1979. *On Having Your Cake and Eating It Too: Econometric Problems in Estimating the Demand for Health Services.* Publication no. R-1149-1-NC. Santa Monica, Calif.: Rand Corporation.

Newhouse, J.P.; Williams, A.P.; Bennett, B.W.; and Schwartz, W.B. 1982a. *How Have Location Patterns of Physicians Affected the Availability of Medical Services?* Publication no. R-2872-HJK/HHS/RWJ. Santa Monica, Calif.: Rand Corporation.

_____. 1982b. "Where Have All the Doctors Gone?" *Journal of the American Medical Association* 247 (May 7):2392–96.

Newhouse, J.P.; Williams, A.P.; Schwartz, W.B.; and Bennett, B.W. 1982c. *The Geographic Distribution of Physicians: Is the Conventional Wisdom Correct?* Publication no. R-2734-HJK/RWJ/RC. Santa Monica, Calif.: Rand Corporation.

Notman, M.T., and Nadelson, C.C. 1973. "Medicine: A Career Conflict for Women." *American Journal of Psychiatry* 10 (October):1123–27.

Oates, R.P., and Feldman, H.A. 1971. "Medical Career Patterns: Choices among Several Classes of Medical Students." *New York State Journal of Medicine* 71 (October 15):2437–40.

_____. 1974. "Patterns of Change in Medical Student Career Choices." *Journal of Medical Education* 49 (June):563–69.

Olmstead, A.L., and Sheffrin, S.M. 1981. "The Medical School Admissions Process: An Empirical Investigation." *Journal of Human Resources* 16 (Summer):459–67.

Onion, D.K. 1978. "A Rural Primary Care Student Preceptorship." *Journal of the Maine Medical Association* 69 (April):124–28.

Orso, C.L. 1979. "Delivering Ambulatory Health Care: The Successful Experience of an Urban Neighborhood Health Center." *Medical Care* 17 (February):111–26.

Otis, G.D.; Graham, J.R.; and Thacker, L. 1975. "Typological Analysis of U.S. Medical Schools." *Journal of Medical Education* 50 (April):328–38.

Otis, G.D., and Weiss, J. 1972. "Explorations in Medical Career Choice." Report on Contract No. (NIH) 71-4066, U.S. Department of Health, Education, and Welfare, May. (Processed.)

_____. 1973. "Patterns of Medical Career Preference." *Journal of Medical Education* 48 (December):1116–23.

_____; Albert, M.; Offir, J.; and Richardson, C. 1973. "Medical Specialty Selection: A Review." Final Report on DHEW Contract No. 72-4197, U.S. Department of Health, Education, and Welfare, February. (Processed.)

Page, R.G., and Herron, M.D. 1969. "Analysis of Preparation for the Study of Medicine Questionnaire Given to Selected Students." In *Preparation for the Study of Medicine*, ed. R.G. Page and M.H. Littlemeyer. Chicago: University of Chicago Press.

Paiva, R.E.A., and Haley, H.B. 1971. "Intellectual, Personality, and Environmental Factors in Career Specialty Preferences." *Journal of Medical Education* 46 (April):281–89.

Paiva, R.E.A., Juan, I.R.; and Haley, H.B. 1974. "Factors in Internship Choice." *Journal of Medical Education* 69 (April):343–50.

Paringer, L. 1980. "Medicare Assignment Rates of Physicians: Their Responses to Changes in Reimbursement Policy." *Health Care Financing Review* 1 (Winter):75–89.

Parker, R.C. 1970. "The Vanishing Rural Physician." *Bulletin of the Medical Society, County of Monroe and Seventh District Branch, Medical Society of the State of New York* 28 (December):546–47.

––––––, and Sorensen, A.A. 1978. "The Tides of Rural Physicians: The Ebb and Flow, or Why Physicians Move Out of and Into Small Communities." *Medical Care* 16 (February):152–66.

Parker, R.C., and Tuxill, T.G. 1967. "The Attitudes of Physicians toward Small-Community Practice." *Journal of Medical Education* 42 (April):327–44.

Pashigian, P.B. 1973. "The Hill-Burton Program: The Effects of Federal Subsidy in Kind on the Hospital Industry." Report No. 7346, Center for Mathematical Studies in Business and Economics, University of Chicago. (Processed.)

Paul, D.W. 1978. "Regional Physician Maldistribution." *Texas Medicine* 74 (May):116–22.

Pauly, M.V. 1980. *Economic Models of Physician Behavior.* Chicago: University of Chicago Press.

––––––, and Redisch, M. 1973. "The Not-for-Profit Hospital as a Physicians' Cooperative." *American Economic Review* 63 (March):87–100.

Pauly, M.V., and Satterthwaite, M.A. 1980. "The Effect of Provider Supply on Price." In *The Target Income Hypothesis and Related Issues in Health Manpower Policy.* DHEW Publication No. (HRA) 80-27. Washington, D.C.: U.S. Department of Health, Education, and Welfare.

––––––. 1981. "The Pricing of Primary Care Physicians' Services: A Test of the Role of Consumer Information." *Bell Journal of Economics* 12 (Autumn):488–506.

Paxton, G.S.; Sbarbaro, J.A.; and Nossaman, H. 1975. "A Core City Problem: Recruitment and Retention of Salaried Physicians." *Medical Care* 13 (March): 209–18.

Perlstadt, H. 1972. "Internship Placements and Faculty Influence." *Journal of Medical Education* 47 (November):862–68.

––––––. 1975. "MCAT: A Gate in Admissions and Internship Placements." *Journal of Medical Education* 50 (February):78–81.

Petersdorf, R.G. 1975. "Issues in Primary Care: The Academic Perspective." *Journal of Medical Education* 50 (December, Part 2):5–13.

Peterson, G.R. 1968. "A Comparison of Selected Professional and Social Charac-
teristics of Urban and Rural Physicians in Iowa." Iowa City, Iowa: Graduate
Program in Hospital and Health Administration, University of Iowa.
(Processed.)

Peterson, O.L., and Bendixen, H.H. 1969. "A Critique of Graduate Medical Education in Community Hospitals." *Journal of Medical Education* 44 (September):762–67.

Peterson, O.L.; Lyden, F.J.; Geiger, H.J.; and Colton, T. 1963. "Appraisal of
Medical Students' Abilities as Related to Training and Careers after Graduation." *New England and Journal of Medicine* 269 (November 23):1174–82.

Peterson, P.Q., and Pennell, M.Y. 1962. "Section 14: Medical Specialists." In
Health Manpower Source Book. Public Health Service Publication No. 263.
Washington, D.C.: Government Printing Office.

Petty, R. 1976. "New Admissions Test Readied." *American Medical News*
(March 29):3.

Phillips, T.J.; Gordon, M.J.; Leversee, J.H.; and Smith, C.K. 1978. "Family Physician Pathway and Medical Student Career Choice: Ten Years after Curriculum Change at the University of Washington." *Journal of the American Medical Association* 215 (October 13):1736–41.

Powers, L.; Parmelle, R.D.; and Wiesenfelder, H. 1969. "Practice Patterns of
Women and Men Physicians." *Journal of Medical Education* 44
(June):481–91.

Powers, L.; Whiting, J.F.; and Oppermann, K.C. 1962. "Trends in Medical
School Faculties." *Journal of Medical Education* 37 (October):1065–91.

Pozen, J.T.; Sorenson, J.R.; and Alpert, J.J. 1979. "Stability and Change in Primary Care and Traditional Residency Programs: A Case Study." In *Becoming
a Physician: Development of Values and Attitudes in Medicine,* ed. E.C. Shapiro and L.M. Lowenstein. Cambridge, Mass.: Ballinger Publishing Company.

Preiss, J.J., and Jackson, R.A 1978. "Student Attitudes and Curriculum Change:
A Longitudinal Study of Selected Variables." In *Undergraduate Medical Education and the Elective System: Experience with the Duke Curriculum,
1966–75,* ed. J.F. Gifford. Durham, N.C.: Duke University Press.

Quenk, N. 1976. "A Retrospective Study of Past Participants in AMSA Foundation Programs. Final Report: AMSA Foundation-National Health Service
Corps Primary Care Preceptorship Project." Report to the Bureau of Health
Manpower, U.S. Department of Health, Education, and Welfare, under Contract No. 231-76-0070 by the AMSA Foundation. (Processed.)

———, and Albert, M. n.d. "A Taxonomy of Physician Work Settings." Study
Report No. 2 to the Bureau of Health Resources Development, U.S. Depart-
ment of Health, Education, and Welfare under Contract No. 1-MI-24197,
University of New Mexico. (Processed.)

Ramsey, J.B. 1980. "An Analysis of Competing Hypotheses of the Demand for
and Supply of Physician Services." In *The Target Income Hypothesis and Related Issues in Health Manpower Policy.* DHEW Publication No. (HRA) 80-
27. Washington, D.C.: U.S. Department of Health, Education, and Welfare.

Redisch, M.; Gabel, J.; and Blaxall, M. 1977. "Physician Pricing, Costs, and Income." Paper presented at the Western Economic Association Meetings, Anaheim, Calif., July.

Reed, D.E. 1970. "Twelve Years' Experience with a Comprehensive Ambulatory Care Program." *Journal of Medical Education* 45 (December):1041–46.

Reinhardt, U.E. 1978. "Comment on 'Competition among Physicians.'" In *Competition in the Health Care Sector*, ed. W. Greenberg. Germantown, Md.: Aspen Systems.

Reitzes, D.C., and Elkhanialy, H. 1976. "Black Physicians and Minority Group Health Care—The Impact of NMF." *Medical Care* 14 (December):1052–60.

Renner, W.F. 1964. "The Community Hospital Internship." *Journal of the American Medical Association* 189 (July 27):290–93.

Renshaw, J.E., and Pennell, M.S. 1971. "Distribution of Women Physicians, 1969." *Woman Physician* 26 (April):187–98.

Reskin, B., and Campbell, F.L. 1974. "Physician Distribution across Metropolitan Areas." *American Journal of Sociology* 79 (January):981–98.

Rezler, A.G. 1974. "Attitude Changes during Medical School: A Review of the Literature." *Journal of Medical Education* 49 (November):1023–30.

Richards, J.M.; Rand, L.M.; and Rand, L.P. 1968. "A Description of Medical College Environments." *American Educational Research Journal* 5 (November):647–58.

Riley, G.J.; Wille, C.R.; and Haggerty, R.J. 1969. "A Study of Family Medicine in Upstate New York." *Journal of the American Medical Association* 208 (June 23):2307–14.

Rimlinger, G.V.; and Steele, H.B. 1963. "An Economic Interpretation of the Spatial Distribution of Physicians in the U.S." *Southern Economic Journal* 30 (July):1–12.

Rising, J.D. 1962. "The Rural Preceptorship: A Ten-Year Report on the Kansas University Program." *Journal of the Kansas Medical Society* 63 (March):847–49.

Rodgers, J. 1981. "Long Run Forecasts of Prices and Expenditures for Physician and Hospital Services." In *Profile of Medical Practice, 1981*, ed. D.L. Goldfarb. Chicago: American Medical Association.

Rodgers, S.A., and Elton C.F. 1974. "An Analysis of the Environment of Medical Schools." *Research on Higher Education* 2:239–49.

Roleston, K.I. 1973. *Michigan Medical Manpower Study: An Investigation of the Decision-Making Factors Among Medical Students, Interns, and Residents, and an Evaluation of Proposed Loan Programs for Retaining Medical Manpower.* Detroit: Blue Shield of Michigan.

Roos, N.P., and Fish, D.G. 1974. "Change in Career Preferences: Students as a Group versus Students as Individuals." *Journal of Medical Education* 49 (November):1057–59.

Rosenberg, M.L. 1973. "Increasing the Efficiency of Medical School Admissions." *Journal of Medical Education* 48 (August):707–17.

Rosenblatt, R., and Moscovice, I. 1978a. "Establishing New Rural Family Practices: Some Lessons from a Federal Experience." *Journal of Family Practice* 7 (October):755–63.

_____. 1978b. "The Growth and Evolution of Rural Primary Care Practice: The National Health Service Corps Experience in the Northwest." *Medical Care* 16 (October):819–27.

_____. 1980. "The National Health Service Corps: Rapid Growth and Uncertain Future." *Milbank Memorial Fund Quarterly/Health and Society* 58 (Spring):283–309.

Rosenlund, M.L., and Oski, F.A. 1967. "Women in Medicine." *Annals of Internal Medicine* 46 (May):1008–12.

Rosenthal, J. 1980. "State Funds in Support of Public and Private Medical Schools, 1979." *Journal of Medical Education* 55 (October):885–87.

Rosett, R.N. 1974. "Proprietary Hospitals in the United States." In *The Economics of Health and Medical Care*, ed. M. Perlman. New York: John Wiley and Sons.

Rothman, A.I. 1972. "Longitudinal Study of Medical Students: Long-Term versus Short-Term Objectives." *Journal of Medical Education* 47 (November):901–2.

_____. 1973. "A Comparison of Persistent High and Low Achievers through Four Years of Undergraduate Medical Training." *Journal of Medical Education* 48 (February):180–82.

_____; Byrne, P.M.; Fruen, M.A.; Parlow, J.; and Steiner, J.W. 1974. "An Empirical Definition of a Medical School's Admission's Procedures." *Journal of Medical Education* 49 (January):71–73.

Rothman, A.I., and Flowers, J.F. 1970. "Personality Correlates of First-Year Medical School Achievement." *Journal of Medical Education* 45 (November):901–5.

Royce, P.C. 1972. "Can Rural Health Education Centers Influence Physician Distribution?" *Journal of the American Medical Association* 220 (May 8): 847–49.

Rushing, W.A. 1975. *Community, Physicians, and Inequality.* Lexington, Mass.: D.C. Heath.

_____, and Wade, G.T. 1973. "Community Structure Constraints and Distribution of Physicians." *Health Services Research* 8 (Winter):283–97.

Sanazaro, P.J. 1965. "Research in Medical Education: Exploratory Analysis of a Blackbox." *Annals of the New York Academy of Sciences* 128 (September):519–31.

_____, and Hutchins, E.B. 1963. "The Origin and Rationale of the Medical College Admission Test." *Journal of Medical Education* 38 (December):1044–50.

Saunders, R.H. 1961. "The University Hospital Internship in 1960: A Study of the Programs of 27 Major Teaching Hospitals." *Journal of Medical Education* 36 (June):561–659.

_____. 1964. "The Dilemma of Internship." *Journal of Medical Education* 39 (May):437–43.

Schaffner, R., and Butter, I. 1972. "Geographic Mobility of Foreign Medical Graduates and the Doctor Shortage: A Longitudinal Analysis." *Inquiry* 9 (March):24–33.

Schaupp, F.W. 1969. "A Study of Factors Influencing Outmigration of M.D. Graduates of West Virginia University, 1926–66." Morgantown, W.Va.: West Virginia University, Bureau of Business Research, January. (Processed.)

Scheffler, R.M. 1971a. "An Empirical Investigation into the Geographic Distribution of Physicians and Specialists." Ph.D. dissertation, New York University.

_____. 1971b. "The Relationship between Medical Education and the Statewide Per Capita Distribution of Physicians." *Journal of Medical Education* 46 (November):995–98.

_____. 1972. The Regional Distribution of Physicians and Specialists." *Review of Regional Studies* 2 (Winter) 63–80.

_____; Yoder, S.G.; Weisfeld, N.; and Ruby, G. 1979. "Physicians and New Health Practitioners: Issues for the 1980s." *Inquiry* 16 (Fall):195–229.

Scher, M. 1973. "Women Psychiatrists in the United States." *American Journal of Psychiatry* 10 (October):1118–22.

Schmidt, P., and Strauss, R.P. 1975a. "Estimation of Models with Jointly Dependent Qualitative Variables: A Simultaneous Logit Approach." *Econometrica* 43 (July):745–55.

_____. 1975b. "The Prediction of Occupation Using Multiple Logit Models." *International Economic Review* 16 (June):471–86.

Schofield, W. 1970. "A Modified Actuarial Method in the Selection of Medical Students. *Journal of Medical Education* 45 (October):740–44.

_____, and Garrard, J. 1975. "Longitudinal Study of Medical Students Selected for Admission to Medical School by Actuarial and Committee Methods." *British Journal of Medical Education* 9 (June):86–90.

Schofield, W., and Merwin, J.C. 1966. "The Use of Scholastic Aptitude, Personality, and Interest Test Data in the Selection of Medical Students." *Journal of Medical Education* 41 (June):502–9.

Schroeder, S.A.; Werner, S.M.; and Piemme, T.E. 1974. "Primary Care in the Academic Medical Centers: A Report of a Survey by the AAMC." *Journal of Medical Education* 49 (September):823–33.

Schumacher, C.F. 1963. "Interest and Personality Factors as Related to Choice of Career." *Journal of Medical Education* 38 (November):932–42.

_____. 1964. "Personal Characteristics of Students Choosing Different Types of Medical Careers." *Journal of Medical Education* 39 (March):278–88.

Schwartz, L.E., and Cantwell, J.R. 1976. "Weiskotten Survey, Class of 1960: A Profile of Physician Location and Specialty Choice." *Journal of Medical Education* 51 (July):533–40.

Schwartz, W.B.; Newhouse, J.P.; Bennett, B.W.; and Williams, A.P. 1980. "The Changing Geographic Distribution of Board-Certified Physicians." *New England Journal of Medicine* 303 (October 30):1032–38.

Schwarz, M.R. 1979. "The WAMI Program: A Progress Report." *Western Journal of Medicine* 130 (April):384–90.

_____, and Flahault, D. 1978. "The WAMI Programme, University of Washington School of Medicine, Seattle, WA, United States of America." In *Personnel for Health Care: Case Studies of Educational Programmes*, ed. F.M. Katz and T. Fulop. Geneva, Switzerland: World Health Organization.

Shalit, S.S. 1977. "A Doctor-Hospital Cartel Theory." *Journal of Business* 50 (January):1–20.

Shapiro, C.S.; Stibler, B.; Zelkovic, A.A.; and Mausner, J.S. 1968. "Careers of Women Physicians: A Survey of Women Graduates from Seven Medical Schools, 1945–51." *Journal of Medical Education* 43 (October):1033–40.

Sheps, C.G., and Seip, C.G. 1972. "The Medical School, Its Products and Its Problems." *Annals of the American Academy of Political and Social Science* 399 (January):38–49.

Sherman, S.N. 1982. "Applicants to U.S. Medical Schools, 1977–78 to 1981–82." *Journal of Medical Education* 59 (November):882–84.

Silberstein, E.B., and Scott, C.J. 1978. "An Evaluation of Undergraduate Family Care Programs." *Journal of Community Health* 3 (Summer):369–79.

Simon, R., and Shriver, B.M. 1964. "Impact of the Undergraduate Psychiatry Program on Choice of Specialty: A Survey of 1957 and 1958 Stipend Recipients." *Journal of Medical Education* 39 (December):1114–17.

Sloan, F.A. 1968. "Economic Models of Physician Supply." Ph.D. dissertation, Harvard University.

———. 1970a. "Hospital Demand for Residents," *Inquiry* 7 (September):65–68.

———. 1970b. "Lifetime Earnings and Physicians' Choice of Specialty." *Industrial and Labor Relations Review* 24 (October):47–56.

———. 1974. "Effects of Incentives on Physician Performance." In *Health Manpower and Productivity*, ed. J. Rafferty. Lexington, Mass.: D.C. Heath.

———. 1976a. "Physician Fee Inflation: Evidence from the Late 1960s." In *The Role of Health Insurance in the Health Services Sector*, ed. R.N. Rosett. New York: National Bureau of Economic Research.

———. 1976b. "Real Returns to Medical Education: A Comment." *Journal of Human Resources* 11 (Winter):118–26.

———. 1980. "Patient Care Reimbursement: Implications for Medical Education and Physician Distribution." In *Medical Education Financing: Policy Analyses and Options for the 1980s*, ed. J. Hadley. New York: Prodist.

———. 1982. "Effects of Health Insurance on Physicians' Fees." *Journal of Human Resources* 17 (Fall):533–57.

———, and Feldman, R. 1978. "Competition among Physicians." In *Competition in the Health Care Sector*, ed. W. Greenberg. Germantown, Md.: Aspen Systems.

Sloan, F.A., and Yett, D.E. 1970. "Incomes and Other Factors Affecting Physician Location Decisions: An Econometric Analysis." Final report on subcontract with New York University in relation to prime contract HEW-OS-69-94 with the U.S. Department of Health, Education, and Welfare. (Processed.)

———. 1971. "Analysis of Migration Patterns of Recent Medical School Graduates." Paper presented at the Health Services Research Conference on Factors in Manpower Performance and the Delivery of Health Care, Chicago, December.

Smith, L.C.R., and Crocker, A.R. 1970. *How Medical Students Finance Their Education*. Public Health Service Publication No. 1336-1. Washington, D.C.: Government Printing Office.

Snyder, D.S. 1967. "The Relationship of Students' Experiences before and during Medical School to Their Conceptions of Professional Responsibility." *Journal of Medical Education* 42 (March):213–18.

Stead, E.A. 1969. "The Role of the University in Graduate Training." *Journal of Medical Education* 14 (September):739–44.

Steele, H.B., and Rimlinger, G.V. 1965. "Income Opportunities and Physician Location Trends in the United States." *Western Economic Journal* 3 (Spring):182–94.

Stefanu, C., and Pate, M.L. 1978. "Location of Residency: Analysis of a Critical Determinant in Keeping Physicians in Texas." *Texas Medicine* 74 (June):61–65.

———, and Chapman, J.S. 1979. "Hospitals and Medical Schools as Factors in the Selection of Location of Practice." *Journal of Medical Education* 54 (May):379–83.

Stefanu, C.; Pate, M.L.; Zetzman, M.R.; Goldman, W.W.; and Brandt, E.N. 1980. "Impact of a Family Practice Residency Program on Physician Location in Small Communities." *Southern Medical Journal* 73 (October):1372–74.

Steinwald, B., and Sloan, F.A. 1974. "Determinants of Physicians' Fees." *Journal of Business* 47 (October):493–507.

Steinwald B., and Steinwald, C. 1975. "The Effect of Preceptorship and Rural Training Programs on Physicians' Practice Location Decisions." *Medical Care* 13 (March):219–29.

Steinwachs, D.M.; Levine, D.M.; Elzinga, D.J.; Salkever, D.S.; Parker, R.D.; and Weisman, C.S. 1982. "Changing Patterns of Graduate Medical Education: Analyzing Recent Trends and Projecting Their Impact." *New England Journal of Medicine* 306 (January 7):10–14.

Stevens, R. 1971. *American Medicine and the Public Interest.* New Haven, Conn.: Yale University Press.

———. 1978. "Graduate Medical Education: A Continuing History." *Journal of Medical Education* 53 (January):1–18.

———; Goodman, L.W.; and Mick, S.S. 1978. *The Alien Doctors: Foreign Medical Graduates in American Hospitals.* New York: John Wiley and Sons.

Stevens, R., and Vermeulen, J. 1972. *Foreign Trained Physicians and American Medicine.* DHEW Publication No. (NIH) 73-325. Washington, D.C.: Government Printing Office.

Stewart, T.J.; Miller, M.C.; and Spivey, L. 1980. "Community of Origin of Spouse and Physician Location in Two Southwestern States." *Journal of Medical Education* 55 (January):53–54.

Stewart, W.H., and Pennell, M.Y. 1960. "Section 10: Physicians' Age, Type of Practice, and Location." In *Health Manpower Source Book.* Public Health Service Publication No. 263. Washington, D.C.: Government Printing Office.

Student American Medical Association. 1972. *A Handbook for Change: Recommendations of the Joint Commission on Medical Education.* Philadelphia: William B. Fell.

Super, D.E. 1957. *The Psychology of Careers: An Introduction to Vocational Development.* New York: Harper.

Sweeney, G.H. 1982. "The Market for Physicians' Services: Theoretical Implications and an Empirical Test of the Target Income Hypothesis." *Southern Economic Journal* 48 (January):594–613.

Taylor, J.M., and Johnson, K.G. 1973. "A Residency Program in Primary Care: The Physician as Provider-Manager." *Journal of Medical Education* 48 (July):654–60.

Taylor, M.; Dickman, W.; and Kane, R. 1973. "Medical Students' Attitudes toward Rural Practice." *Journal of Medical Education* 48 (October):885–95.

Theodore, C.N., and Sutter, G.E. 1967a. *Distribution of Physicians in the U.S., 1963. Vol. 1: Regional, State, County.* Chicago: American Medical Association.

_____. 1967b. *Distribution of Physicians in the U.S., 1965: Regional, State, County Metropolitan Areas.* Chicago: American Medical Association.

_____, and Jokiel, E.A. 1967. *Distribution of Physicians, Hospitals, and Hospital Beds in the U.S. Vol. 1: Regional, State, and County.* Chicago: American Medical Association.

Thompson, T. 1974a. "Curbing the Black Physician Manpower Shortage." *Journal of Medical Education* 49 (October):944–49.

_____. 1974b. "Selected Characteristics of Black Physicians in the United States, 1972." *Journal of the American Medical Association* 229 (September 23):1758–61.

Thurow, L. 1970. *Investment in Human Capital.* Belmont, Calif.: Wadsworth.

Tilson, H.H. 1973a. "Characteristics of Physicians in OEO Neighborhood Health Centers." *Inquiry* 10 (June):27–38.

_____. 1973b. "Stability of Physician Employment in Neighborhood Health Centers." *Medical Care* 11 (September-October):384–400.

Todd, C., and McNamara, M.E. 1971. *Medical Groups in the U.S., 1969.* Chicago: American Medical Association.

Trzebiatowski, G.L., and Peterson, S. 1979. "A Study of Faculty Attitudes toward Ohio State's Three-Year Medical Program." *Journal of Medical Education* 54 (March):205–9.

Turner, E.V.; Helper, M.M.; and Kriska, S.D. 1974. "Predictors of Clinical Performance." *Journal of Medical Education* 49 (April):338–42.

U.S. Department of Health, Education, and Welfare. 1973. *The Health Professions Educational Assistance Program, FY 1963-1972.* Washington, D.C.: U.S. Department of Health, Education, and Welfare.

_____. 1974. *How Medical Students Finance Their Education.* DHEW Publication No. 75-13. Washington, D.C.: U.S. Government Printing Office, June.

_____. 1976. *Forward Plan for Health, FY 1978-82.* Washington, D.C.: Government Printing Office.

U.S. Department of Health and Human Services. 1982. *Third Report to the President and Congress on the Status of Health Professions Personnel in the United States.* DHHS Publication No. (HRA) 82-2. Washington, D.C.: U.S. Department of Health and Human Services.

Verby, J.E. 1977. "The Minnesota Rural Physician Redistribution Plan, 1971 to 1976." *Journal of the American Medical Association* 238 (August 29):960–64.

Wacht, R.F. 1972. "Economic Determinants of Physician Distribution within the Southeastern Region of the United States." Atlanta: Georgia State University, November. (Processed.)

Waldman, B. 1977. "Economic and Racial Disadvantage as Reflected in Traditional Medical School Selection Factors." *Journal of Medical Education* 52 (December):961–70.

Walsh, R.J.; Aherne, P.; and Ryan, G.A. 1972. *1972 Reference Data on the Profile of Medical Practice.* Chicago: American Medical Association.

Walton, H.J. 1969. "Personality Correlates of a Career Interest in Psychiatry." *British Journal of Psychiatry* 21 (November):529–35.

Warner, J. 1975. "Programs to Influence Physicians' Specialty Choice Decisions." Chicago: Center for Health Services Research and Development, American Medical Association. (Processed.)

———, and Aherne, P., eds. 1974. *1974 Edition Reference Data on Profile of Medical Practice.* Chicago: American Medical Association.

Wasserman, E.; Yufit, R.I.; and Pollack, G.H. 1969. "Medical Specialty Choice and Personality: Outcome and Post-graduate Followup Results." *Archives of General Psychiatry* 21 (November):529–35.

Watson, C. J. 1980a. "An Empirical Model of Physician Practice Location Decisions." *Computers and Biomedical Research* 13 (August):363–81.

———. 1980b. "The Relationship between Physician Practice Location and Medical School Area: An Empirical Model." *Social Science & Medicine* 14 (March):63–69.

Webster, T.G. 1975. "Student Decisions and Self-Images in Medical School." In *Medical Behavioral Science*, ed. T. Millon. Philadelphia: W.B. Saunders.

Wechsler, H.; Dorsey, J.L.; and Bovey, J.D. 1978. "A Follow-Up Study of Residents in Internal Medicine, Pediatrics, and Obstetrics-Gynecology Training Programs in Massachusetts: Implications for the Supply of Primary-Care Physicians." *New England Journal of Medicine* 298 (January 5):15–21.

Weil, P.A., and Schleiter, M.K. 1981. "National Study of Internal Medicine Manpower: VI. Factors Predicting Preferences of Residents for Careers in Primary Care and in Clinical Practice or Academic Medicine." *Annals of Internal Medicine* 94 (May):691–703.

———, and Tarlov, A.R. 1981. "National Study of Internal Medicine Manpower: V. Comparison of Residents in Internal Medicine—Future Generalists and Subspecialists." *Annals of Internal Medicine* 94 (May):678–90.

Weiskotten, H.G.; Wiggins, W.S.; Altenderfer, M.E.; Gooch, M.; and Tipner, A. 1960. "Trends in Medical Practice: An Analysis of the Distribution and Characteristics of Medical College Graduates, 1915–50. *Journal of Medical Education* 35 (December):1071–121.

———. 1961. "Changes in Professional Careers of Physicians: An Analysis of a Resurvey of Physicians Who Were Graduated from Medical College in 1935, 1940, and 1945." *Journal of Medical Education* 36 (November):1565–85.

Weisman, C.S.; Levine, D.M.; Steinwachs, D.M.; and Chase, G.A. 1980. "Male and Female Physician Career Patterns: Specialty Choices and Graduate Training." *Journal of Medical Education* 55 (October):813–25.

Weiss, J.E. 1971. "Socioeconomic and Technological Factors in Trends of Physicians to Specialize." *HSMHA Health Reports* 86 (January):46–51.

Wennberg, J.E., and Gittleson, A. 1975. "Health Care Delivery in Maine: Patterns of Use of Common Surgical Procedures." *Journal of the Maine Medical Association* 66 (May):123–49.

Werner, J.L.; Wendling, W.; and Budde, N. 1978. "The Physician's Location and Specialty Choice: A Simultaneous Logit Approach." Paper presented at the Midwest Economic Association Meetings, Chicago, April.

Westling-Wilkstrand, H.; Monk, M.A.; and Thomas, C.B. 1970. "Some Characteristics Related to the Career Status of Women Physicians." *Johns Hopkins Medical Journal* 127 (November):273–86.

Wiggins, W.S.; Green, F.; and Altenderfer, M.E. 1970. *Trends in Medical Practice —An Analysis of the Distribution and Characteristics of Medical College Graduates, 1915–1955.* Chicago: American Medical Association.

Wilensky, G.R. 1979. "Retention of Medical School Graduates: A Case Study of Michigan." In *Research in Health Economics*, ed. R.M. Scheffler. Greenwich, Conn.: JAI Press.

Willard, W.R. 1964. "Achievement of Reasoned Goals for the First Hospital Year." *Journal of the American Medical Association* 189 (July 27):279–82.

Williams, A.P.; Carter, G.M.; Chu, D.S.C.; Coleman, S.B.; Massel, A.P.; Neu, C.R.; Rasmussen, R.L.; and Rogers, W.H. 1976. *The Effect of Federal Biomedical Research Programs on Academic Medical Centers.* Publication no. R-1943-PBRP. Santa Monica, Calif.: Rand Corporation.

Williams, G. 1980. *Western Reserve's Experiment in Medical Education and Its Outcome.* New York: Oxford University Press.

Williams, P.A. 1971. "Women in Medicine: Some Themes and Variations." *Journal of Medical Education* 46 (July):584–91.

Williams, R.C., and Uzzell, W.E. 1960. "Attracting Physicians to Smaller Communities." *Hospitals* 34 (July):49–51.

Wing, P., and Blumberg, M.S. 1971. "Expenditures and Sponsored Research at U.S. Medical Schools: An Empirical Study of Cost Patterns." *Journal of Human Resources* 6 (Winter):75–102.

Wingert, W.A. 1966. "The Utilization of the Intern in a Pediatric Outpatient Setting." *Journal of Medical Education* 41 (August):756–65.

Wise, H.B.; Spear, P.W.; and Silver, G.A. 1966. "A Program in Community Medicine for the Medical Resident." *Journal of Medical Education* 41 (November):1071–76.

Woods, B.T.; Jacobson, M.D.; and Netsky, M.G. 1967. "Social Class and Academic Performance by Medical Students." *Journal of Medical Education* 42 (March):225–30.

Wooldridge, J. 1976. "Differences in Pricing Policy. Modes of Practice and Location between White Male and Minority Physicians." Paper presented at the Annual Meeting of the Western Economic Association, San Francisco, June.

Woolf, M.A. 1978. *Demographic Factors Correlated with the Maintenance of Physician Manpower in Rural Communities: A Study of NHSC Sites.* Washington, D.C.: U.S. Department of Health, Education, and Welfare.

————; Uchill, V.L.; and Jacoby, I. 1981. "Demographic Factors Associated with Physician Staffing in Rural Areas: The Experience of the National Health Service Corps." *Medical Care* 19 (April):444–51.

Wunderman, L.E. 1979. *Physician Distribution and Medical Licensure in the U.S., 1978.* Chicago: American Medical Association.

————. 1980. "Female Physicians in the 1970s: Their Changing Roles in Medicine." In *Profile of Medical Practice, 1980,* ed. G.L. Glandon and R.J. Shapiro. Chicago: American Medical Association.

Yancik, R. 1977. "Time of Decision to Study Medicine: Its Relation to Specialty Choice." *Journal of Medical Education* 52 (January):78–81.

Yett, D.E. 1975. *An Economic Analysis of the Nurse Shortage.* Lexington, Mass.: D.C. Heath.

————. 1978. "Comment on 'Competition among Physicians.'" In *Competition in the Health Care Sector,* ed. w. Greenberg. Germantown, Md.: Aspen Systems.

————; Der, W.; Ernst, R.L.; and Hay, J.W. 1982. "A Model of Physician Pricing, Output, and Health Insurance Reimbursement: Findings from a Study of Two Blue Shield Plans." In *Economics of Health Care,* ed. J. van der Gaag, J. Neenan, and T. Tsukahara. New York: Praeger.

Yett, D.E.; Drabek, J.L.; Intriligator, M.D.; and Kimbell, L.J. 1973. "The Preliminary Operational HRRC Microsimulation Model." Final Report to the Division of Manpower Intelligence, U.S. Department of Health, Education, and Welfare, on Contract No. NIH 71-4065.

Yett, D.E., and Sloan, F.A. 1974. "Migration Patterns of Recent Medical School Graduates." *Inquiry* 11 (June):125–42.

Yufit, R.I.; Pollack, G.H.; and Wasserman, E. 1969. "Medical Specialty Choice and Personality." *Archives of General Psychiatry* 20 (January):86–92.

Zabarenko, R.N., and Zabarenko, L.M. 1978. *The Doctor Tree: Developmental States in the Growth of Physicians.* Pittsburgh: University of Pittsburgh Press.

Zetzman, M.R., and Stefanu, C. 1977. "Selecting a Community for Medical Practice: A Study of Factors, Characteristics, and Preferences among Practicing Physicians, Family Practice Residents, and Medical Students." *Texas Medicine* 73 (January):86–92.

Zimet, C.N., and Held, M.L. 1975. "The Development of Views of Specialties during Four Years of Medical School." *Journal of Medical Education* 50 (February):157–65.

Zimny, G.H. 1980. "Predictive Validity of the Medical Specialty Inventory." *Medical Education* 14 (November):414–18.

————, and Senturia, A.G. 1973. "Medical Specialty Counseling: A Survey." *Journal of Medical Education* 48 (April):337–42.

————. 1974. "A Longitudinal Study of Consistency of Medical Student Specialty Choice." *Journal of Medical Education* 49 (December):1179–81.

Zimny, G.H., and Thale, T.R. 1970. "Specialty Choice and Attitudes toward Medical Specialists." *Social Science & Medicine* 4:257–64.

Zuckerman, H.S. 1978. "Structural Factors as Determinants of Career Patterns in Medicine." *Journal of Medical Education* 53 (June):453–63.

Index

About the Authors

RICHARD L. ERNST, PH.D., is a research associate at the Human Resources Research Center, University of Southern California in Los Angeles. He has taught economics at The University of Illinois and The University of California, Berkeley. Dr. Ernst earned his Ph.D. at The University of California, Berkeley. He has published in both books and journals and presented several papers at association meetings.

DONALD E. YETT, PH.D., is the director of The Human Resources Research Center, University of Southern California and Professor of Economics in the Department of Economics at The University of Southern California. He also taught at The University of California, Los Angeles; Washington University in St. Louis; and Ohio State University. His Ph.D. is from The University of California, Berkeley. Dr. Yett has directed research projects, acted as a consultant often, published widely, and been active in professional organizations.